TAREEN'S UNDERSTANDING PSYCHIATRY

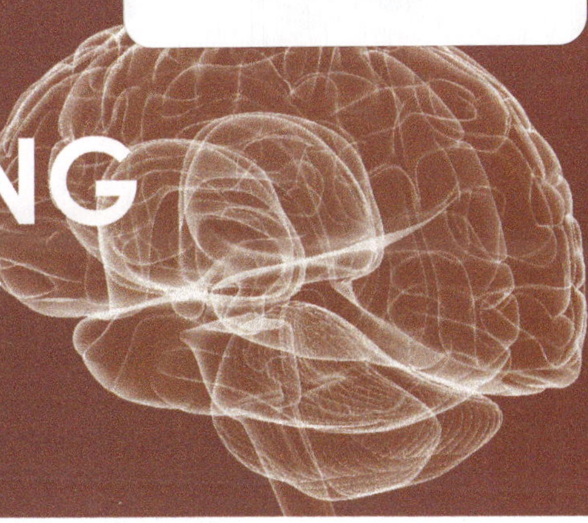

Fourth Edition

Tanvir Ahmad Rana

MBBS (Lahore), DPM (Wales), FRCPsych (London)

Fellow and Diplomate American Board of Medical Psychotherapists

Paramount Books (Pvt.) Ltd.

Karachi | Lahore | Islamabad | Hyderabad | Faisalabad | Peshawar | Abbottabad

Tareen's Understanding Psychiatry

by

Tanvir Ahmad Rana

First Edition 1998
Second Edition 2004
Third Edition 2016
Fourth Edition 2022

Notice
This is a POD edition by **Paramount Books (Pvt.) Ltd.,**
in collaboration with Ingram Content Group

Paramount Books (Pvt.) Ltd.

152/O, Block-2, P.E.C.H.S., Karachi-75400.
Tel: +92-21-34310030, info@paramountbooks.com.pk
www.paramountbooks.com.pk

ISBN: 978-969-210-788-4

Printed in Pakistan

DEDICATION

To

Amera

Dedicating this book to her is an inadequate expression of my love and gratitude.

BOOK REVIEWS

Tareen's Understanding Psychiatry is a true teacher's 'work of art'. It simultaneously is both impressive in its depth of knowledge and simplicity of explanation. As one reads through the book, one feels the patient guidance of the professor. The student is taken by the hand and calmly led through the complex labyrinth of the field of psychiatry. Without compromise on depth and breadth, the principles of psychiatry are simply and clearly laid out, and psychiatric disorders are distinctly presented and discussed. What is most impressive about this book is that throughout the learning process, the humanity of patients is brought forth. I would heartily recommend this book to the students of Wagner College.

Dr Nora Lowy, Program Director, Wagner College, New York.

Tareen's Understanding Psychiatry is a superb textbook on psychiatry. Its strengths lie in that it is very well written, clear and covers all the important areas of psychiatry. The contents are up-to-date and, importantly, in addition to a theoretical discussion, there is much clinical wisdom and experience distilled in the pages. The book is intended for medical students and trainee psychiatrists alike, since both groups would benefit from this book; moreover, experienced psychiatrists and allied clinicians would also find this book useful for reference and review.

Dr Matthew Broome, Associate Editor British Journal of Psychiatry, Senior Clinical Research Fellow, Department of Psychiatry, University of Oxford.

Tareen's Understanding Psychiatry is a clear, pleasant to read, practical and scientifically sound comprehensive psychiatry book. Grounded in the author's scholarly expertise and clinical experience, this textbook is an excellent tool for medical students and trainee doctors in psychiatry, as well as for other mental health professionals. The book provides up-to-date, scientific and concise information with practical insights into the field of psychiatry. It is an accessible and authoritative educational reference and clinical compendium.

Professor Andrea Fagiolini, Chairman and Residency Training Director, Division of Psychiatry, University of Siena, Italy

Tareen's Understanding Psychiatry is a great project. I like it, and I wish we had such a well-written, clear and systematic textbook here in Germany.

Professor Oliver Pogarell, Dept. of Psychiatry and Psychotherapy, Ludwig-Maximilians- University of Munich

PREFACE TO THE THIRD EDITION

When the first edition of *Understanding Psychiatry* was published in 1998, it immediately became a popular book for medical students and junior doctors. The second edition was published in 2004 and likewise was widely regarded as a comprehensive psychiatry book.

Since then, there have been lots of changes and research developments in psychiatric practice. These advancements have been taken into account and incorporated in this third edition, which has been completely updated and revised. Like the previous two editions, this book has been written primarily for medical students and trainee doctors in psychiatry. Other professionals like mental health nurses, social workers, psychologists, occupational therapists, physician assistants and general practitioners will also find this book useful.

I am hopeful that I have produced a book that lives up to the high standards of the first two editions written by Professor I. A. K. Tareen and Professor Khalida I. Tareen. I have also attempted to write this text at a level which is readable, appropriate and outlines the essentials of psychiatry.

This book contains and reflects the extensive clinical and teaching experience of the original authors and the current author.

Teaching undergraduate medical students and psychiatric trainees has been a great learning experience for me. I, just like the authors of the previous editions, believe that it is not enough to teach them the aetiology, psychopathology and symptomatology of the various psychiatric illnesses, or give them a checklist of questions to complete. It is essential that they understand that mentally unwell patients are individual human beings with unique personal narratives. They need to realise the extent to which these patients are unfortunately stigmatised, and learn to deal with them in an empathic way. Moreover, they ought to be trained in phrasing their questions sensitively, and in the light of the information obtained, to arrive at an accurate diagnosis and consequently formulate a comprehensive management plan. Just like the previous editions, this book also contains succinct lists of helpful questions for eliciting various aspects of history and for mental state examination.

Victor Frankl, in *Man's Search for Meaning*, said: 'Ultimately, man should not ask what the meaning of his life is, but rather must recognise that it is he who is asked. In a word, each man is questioned by life; and he can only answer to life by answering for his own life; to life he can only respond by being responsible'.

If readers of this book will be able to help and alleviate the sufferings of some psychiatric patients and their families, I would consider that my humble effort and the five years spent in writing this book have been worthwhile.

I would then have, hopefully, responded to my life's question.

Tanvir Ahmad Rana
Sutton Coldfield, UK

PREFACE TO THE FOURTH EDITION

This edition was prompted by the immense and widespread response to the third edition. The publishers informed me that the third edition had literally run out of print, and asked for the fourth edition. Keeping in view the huge demand, the publishers wanted it to be published as soon as possible. Moreover, psychiatry, just like other branches of medicine, is an ever-changing speciality. Due to new research and clinical experience, changes in diagnosis, treatment and drug therapy are required. I, therefore, agreed and decided to revise this book.

This book has been written primarily for students and trainee doctors. However, I am hopeful that it will also be useful to higher or specialist trainees in psychiatry, and individuals from other disciplines such as psychologists, psychotherapists, physicians, nurses, occupational therapists, social workers, counsellors and legal specialists. I considered it essential that this book includes the most current information on psychiatric diagnosis and treatment. In the chapter on psychopathology, I have highlighted the main differences between ICD-10 and ICD-11.

Keeping in mind the developments in psychiatry, most of the chapters in the Fourth Edition have been thoroughly revised, updated and enlarged.

The main purposes of psychiatry are to recognise mental illnesses, discover their causes, treat them and attempt to develop preventive measures. Although psychiatry is a very clinical and human branch within medicine, not infrequently the public images and associations tend to cloak it with an aura of vagueness and imprecision. Psychiatric diagnoses are associated with stigma and misunderstandings. These are mainly due to the misconception that psychiatric illnesses do not have established physical causes, and mental illnesses are not real, or are the patients' own faults. Sometimes these misconceptions are quite pervasive, and evoke a mixture of associations, e.g., Freud treating his patients on the couch, Jack Nicholson receiving electroconvulsive therapy in *One Flew Over the Cuckoo's Nest*, Russel Crow overpowering schizophrenia by sheer will power in *The Beautiful Mind*, and Ralph Fieness in *Red Dragon* killing people because of his very disturbed childhood.

Irrespective of the various misconceptions about psychiatry, there are several reasons why this speciality may be the most exciting discipline within medicine. First, psychiatrists are specialists who work with the most interesting organ within the body, the brain. The brain controls nearly all aspects of functioning within the rest of the body as well as the way people interact with and relate to one another. Psychiatry, in contrast to popular belief, can be very scientific and technical, but at the same time it can also be very human and personal. For example, when the psychiatrist listens to a patients' stories, those experiences can be very rewarding because of the pleasure of being able to provide help and alleviate their sufferings.

My first trainers and teachers in psychiatry, Professor I. A. K. Tareen and Professor Khalida Ijaz Tareen always emphasise that the best book of psychiatry is actually the patient himself or herself, and the more time one spends with the patient the more beneficial it is for the psychiatrist's learning and clinical practice. While not disputing their remarkable insight and advice, I still hope that this book will at least add some additional knowledge, colour and flavour to the vast existing psychiatric literature, and will also enable readers to improve the mental health and happiness of their psychiatric patients. In that optimistic belief, I once again present to you *Tareen's Understanding Psychiatry*.

Tanvir Ahmad Rana
Sutton Coldfield, UK

AUTHORS' BIOGRAPHIES

Author of the first and second editions: **PROFESSOR KHALIDA IJAZ TAREEN**

Professor Khalida Ijaz Tareen is Professor Emeritus of Child Psychiatry, King Edward Medical University, Lahore and Visiting Professor of Child Psychiatry at The Institute of Child Health, Lahore. She established the Child and Family Psychiatry Department of K.E.Medical College; the first and the only one of its kind in the country. She developed these services to cover a wide range of programmes including teaching and training of undergraduate and postgraduate students in child psychiatry as well as paediatrics.

As a member of the World Health Organisation Expert Advisory Panel on Mental Health for 16 years and a member of the Punjab Commission on Child Welfare, her main contribution involves her incessant struggle to create awareness regarding mental health problems in children and the need for the provision of mental healthcare services for the children.

Prof. Tareen is the founding member and secretary-general of the National Society for Mentally and Emotionally Handicapped Children. As project director, she runs the Special Education and Training Centre, a charitable organisation providing free educational and vocational services for the learning children with disabilities and an outreach community-based programme for disadvantaged women and children. Author of a number of research papers, booklets and books, Prof. Khalida Tareen has translated and modified WISC-R and Portage Guide to early stimulation into Urdu and easy usage in various clinical settings.

Prof. Tareen has been an Honorary Member of the World Psychiatric Association, Founder Member of the Section of World Psychiatric Association on Psychiatric Disorders in Women, President of Pakistan Psychiatric Society and is listed in the World Directory of Resource Persons on learning disability. Prof. Tareen has chaired numerous scientific sessions at national and international psychiatric conferences, and also chaired the regional meetings of the World Psychiatric Association, in Pakistan.

She has collaborated with WHO and UNICEF on many research projects, and also established international links with world-renowned research centres in Sweden and New York. She has received lifetime achievement awards from the Pakistan Psychiatric Society and British Pakistani Psychiatrists Association. Prof. Tareen was honoured as the chief guest at the 150 years celebrations of King Edward Medical College Alumni Association of the UK. She is a recipient of Hazrat Khadija tul Kubra Gold Medal and has also been awarded Sitara-e-Imtiaz by the Government of Pakistan.

Author of the first and second editions: **PROFESSOR I. A. K. TAREEN**

Professor I. A. K. Tareen graduated from King Edward Medical College, Lahore, Pakistan, and has held different consultant and teaching posts, in both UK and Pakistan. Formerly, he was the Head, Academic Department of Psychiatry and Behavioural Sciences, KEMU. This was his own brain child and was the first and the only purpose-built, multi-disciplinary teaching psychiatry department in the country.

His unique contribution to the mental health services in Pakistan is bringing Psychiatry out of the mental hospital into the setting of a general teaching hospital. He has been instrumental in bringing about constructive changes in the academic curricula of undergraduate and postgraduate medical courses as well as advanced university courses in clinical psychology. As Project Director UN/PAK Drug Abuse Control Programme, he established a model drug abuse treatment and rehabilitation centre at Mayo Hospital, Lahore, Pakistan, which was visited by the late Lady Diana, Princess of Wales, in 1991.

As Dean of the Faculty of Psychiatry, College of Physicians and Surgeons, Pakistan, he has assisted the college in the development of the curriculum for Fellowship in Psychiatry. He has also been an examiner for this college for Fellowship in Neurology and Psychiatry, and has also been an examiner for MD and M.Phil in Psychiatry, University of Punjab. Prof. Tareen is on the editorial board of a number of scientific journals and has authored various books and numerous research papers and articles.

A link in the same chain of his personal achievements has been the initiation of the Overseas Doctors Training Scheme by the Royal College of Psychiatrists, UK. A number of his trainees have academic affiliations with universities in Pakistan, UK, Canada, and USA, and many others are working as consultant psychiatrists.

He has been President of Mental Health Federation of Pakistan, Member National Coordinating Group for Mental Health Government of Pakistan, Adviser Federal Ministry of Health for Registration of Psychotropic Substances, Chairman of the committee for drugs across the counter at the chemists, Founder of the first lending library for medical students at KEMC, Founder Member Patients Welfare Association Mayo Hospital, President Students-Patients Welfare Society, and President Pakistan Psychiatric Society.

Prof. Tareen was Chairman Scientific Committee, a regional meeting of World Psychiatric Association, and Chairman Scientific Committee 18th International Conference on Medical and Health Sciences. He is currently member of the Punjab Mental Health Authority. He collaborated with WHO in field trials of ICD-10 classification, and in the development of The Lahore Somatic Inventory with the University of Leeds.

He represented Pakistan at the 150 years celebrations of the Royal College of Psychiatrists, London, and at SAARC Workshop on Treatment, Rehabilitation and Detoxification of Drug Dependents. He, along with Prof. Khalida Tareen, established Tareen Mental Health Centre, which has been disseminating information about mental illness through various booklets and brochures, etc. Moreover, this centre has organised numerous educational events for psychiatrists, general practitioners as well as the public. A free clinic for poor psychiatric patients has also been established, which provides not only free consultation but medicines as well. It has played important role in highlighting the importance of mental health and reducing the stigma.

For his unflagging commitment to excellence and rendering unparalleled services, he received lifetime achievements awards from the Pakistan Psychiatric Society and British Pakistani Psychiatrists Association. The KEMU Alumni Association of North America and Association of Pakistani Physicians of North America, likewise acknowledging his distinguished accomplishments, awarded him special Shields.

Author of the third and current edition: **PROFESSOR TANVIR AHMAD RANA**

Professor Tanvir Ahmad Rana is currently working as a Consultant Psychiatrist in the UK. He has been a psychotherapy tutor for the past five years and has trained numerous doctors in psychodynamic psychotherapy as well as cognitive behavioural therapy. His past academic affiliations have been with Warwick, Birmingham, Wolverhampton and Keele universities. He is a Visiting Professor at Wagner College, New York and Staffordshire University. He regularly delivers presentations across England and has been invited as a guest speaker in many countries. Professor Rana has reviewed grant applications for England's National Institute for Health Research and has been the principal and co-investigator of many clinical trials. His original research publications are on Assertive Outreach and Non-Medical Prescribing.

He is a member of the Appointments Advisory Committee of the RCPsych, London. He has co-authored *Psychology for MRCPsych Examination* and co-edited *Understanding Psychology*.

He is currently working on various books: *In Search of Happiness, From Socrates to Sartre: An Outline of Philosophy,* and *From Homer to Hemingway: A Brief History of Western Literature. Besides Neckar's Bank,* his second collection of essays (on literature, philosophy, history, music and art), is being published very soon.

ACKNOWLEDGEMENTS

This book, like my other books, is the result of support from other people. Some people contributed directly to this book, while others helped me in my personal and professional life, and thereby made the publication of this book possible. I want to express my deep-felt thanks to the following people: -

Professor I. A. K. Tareen and Professor Khalida Ijaz Tareen. Just like for the Third Edition, there has been active participation and significant contribution by them for this edition.

Late Chaudhry Ali Asghar, Late Professor Zahida Mir, and Late Gul Mohammad for their immense support in my professional career while I was in Pakistan.

Dr Rana Azkar Hussain, for his consistent and generous guidance in my clinical and academic career.

Kaneez Shahid, Munir Ahmad Rana, Nargis Munir, Tazeem Nazir Bhatti, Nasir Ahmad Rana, Naureen Nasir, Saima Shabbir, Yahsab Ahmad Rana, Akif Ahmad Rana and Areesha Rana for their extreme care while I stayed at Lahore and completed this book. All of them looked after me which made the writing project very conducive.

Dr Maqsood Ahmad, Dr Anjum Bashir, Dr Mateen Durrani, Dr Rais Ahmed, Dr Eaisha Tareen, Dr Ilyas Q. Mirza, Dr Amina Tareen, Dr Qayyum Naz, and Dr Asma Tareen, for their helpful suggestions and assistance.

Dr Saifuddin Jahangir Akbar, Dr Tahir Suleman, Dr Tanvir Akhtar Butt, Dr Tanveer Ahmad Butt, Dr Zubair Ahmed, Dr Sultan Mehmood Lali, Zia Ullah Khan, Mohammed Amir, Aslam Naz, and Abbas Ali Mian, for their incessant encouragement and motivation.

Dr Tasneem Shahid, Dr Shabbir Ahmad Rana, Dr Mahwash Rana and Dr Fahaddas Rana for taking the responsibility of reading the main chapters, and making very helpful and critical suggestions.

Huzaifa, Laraib, Arsal, Sana, and Anzal, for helping me on many occasions with my PC, dictation, transcription and typing issues.

Arwa, Hiba, and Maham for their innocent smiles and laughter, which relaxed and motivated me to work harder on this project

Most importantly, special thanks to Amera. This work could not have been accomplished without support and encouragement from my wife, who once again, with understanding and good humour, endured countless hours of evenings and weekends of my being devoted to this book, hours which otherwise would have been spent with my family.

CONTENTS

CHAPTER

Psychopathology: Signs and Symptoms of Psychiatric Disorders

01

Although psychopathology is commonly defined as the study of abnormalities in the mental state, the definitions or conceptions of psychopathology have been the focus of heated debate throughout the history of psychology and psychiatry. Some authors continue to insist that this controversy is not over.

Various conceptions of psychopathology have been offered over the years. One main aspect of psychopathology is that pathological phenomena are those that are abnormal or statistically deviant or infrequent. However, many people think of psychopathology as behaviour and experience that are not just statistically abnormal but also maladaptive (dysfunctional). Normal and abnormal are statistical terms that do not refer to statistical norms and deviations, but to the effectiveness or ineffectiveness of a person's behaviour. Some other conceptions of psychopathology lay stress on subjective distress and disability, or behaviour that deviates from social or cultural norms. Another school of thought defines psychopathology as harmful dysfunction.

Finally, any conceptions of psychopathology should include a discussion of the two-current classification of mental disorders, DSM 5 and ICD 11. DSM 5 involved hundreds of people working over a 12-year process and was published in 2013. ICD 11 was released in 2018, as a preliminary version and will be implemented later this year. It was not available in hard copy at the time of publication of this book. ICD 11 has been completed over the course of a decade involving 300 specialists across 55 countries. It is important to mention some significant changes to the mental health disorders in ICD 11. The ICD-11 added diagnoses of Attention-deficit Hyperactivity Disorder (ADHD), Complex PTSD, Compulsive Sexual Behaviour Disorder, Gaming Disorder and Prolonged Grief Disorder. ICD-11 has deleted diagnoses of Acute Stress Disorder, and Gender Incongruence. The section on personality disorders has been completely overhauled. There is now one diagnosis of "personality disorder" as it was found that there was much overlap in clinical practice. Personality disorder is labelled as mild, moderate, or severe, and measured in terms of six trait domains to retain some of the earlier specificity of the diagnosis.

Psychiatrists are sometimes blamed regarding diagnoses of psychiatric illnesses. Actually, diagnoses in psychiatry serve a variety of important purposes and are not just a "label", a misunderstanding that is propagated by the critics. It is certainly true that stigma, although to a comparatively lesser extent now, continues to exist all over the world. However, making a careful diagnosis is as essential and fundamental in psychiatry, as it is in the remainder of medicine. Diagnoses are important because of various reasons. The symptoms of mental illness encompass a wide range of emotional, cognitive, and behavioural abnormalities. The use of diagnoses introduces order and structure to this complexity. Diagnoses are used to choose an appropriate treatment, formulate a comprehensive management and help psychiatrists predict the outcome. Moreover, diagnoses have medico-legal relevance and facilitate communication among clinicians, healthcare providers and policy makers for mental health service planning.

In psychiatry, one has to be apt at sharp observation and precise description. Before any patient is examined, it is essential that the interviewer has a firm grasp of the abnormal mental phenomena. Although there are some disagreements between the two classification systems, these salient differences do not reflect real scientific differences, but rather represent historical by-products of independent committee processes. Irrespective of the disagreements, a thorough understanding of psychopathology and classification criteria, is a prerequisite before one can make an accurate diagnosis and management plan.

Descriptive psychopathology, also called phenomenological psychopathology, is the objective description of conscious and observable behaviours. Abnormalities of mental state are viewed as signposts that point towards particular diagnoses. However, these abnormalities should not be considered just as fragments of a disordered mind but as reflections of the whole personality and mental functioning of that individual. In this chapter, the signs and symptoms of various psychiatric disorders are defined. Signs are the objective manifestations of a pathology that are observed by the interviewer whereas symptoms are subjective experiences reported by the patients. However, signs and symptoms in psychiatry can overlap and because of this, psychiatric disorders are often described as syndromes. A syndrome is a group of recognizable signs and symptoms that is less specific than a disorder or disease.

Many books have given lists of signs and symptoms in alphabetical order. Although these glossaries are helpful, the author of this book is of the view that it is even more helpful to define these terms according to various headings of the mental state examination, and that pattern has been followed here.

Form and Content

The distinction between form and content is best explained by examples. If a patient says that he is hearing a voice calling him a bad person, the form is an auditory hallucination while the content is that he is a bad person. Another patient may complain that she is being disturbed by intrusive thoughts that she is an evil person. Here the form is different and suggests obsessive-compulsive disorder. Form is more important when making a diagnosis but content can be significant in the management. Moreover, patients are more concerned with the content.

The Role of Cultures

Before one can be sure of a patient suffering from specific symptoms, it is imperative to be aware of the influence of cultures in presentation of various symptoms. In many eastern cultures, people with depressive disorder may somatise their symptoms. Similarly, particular care is needed regarding religious delusions as some people believe that they are close to God because of their good deeds and their prayers are being answered, etc. Like other delusions, it would be the reasoning that the patient will put forward to explain the beliefs, which will determine whether it is a delusion or not.

DISTURBANCES OF MOOD

The term mood is sometimes used as a broad term to describe all emotions, e.g., anxious mood. On the other hand, it is also used in a limited way to imply an emotion which is depressed at one end of the spectrum and elated at the other. Mood and affect are sometimes used interchangeably and efforts have been made to distinguish between them.

Mood: It is now in a more general use and is defined as a prolonged and pervasive emotional state.

Affect: This is a momentary and short-term experience of emotion. Common examples of affect are euphoria, anger, and sadness. Affect is variable over time, in response to changing emotional states, whereas mood refers to a sustained emotion.

Subjective mood: It is important to ask about the mood from the patient directly, and write in verbatim.

Objective mood: Apart from general observation, the depth and breadth (variation of emotional display) of mood has to be noted down as well.

Euthymic: This is normal range of mood.

Depressed mood: Pathological feeling of sadness, out of proportion or unduly prolonged. Questions about feelings of despair and hopefulness will give an idea of the severity.

Dysphoric: Is an unpleasant mood.

Dysthymic: Mood which is tending to be sad and miserable, but not enough in intensity to qualify as being depressed.

Anhedonia: There is loss of feelings, and interest in all regular and pleasurable activities is lost. Some writers have further divided this into social anhedonia (loss of pleasure with people) and physical anhedonia (eating and drinking, etc). This is a central and diagnostic feature of depressive disorder but occurs in residual schizophrenia as well. However, in some people with depressive disorder irritability can mask the underlying low mood.

Hyperthymic: Tending to be over cheerful and unrealistically optimistic.

Cyclothymic: It is the tendency of marked swings of mood from being cheerful to unhappy over a period of time, but not sufficient to qualify as having bipolar mood swings. It is usually present in cyclothymic personality disorder.

Alexithymia: It is the inability or difficulty in describing or being aware of one's emotions.

Lability of mood: It is an increased, sudden and unstable variation in mood from cheerfulness to sadness or tearfulness. It is short-lived but is often an intense change in feeling in response to either a minor event or an unrelated external stimulus. This is often encountered in mania but may be seen in depressive disorder, cerebrovascular syndromes, dementia and rarely in acute schizophrenia

Emotional incontinence: This is an extreme form of lability of mood, when emotions get out of control.

Elevated mood / Elation: More cheerfulness than usually warranted in the situation or circumstances.

Euphoria: Intense elation with feelings of grandeur.

Expansive: Unreserved expression of one's positive feelings without restraint.

Ecstasy: Feeling of intense euphoria and rapture.

Irritability and anger: Irritability is a state of an increased propensity for anger. Irritability and anger are not helpful in diagnosis as both of these can be present in all psychiatric disorders. However, as mentioned above irritability can mask the underlying low mood in depressive disorder. Irritability may also take the place of the usual euphoria in hypomania.

Diurnal variation of mood: In depressive disorder, the mood is typically and regularly worse in the morning and improves as the day progresses. Although it is one of the diagnostic features of depressive disorder, its absence does not rule out depressive disorder.

Flattening of affect: Affective flattening manifests itself as a characteristic impoverishment of emotional expression, reactivity, and feeling. Affective flattening can be evaluated by observation of the patient's behaviour and responsiveness during a routine interview. However, the evaluation of affective expression may be influenced by the patient's use of prescription drugs, as the parkinsonian side effects of antipsychotics may lead to mask-like facies and diminished associated movements. Other aspects of affect, such as responsivity or appropriateness, are not affected.

There is a clear reduction in display of emotions and both range and depth are adversely affected. The voice is monotonous, the face is immobile, there is less eye contact, decreased spontaneous movements, and increased latency of response. It is usually associated with schizophrenia but a depressed patient can also present with this reduction in emotional modulation and reactivity.

Blunting of affect: Is sometimes used synonymously with flattening of affect but strictly speaking this is a more severe form of flattening of affect. It refers to coarsening of emotions and also an insensitivity to social context.

Apathy: It is indifference and absence of all feelings.

Perplexity: Is anxious and puzzled bewilderment.

Histrionicity: An exaggerated expression of emotions which are shallow.

Disassociation of affect (denial): Seen in conversion disorders (la belle indifference). The person fails to experience and display the expected emotional distress about the disability being mentioned.

Inappropriate or incongruous affect (parathymia): There is discordance between the emotional feeling and the content of the talk or event accompanying it. For example, a patient may laugh while talking about death. Usually a symptom of schizophrenia.

Other Emotions

Anxiety: Anxiety is a normal feeling of apprehension in response to a threat but becomes abnormal when it is so severe that it is out of proportion to the danger. The components of anxiety are psychological, somatic and autonomic features. Anxiety may be focused on an object, situation or activity which is avoided (phobia) or it may be free-floating.

Free-floating anxiety: Pervasive, unfocused fear not attached to any particular situation or idea. This is a hallmark of generalised anxiety disorder.

Agitation: Severe anxiety with motor restlessness.

Panic: Acute, episodic, and intense attack of anxiety.

Phobia: Persistent irrational fear of, and wish to avoid, a specific object or situation.

Tension: Increased motor and psychological activity that is unpleasant.

Ambivalence: Co-existence of two opposing impulses toward the same thing simultaneously.

Abreaction: Emotional release or discharge after recalling a painful experience.

Physiological disturbances associated with mood

Vegetative signs: Signs of somatic dysfunction, are associated with depressive disorder.

Anorexia: Loss or decrease in appetite, which can consequently result in weight loss.

Hyperphagia: Increase in appetite.

Insomnia: Lack of adequate sleep. It can be having difficulty sleeping in the early or middle part of the night or can be early morning awakening.

Hypersomnia: Excessive sleep. Some patients with depressive disorder may have this problem.

Diurnal variation of mood: See above.

Decreased libido: Diminished sexual desire.

Constipation: Inability or difficulty in defecating.

Disturbances of Perception

Perception is the process of transferring stimulation into psychological information. In other words, it is becoming aware of what is presented through the sense organs. Disorders of perception are divided into sensory distortions and false perceptions (illusions, pseudohallucinations, and hallucinations).

Sensory Distortions

Disturbances in the sensory modalities themselves generally occur in organic lesions, for example in parietal lobe lesions there is sometimes a change in the perceived shape of the objects. However, in non-organic states, a person can also perceive the objects in a distorted way. For example, the intensity of the perceived objects is either enhanced (in hypomania/mania) or diminished (in depressive disorder). These changes can appear to be in the size, shape, colour and location of those objects. These distorted perceptions can occur in epilepsy, and rarely in schizophrenia.

Visual hyperaesthesia: The intensity of the colours is heightened. This can occur in ecstasy experiences, LSD intake, mania and epileptic aura.

Micropsia: The size of the perceived object is smaller than the actual size.

Macropsia: The size of the perceived object is larger than the actual size.

Dysmegalopsia: Objects appear larger on one side than the other.

Hyperacusis: The intensity of perception is heightened in the auditory modality. It results because of lowering of the threshold when even small noises or voices become very unpleasant. This can happen in depressive disorder, migraine and alcohol hangover.

Hypoacusis: Diminishing of the intensity of perception in the auditory modality.

Splitting of perception: Inability to form the usual, assumed links between two or more perceptions. Links between different sensory modalities fail to be made. Occurs in organic states and schizophrenia.

Imagery (fantasy): Is the awareness of a perception which the mind creates and terminates at will.

Eidetic imagery: It is an intense and detailed visual imagery that has a photographic quality. It is considered a normal phenomenon and occurs frequently in children. It is an image of something once perceived, which can be conjured up with almost all the original details intact.

Illusion: Misinterpretation of external stimuli, usually when the general level of sensory stimulation is low and the person is tired or anxious.

Pareidolic illusion (pareidolia): Is a common and normal phenomenon. The perception is conjured up by ill-defined sense impressions, so the imagery persists despite the presence of perception.

Hallucinations: These are sensory perceptions in the absence of an external stimulus. In other words, these are actual perceptual abnormalities, and not just believing something. Hallucinations have the qualities and force of the corresponding normal perceptions, being just as vivid, whole and immediate. They are independent of the will; in that, they cannot be conjured up or dismissed and they will continue to force themselves to the patient's attention. Hallucinations are usually experienced alongside and simultaneously with normal perception. Patients frequently find no difficulty in discriminating between their hallucinations and true perceptions. Auditory hallucinations are the most common type of hallucinations in schizophrenia. Their content is usually bizarre, insulting, threatening or commanding. In major depressive disorder, the voices usually have derogatory or nihilistic content.

Pseudohallucinations: They do not have any diagnostic value as they are found across a wide range of psychopathological states, from severe personality disorders to toxic confusional states. The term pseudohallucination has led to a tendency to approach the phenomenon as something to be dismissed as having no inherent interest. In reality, it is an abnormal experience in spite of little diagnostic value, and is indicative of a significant disturbance of mental state.

There are different definitions in psychopathological literature. Two distinct meanings (and terms):

- **Imaged pseudohallucinations:** Sensory experience that differs from hallucination in not seeming to represent external reality. Percepts seem to be located within the mind rather than in external space. Resemble imagery though, unlike imagery, cannot be dismissed by will.
- **Perceived pseudohallucinations:** Sen-sory experience appears to originate in the external world, but it seems unreal.

Elementary hallucinations: Bangs, whistles and flashes.

Complex hallucinations: Voices, music, faces and scenes.

Auditory hallucinations (voices called phenomes):

- **Second person auditory hallucinations:** Voices speak directly to the person. They can occur in all psychiatric illnesses and are therefore not very helpful in diagnosis.
- **Third person auditory hallucinations:** Voices talk among themselves which the patient hears. These types of hallucinations are comparatively more important in diagnosis. Voices can take many forms.
    1. **Voices doing running commentary:** They are usually derogatory but can rarely have positive content.
    2. **Voices speak the patient's thoughts** (Gedankenlautwerden) as the patient is thinking.
    3. **Thought echo** (echo de pensee): Voices immediately repeat thought of the patient. According to some authors this repetition is in the form of thought and not a voice.

Mood congruent hallucinations: Hallu-cinations whose content is consistent with either depressed or a manic mood.

Mood incongruent hallucinations: Hallucinations whose content is not consistent with either depressed or a manic mood.

Visual hallucinations: They vary from ill- defined shapes and colours through clear objects and persons to the complex visions which may, for example, accompany ecstatic states. They characteristically occur in organic states e.g., delirium tremens, post-concussional state, epileptic twilight state, hepatic failure, glue-and petrol-sniffing, mescalin and LSD abuse.

Lilliputian hallucinations: Visual hallucinations of dwarf figures.

Teichopsia: Visual hallucinations of geometrical shapes.

Autoscopic hallucinations (phantom mirror image): Seeing one's own body projected into external space.

Negative Autoscopy: Patient fails to see oneself in the mirror.

Olfactory hallucinations: Are frequently experienced together with gustatory hallucinations. They occur in schizophrenia, depressive disorder, and temporal lobe epilepsy.

Gustatory hallucinations: Are usually of unpleasant tastes occur in schizophrenia, depressive disorder and temporal lobe epilepsy.

Tactile hallucinations (haptic hallucinations): Hallucinations of being touched, pricked or strangled. Hallucinations of deep sensation are experienced as if viscera are being pulled out. Tactile and somatic hallucinations need careful attention as some patients may have odd ways of expressing true sensory disturbances from the delusional elaborations.

Formication: A tactile hallucination in which there is a sensation of something creeping or crawling under the skin. Occurs characteristically in delirium tremens and cocaine withdrawal.

Hypnogogic hallucinations: Hallucinations experienced while going to sleep.

Hypnopompic hallucinations: Hallucinations experienced while waking up. Both hypnogogic and hypnopompic hallucinations occur in narcolepsy, cataplexy, sleep paralysis and in normal people as well.

Extracampine hallucinations: Experienced outside the limits of the sensory field. For example, the patient may say he or she is hearing voices from many miles away.

Reflex hallucinations (synaesthesia): Stim-ulus in one sensory modality results in a hallucination in another sensory modality. In other words, perceptions in one modality are simultaneously experienced as if they were also present in another modality. This phenomenon is experienced in some drug intoxications. In cannabis intoxication, for example, the visual effects occur concomitantly with music.

Functional hallucinations: Sometimes external stimuli provoke hallucinations in the same sensory area. In other words, normal perception of the stimulus and the hallucination in the same modality are experienced simultaneously. These hallucinations are sometimes confused with illusions, but are rare phenomena.

Disturbances of Thought

For convenience's sake, these are grouped under four headings:

1. Disturbance of stream of thought
2. Disturbance of form of thought
3. Disturbance of content of thought
4. Disturbance of possession of thought

1. Disturbances of Stream of Thought

Pressure of speech (tachyphasia): There is excessive increase in the amount of speech which is loud and accelerated. The person continues to talk without any social stimulation and it is difficult to interrupt. Ideas and thoughts arise in abundance, have a lot of variety and accelerate through the mind. Usually, occurs in hypomania/mania. The pressure of speech. The patient has an increase in the amount of spontaneous speech as compared with what is considered ordinary or socially customary. The patient talks rapidly and is difficult to interrupt. Pressured speech is often seen in mania but can be found in other syndromes as well. Some sentences may be left uncompleted because of eagerness to get on to a new idea. Simple questions that could be answered in only a few words or sentences are answered at great length so that the answer takes minutes rather than seconds and indeed may not stop at all if the speaker is not interrupted. Even when interrupted, the speaker often continues to talk. Speech tends to be loud and emphatic. Sometimes speakers with severe pressure will talk without any social stimulation and talk even though no one is listening. This disorder may be accompanied by derailment, tangentiality, or incoherence, but it is distinct from them.

Logorrhoea (verbosity): Implies increased amount rather than the speed of speech. More words are used than needed (wordiness).

Poverty of speech: There is very limited speech so the spontaneous speech and responses to questions are very brief. Sometimes answers can be monosyllabic. Usually occur in schizophrenia, although some patients with depressive disorder may also exhibit this.

Poverty of content of speech: Patient's speech lacks richness and variety. Speech can be adequate in amount but it conveys very little information as it is vague, has empty repetitions or there are obscure phrases. Occurs in residual schizophrenia.

Thought block (snapping off): There is an abrupt interruption in the chain of thoughts and the patient reports complete emptying of the mind. The thought is never recalled. The reason for this is not distraction by other thoughts. After a period of silence, which may last from a few seconds to minutes, the person indicates that he or she cannot recall what he or she has been saying or meant to say. Thought block is difficult to elicit but as it is almost diagnostic of schizophrenia, however, the clinician needs to be very careful and sure about it.

2. Disturbances of Form of Thought (Formal Thought Disorder)

Formal thought disorder, sometimes called schizophrenic language disorder, is characterised by disturbance in the area of semantics, although in chronic and advanced cases, the syntax may also be disrupted. According to some writers, in the absence of coarse brain disease, the presence of formal thought disorder is diagnostic of schizophrenia. However, as these symptoms do not occur in isolation and there are symptoms in other areas as well, this makes the diagnosis more reliable. Most patients suffering from schizophrenia exhibit some formal thought disorder at some stage of their illness. There is not only some overlap of meaning between some of the following terms but also some concepts have different meanings for some writers. This is because they have been described historically by different psychiatrists from various countries, who have written in different languages.

Akataphasia: A disorder in the expression of thought in speech.

Bradyphasia: Is a speech that is reduced in the rate but not necessarily in content.

Perseveration: Persistent and inappropriate repetition of the same words or thoughts. Perseveration differs from the repetitive use of stock words or interjections such as, 'you know', or 'like'. Occurs usually in frontal lobe dysfunction, and also in schizophrenia.

Echolalia: Repeating of words or sentences of one person by the other.

Palilalia: The perseverated word is repeated with increasing frequency.

Logoclonia: Perseveration of the last syllable of the last word.

Flight of ideas: Thoughts move quickly from one topic to another but logical sequence and connection of ideas is preserved. Characteristically occurs in hypomania/mania.

Desultory speech: In this there are no logical connections.

Asyndesis (asyndetic thinking): There is a lack of causal links between thoughts. In other words, breakdown of connection between thoughts.

Fragmentation: An idea is broken into many parts which are in themselves not understandable.

Interpenetration: There is inappropriate intrusion of unrelated ideas into a thought which was comprehensible in the beginning.

Clang associations: This occurs in schizophrenia and mania. The sounds of the words rather than their meaning determine the choice of words. There is no connection in the meaning of the two words. Clanging includes puns (a second meaning of the first word), rhymes, assonance and alliteration.

Loosening of associations: Loss of the normal structure of thinking. It is muddled, illogical and does not become clearer on further questioning.

Knight's move or derailment: Transition between one topic to another with no logical connection between the two topics. There is disruption of the thought content with insertion of other thought contents in place of the true chain of thought.

Omission: Here a thought or a part of the thought is inappropriately omitted from the speech.

Transitory thinking: This is characterised by derailments and omission in the train of thought by which both the semantics and syntax may be disrupted.

Drivelling thinking: In this there is a mixing and muddling of the thoughts (substitution) that obscures the meaning. The patient may initially give the impression that something meaningful is being said but it soon becomes apparent that it is a flow of words and high sounding phrases signifying little or nothing.

Vorbeireden (talking past the point): The speech never reaches the point at hand. It is used interchangeably with Vorbeigehen (going past the point).

Verbigeration: Speech is reduced to senseless repetition of sounds, words or phrases. When this is extreme, it is called word salad.

Self-referential speech: Here there is communications that returns repeatedly to the patients and their highly personal interests and preoccupations.

Overinclusion: This is a tendency to include irrelevant items in a concept. When a patient attempts to convey an idea, he or she is unable to maintain the boundaries of a thought.

Circumstantiality: The language of schizophrenic patients is sometimes weighed down with unnecessary detail. There is loss of goal, and the communication drifts apparently aimlessly. There is an overinclusion of tedious details before reaching the point. It is common in obsessive-compulsive personality disorder but is also present in normal people as well. Circumstantial replies or statements may last for many minutes if the speaker is not interrupted and urged to get to the point. Interviewers will often recognise circumstantiality on the basis of needing to interrupt the speaker to complete the process of history taking within an allotted time. When not called circumstantial, these people are often referred to as long-winded.

Although it may coexist with instances of poverty of content of speech or loss of goal, circumstantiality differs from poverty of content of speech in containing excessive amplifying or illustrative detail and from loss of goal in that the goal is eventually reached if the person is allowed to talk long enough. It differs from derailment in that the details presented are closely related to some particular goal or idea and that the particular goal or idea must, by definition, eventually be reached (unless the patient is interrupted by an impatient interviewer).

Word approximations: Here words are used unconventionally. Words have meanings that are comprehensible but are used to fill the semantic gap.

Tangentiality: Oblique, digressive, or even irrelevant manner of speech in which the central idea is not communicated. Inability to have goal-directed association of thought; patient never gets from desired points to the desired goal. The patient replies to a question in an oblique, tangential, or even irrelevant manner. The reply may be related to the question in some distant way, or the reply may be unrelated and seem totally irrelevant.

Fusion: There is some preservation of the normal chain of association, but bringing together of heterogenous elements.

Condensation: It is similar to fusion. Com-bining various concepts into a single false one. One symbol stands for a number of constituents.

Displacement and substitution: Here one idea is used for an associated idea.

Mixing or muddling: Amalgam of the constituent parts of a single thought process and represent extreme degree of fusion and derailment. The resultant speech disorder is called drivelling.

Metonyms: Use of word or phrase that is related to the proper one but is not the one ordinarily used. Imprecise approximations for a more exact word.

Neologism: New words or phrases invented by the patient. Patients also give new and highly idiosyncratic meanings to existing words. Occurs in schizophrenia. Neologisms need to be differentiated from words or pharases deliberately invented by family members or friends to communicate in a private or funny way.

Cryptolalia: This is the private, spoken language.

Cryptographia: This is the private, written language.

Concrete thinking: Inability to think abstractly. Rather than considering the overall meaning of a concept, the patient selects and focuses on one aspect of the concept and the metaphorical nature is lost.

Alogia (laconic speech): Negative thought disorder, or poverty of thoughts as expressed in words.

Poverty of thought content (empty speech): See above.

Stock words/phrases: As patients with schizophrenia have a limited vocabulary, they repeatedly rely upon, and frequently use certain words or phrases. These have a greater and wider meaning for them than other people.

Paralogia: Is used to describe positive thought disorder, or the intrusion of irrelevant or bizarre thought.

Paraphasia: Is the destruction of words with interpolation of more or less garbled sound. Other terms used synonymously are paraphemia, pseudoagrammatism, and paraphasia.

Literal paraphasia: Is a gross misuse of the meaning of words to such an extent that statements no longer make any sense.

Verbal paraphasia: Describes the loss of the appropriate word but the statements are still meaningful.

Agrammatism: When grammar is altered, the loss of parts of speech is described as agrammatism

Telegramese: When adverbs are also lost, it results in coarsening and poverty of sentences.

Paragrammatism: Literally means wrong use of grammar.

Parasyntax: Wrong use of syntax. In paragrammatism and parasyntax there is inappropriate use of words and there is a mass of complicated clauses which make no sense in achieving the goal of thought. The individual phrases are, however, in themselves, quite comprehensible.

Desultory thinking: Ideas are expressed correctly in terms of syntax and grammatical construction, but are juxtaposed inappropriately. Thoughts jump from one idea to another without having any logical connections.

Dereism: Mental activity not concordant with logic or experience.

Autistic thinking: Preoccupation with the inner, private world; sometimes used simultaneously with dereism.

Magical thinking: A form of dereistic thinking; thinking in which thoughts, words, or actions assume that they can cause or prevent events.

Primary process thinking: This is normally in dreams, it is dereistic, illogical, and magical.

Glossolalia (speaking in tongues): The expression of a revelatory message through unintelligible words.

3. Disturbances of Content of Thought

Overvalued idea: Isolated, preoccupying belief, which is neither delusional nor obsessional in nature, but dominates a person's life. It is understandable when the person's situation and background is known. In anorexia nervosa, the distorted body image is usually an overvalued idea but can reach to a delusional extent.

Delusion: It is a belief, based on incorrect inference about external reality, and is not consistent with the patient's intelligence, education and cultural background. Deluison is not amenable to reason nor modifiable by experience. It is held with such a strong and absolute conviction that it cannot be altered by presenting evidence to the contrary. It is experienced as self-evident reality, not as merely opinion or belief. Delusions are experienced as being of great personal significance and usually preoccupy the person to the point of disrupting social and interpersonal functioning. It is important to note that it is not the falsity of the delusion that determines whether the belief is delusional but the nature of the mental processes that led up to it and the reasoning and explanation put forward by the patient. The content of a delusion is often regarded by others as inherently unlikely. Some other important aspects of delusions are, their emergence in a manner which suggests their pathological origins, and evoking persistent idiosyncratic behaviours which are potentially damageing to oneself and others. However, the patient's behaviour may or may not be influenced by the specific delusions.

In their mildest form delusions may persist for only weeks to months, and the patient may question his or her beliefs or doubt them. The assessment of the severity of delusions should take into account their persistence, their complexity, the extent to which the patient acts on them, the extent to which the patient doubts them, and the extent to which the beliefs deviate from those that non-psychotic people might have.

Double orientation: Delusions do not necessarily influence all the feelings and actions. For example, a patient may firmly believe that he is a king but at the same time is living in poor socio-economic conditions without appreciating this gross reality. This separation of belief from feeling and action is called double orientation.

Partial delusion: When the delusion is being initially formed it is held at first with a degree of uncertainty. Also, during recovery, patients pass through a stage of increasing doubt before finally rejecting the delusions.

Primary delusion (autochthonous): Appears suddenly with full conviction but without any mental events leading up to it. Indicative of schizophrenia.

Secondary delusion: Derived from a preceding morbid experience. The false belief is understandable in present circumstances e.g., a nihilistic delusion subsequent to depressed mood.

Systematised delusions: Accumulation of secondary delusions to form a complicated delusional system. Beliefs are united by a single event or theme.

Mood congruent delusion: A delusion wh-ose content is consistent with either a depressed or elated mood.

Mood incongruent delusion: A delusion whose content is not consistent with either a depressed or elated mood.

Shared delusions (folie à deux): A normal person living with a deluded patient comes to share his delusional belief. When they are separated the normal person usually loses the delusion.

Delusional mood: The preceding mood, a feeling of foreboding, before the full development of the delusion.

Delusional memory: A new significance (delusional belief) is attached to past events.

Delusional perception: Immensely and suddenly, a significant and delusional meaning is given to a normal percept. This is a Schneiderian first-rank symptom (see below).

Delusional Misinterpretation

- **Illusion of doubles:** Belief that a familiar person has been replaced by an imposter who is the exact double of the original. This is a central feature of Capgras syndrome.

- **Fregoli's delusion:** Person sees several different people one after the other and believes that he or she has seen a single person in several disguises.

Delusions According to Their Themes

- **Persecutory delusions:** A delusion in which the central theme is that a person is being persecuted or conspired against. The commonly used term paranoid delusion is not recommended because its meaning is multiple.
- **Paranoid delusions:** Include delusions of persecution, grandeur and reference.
- **Delusions of reference:** The central theme is that remarks, statements, events, objects, or other people have a particular and unusual significance, usually of a negative nature. For example, the patient walks into a room, sees people laughing, and suspects that they were just talking about him or her. Sometimes items read in the newspaper, seen on television, or transmitted over the internet are considered special messages to the person.
- **Ideas of reference:** The patient is suspicious but recognises that his or her idea may be erroneous. When the patient actually and firmly believes that the statements or events refer to him or her, then this is considered a delusion of reference.
- **Grandiose (expansive) delusions:** A delusional belief having an exaggerated sense of one's importance, power, or future plans. The patient believes that he or she has special powers or abilities or is a famous person. Some patients believe that they are writing some great novel, composing a great symphony, or are inventing something wonderful and exceptional.
- **Delusions of guilt (and worthlessness):** Usually found in major depressive disorder. The patient believes that he or she has committed some terrible sin or done something unforgivable. Sometimes the patient is excessively or inappropriately preoccupied with things he or she did as a child that were wrong, such as stealing candy from a store. The patient may feel responsible for causing some disastrous event, such as a fire or an accident, with which he or she in fact has no connection. Sometimes these delusions have a religious flavor, involving the belief that the sin is unpardonable and that the patient will suffer eternal punishment from God. Some patients simply believe that they deserve punishment by society and may spend a good deal of time confessing these sins to whoever will listen.
- **Nihilistic delusions:** A person believes that some person or thing has ceased to exist. Seen in major depressive disorder. Some patients believe that their bodies are rotting and their bowel system has permanently stopped. Such extreme forms of nihilistic delusions are called Cotard's syndrome.
- **Delusions of poverty:** A false belief that one is a bereft or will be deprived of all material possessions.
- **Hypochondriacal delusions:** Contrary to medical evidence, the patient believes he or she suffers from a disease.
- **Religious delusions:** The patient is preoccupied with false beliefs of a religious nature. Sometimes these exist within the context of a conventional religious system, such as beliefs about the Second Coming, the Antichrist, or possession by the Devil. At other times, they may involve an entirely new religious system or a pastiche of beliefs from a variety of religions. Religious delusions may be combined with grandiose delusions (if the patient considers himself or herself a religious leader), delusions of guilt, or delusions of being controlled. Religious delusions must be outside the range of beliefs considered normal for the patient's cultural and religious background.
- **Delusions of jealousy (infidelity):** Belief that one's partner or lover is unfaithful. Usually present in men. Has very high risk for violence especially when alcohol is being abused. Random bits of information are construed as "evidence." The person usually goes to great effort to prove the existence of the affair, searching for hair in the bedclothes, the odour of shaving lotion or smoke on clothing, or receipts or cheques indicating that a gift has been bought for the lover. Elaborate plans are often made to trap the two together.
- **Delusions of love /sexual or amorous delusions (de Clerambault's synd-rome):** A delusional belief, more in women, in which the person believes that someone higher in social status is in love with them. Also called erotomania.
- **Somatic delusions:** The patient believes that somehow his or her body is diseased, abnormal, or changed. For example, the patient may believe that his or her stomach or brain is rotting, that his or her hands have become enlarged, or that his or her facial features are ugly or misshapen. Sometimes somatic delusions are accompanied by tactile or other hallucinations. For example, a patient believes that he has ball bearings rolling about in his head, placed there by a dentist who filled his teeth, and can actually hear them clanking against one another!
- **Lycanthropy:** This is a delusion of turning into an animal.
- **Pseudologia phantastica:** The person appears to believe in the reality of his or her fantasies and acts on them.

4. Disturbances of Possession of Thought

Delusions of control: In which one's will, thoughts and feelings are being controlled and operated by external forces. The central requirement for this type of delusion is an actual strong subjective experience of being controlled. It does not include simple beliefs or ideas, such as that the patient is acting as an agent of God or that friends or parents are trying to coerce him or her into doing something. Rather, the patient must describe, for example, that his or her body has been occupied by some alien force that is making it move in peculiar ways, or that messages are being sent to his or her brain by radio waves and causing him or her to experience particular thoughts and feelings that the person recognises are not his or her own.

Thought broadcasting/Audible thoughts: The patient believes that his or her thoughts are broadcast so that he or she or others can hear them. Sometimes the patient experiences his or her thoughts as a voice outside his or her head; this is an auditory hallucination as well as a delusion. Sometimes the patient feels that his or her thoughts are being broadcast, although he or she cannot hear them. Sometimes he or she believes that his or her thoughts are picked up by a microphone and broadcast on the radio, the television, or through the Internet.

Thought insertion: The patient believes that thoughts that are not his or her own have been inserted into his or her mind against the will. For example, the patient may believe that a neighbor is practising voodoo and planting alien sexual thoughts into his or her mind. This symptom should not be confused with experiencing unpleasant thoughts that the patient recognises as his or her own, such as delusions of persecution or guilt.

Thought withdrawal: The patient believes that thoughts have been taken away from his or her mind against the will. The patient is able to describe a subjective experience of beginning thought and then suddenly having it removed by some alien force. This symptom does not include the mere subjective recognition of alogia.

Schneiderian First-rank Symptoms

Kurt Schneider was of the view that in the absence of brain disease, a clear evidence of one first-rank symptom is diagnostic of schizophrenia (although most psychiatrists emphasise additional symptoms for an accurate diagnosis). Schneiderian symptoms include thought insertion, thought withdrawal, thought broadcast, delusional perception (see above) and the following:

- **Made feelings:** Feelings are attributed to external force or agency.
- **Made impulses:** Drive and impulses seem to be alien
- **Made volitional acts:** Patients report that their actions and movements are not under their control, and are being controlled from outside.
- **Somatic passivity:** Belief that parts of the body are being controlled from outside.

Disturbance of Language and Speech

The functions of thinking and speaking (obviously) overlap and cannot be readily separated from each other.

Psychogenic Anomalies

Mutism: Absence of faculty of speech. This occurs as an abnormal reaction to stress, but can also have an organic basis.

Approximate answers: The patient just avoids giving a correct answer to a simple question.

Paraphasia: It is the production of an inappropriate sound in place of a word or phrase.

Pseudologia fantastica: A condition of fluent, plausible lying, often associated with histrionic personality disorders. The patient believes in the fantastic statements.

Eccentric and pedantic use of words may sometimes be seen in those of anankastic personality.

Speech Disturbances

Aphonia: Loss of the ability to vocalise; the patient only talks in a whisper. May also occur without organic cause (hysterical aphonia).

Dysphonia: Denotes impairment with hoarseness, but without complete loss of function.

Dysarthria: Disorders of articulation may be caused by lesions of the brain stem such as bulbar and pseudobulbar palsy, structural or muscular disorders of the mouth, pharynx, larynx and thorax.

Stuttering: Frequent repetition or prolongation of a sound or syllable, giving rise to markedly impaired speech fluency.

Cluttering: Erratic and dysrhythmic speech, consisting of rapid and jerky spurts.

Dysprosody: Loss of normal speech melody.

Logoclonia: See above.

Echolalia: See above.

Aphasia: Loss of language altogether.

Dysphasia: Impairment of, or difficulty with, language.

Expressive Dysphasia: Difficulty in trying to express verbal language.

Receptive dysphasia: Difficulty in comprehending oral language.

Obsessional and Compulsive Symptoms

Obsessions: Are repetitive thoughts that the patient recognises as his own, but finds them irrational and repugnant, and tries to resist them but is unsuccessful in doing so. Recurrent persistent thoughts, impulses, or images enter the mind despite efforts to exclude them. There is a subjective sense of a struggle—the patient fruitlessly resists the obsessions regarding them as senseless. Central to the experience of an obsession is usually a fear or phobia.

Obsessional ruminations: Are repeated the-mes, usually of worrying nature.

Obsessional doubts: Repeated thoughts expressing uncertainty about previous actions.

Obsessional impulses: Repeated urges to carry out actions that are against social norms. The person, however, is able to resist these urges.

Obsessional phobias: Here the obsessional symptom is associated with avoidance as well as anxiety.

Compulsions: These are repetitive seemingly purposeful stereotyped behaviours. There is a pathological need to act on an impulse that, if resisted, produces anxiety. In practice, compulsions are behavioural responses to obsessions, although not all obsessions lead to compulsions.

Checking rituals: e.g., Repeated checking of locks and doors.

Cleaning rituals: e.g., Repeated hand washing.

Counting rituals: Counting in some special way.

Dressing rituals: e.g., Putting the clothes in special order.

Obsessional slowness: Sometimes slowness is a primary feature of unknown origin (rather the slowness of actions of obsessional people).

Coprolalia: Compulsive utterances of obscene words.

Motor signs and symptoms

Tics: Irregular repeated movements involving a group of muscles. These do not have any apparent purpose or significance.

Static tremor: Can occur in hands, head, or upper limb.

Spasmodic torticollis: Involves spasm of neck muscles with twisting of the head.

Chorea: Abrupt, random jerky movements resembling fragments of goal-directed behaviour.

Athetosis: Slow, semi-rotary writhing movements.

Orofacial dyskinesia: Restless movements of tongue, mouth and facial muscles.

Mannerisms: Repeated involuntary movements that appear to have some social or functional significance. These are ingrained and habitual.

Stereotypies: Repeated movements of a single part of the body that are regular and without obvious significance.

Grimacing: Same meaning as ordinary use.

Schnauzkrampf: Literally snout spasm, a facial expression in which the nose and lips are drawn together in a pout.

Echopraxia: Automatic imitation of movements of another person.

(In **echolalia**, words or phrases are imitated).

Automatic obedience: Subject does whatever is asked without questioning or thinking about the consequences.

Advertence: The patient turns towards the examiner when he addresses him; it has got a bizarre exaggerated and inflexible quality.

Forced grasping: The offered hand is repeatedly grasped and shaken, despite requests not to do so.

Mitmachen: The body can be put into any posture.

Mitgehen: This is extreme form of mitmachen. Excessive compliance in which the patient' s limbs can be moved into any position with the slightest pressure.

Ambitendence: The patient alternates between opposite movements.

Catatonia: Motor anomalies in non-organic disorders. A state of increased muscle tone at rest.

Catalepsy (catatonic posturing): Maint-enance of unusual postures for long periods of time with no sense of discomfort e.g., psychological pillow. Catalepsy is accompanied by waxy flexibility (see below).

Catatonic waxy flexibility (Cerea flexibilitas): Person can be moulded into a position as if she or he is made of wax. This position is then maintained for a long period.

Catatonic excitement: Agitated, purposeless motor activity, uninfluenced by external stimuli.

Catatonic negativism: An apparently motiveless resistance to all instructions or attempts to be moved. When passive, the person may resist any effort to be moved; when active, the person may do the opposite of what is asked.

Catatonic stupor: Markedly slowed motor activity often to a point of immobility and lack of speech and seemingly unawareness of surroundings (presence of full consciousness).

Catatonic rigidity: Voluntary assumption of a rigid posture, held against all efforts to be moved.

Cataplexy: Temporary loss of muscle tone and weakness precipitated by emotional states.

Psychomotor agitation: Excessive motor activity associated with a feeling of inner tension. Mental disturbance causes physical restlessness and increased arousal, but this is non-productive and repetitious.

Psychomotor retardation: Generalised slo-wing down of physical reactions, movements, and speech.

Perseveration: Senseless repetition of a previously requested movement.

Sleepwalking (somnambulism): Motor activity during sleep.

Dipsomania: Compulsion to drink alcohol.

Kleptomania: Recurrent compulsion to steal objects that are not needed for personal use or for their monetary value.

Nymphomania: Excessive and compulsive need for coitus in females.

Satyriasis: Excessive and compulsive need for coitus in males.

Trichotillomania: Compulsion to pull out one's hair.

Ritual: Autonomic activity, compulsive in nature and aiming at reducing anxiety.

Ataxia: Failure of muscle coordination; irregularity of muscle action.

Polyphagia: Pathological overeating.

Acting out: A direct expression of an unconscious wish or impulse in action, without consideration of consequences.

Abulia: A reduced impulse to act and think, associated with indifference about consequences of action (because of a neurological defect).

Disturbances Associated with Cognitive Disorder

Agnosia: An inability to recognise and interpret the significance of sensory impressions. Agnosias may affect different sensory modalities and are usually a reflection of cortical damage.

Anosognosia: Inability to recognise a neurological defect as occurring to oneself.

Somatoagnosia (autotopagnosia): Inability to recognise a body part as one's own.

Visual agnosia: Inability to recognise objects or persons.

Astereognosis: Inability to recognise objects by touch.

Prosopagnosia: Inability to recognise faces.

Apraxia: Inability to carry out specific tasks.

Simultagnosia: Inability to comprehend more than one element of a visual scene at a time or to integrate the parts into a whole.

Adiadochokinesia: Inability to perform rapid alternating movements.

Disturbances Associated with Conversion and Disassociation Phenomena

Hysterical anaesthesia: Loss of sensory modalities resulting from emotional conflicts.

Fugue: Taking on a new identity with amnesia for the old identity.

Multiple personality: One person who appears at different times to be two or more entirely different personalities.

Depersonalisation: Change of self-awareness such that the person feels unreal, detached from his own experience and unable to feel emotion.

Derealisation: Change of awareness about the environment, such that objects appear unreal and people appear as lifeless, two-dimensional 'cardboard' figure. Despite the complaint of inability to feel emotion, both depersonalisation and derealisation are highly unpleasant experiences. Sometimes other accompanying experiences are changes in the experience of time, changes in the body image (such as limbs with altered shape and size) and the feeling of being outside one's own body.

Micropsia and Macropsia: Objects comparatively appear smaller and larger respectively. Occurs in organic conditions e.g., complex partial seizures. Such changes may occur in severe fatigue, sleeplessness, toxic states, and temporal lobe epilepsy.

Types of Memory and Disturbances of Memory

Working memory: A very limited amount of information (e.g., holding a phone number).

Short-term memory: Holds recent memories and experiences. Material can be transferred to long-term memory.

Long-term (remote) memory: This is a sto-re for permanent memories with unlimited capacity.

Episodic memory: Storage area for information. Is for experiences such as meeting a friend.

Procedural memory storage: It is for lear-ned skills.

Semantic memory: Is concerned with factual information, the meaning of words, and the attributes of objects.

Procedural memory: Is for skills such as driving a car. Also called implicit memory.

Explicit memory: In which the learned information can be recalled.

Amnesia (dysmnesia): Partial or total failure of memory. May be organic or emotional in origin. Memory loss caused by organic conditions usually affects recall of recent events more than recall of distant ones, and is not a total loss. Total loss of all memory including that of personal identity strongly suggests psychogenic causes.

Amnestic disorder: Some organic conditions give rise to partial effect, in which the person is unable to remember events occurring a few minutes before, but can recall remote events. This disorder is concerned at least in part with retrieval.

Anterograde amnesia: Loss of memory for events subsequent to the onset of the amnesia; common after trauma.

Retrograde amnesia: Loss of memory for events preceding the onset of the amnesia.

Paramnesia: Falsification of memory by distortion of recall.

Disturbances of Recognition

Jamais vu: Failure to recognise events that have been encountered before.

Déjà vu: Conviction that an event repeats one that has been experienced in the past when in fact it is novel.

Confabulation: A person gives a reply that may sound plausible and which he believes to be true, but that is actually false. Common in frontal lobe syndrome and dementia.

Psychogenic amnesias: Thought to result from an active process of repression that prevents the recall of memories that would otherwise evoke unpleasant emotions.

False memory syndrome: Matter of dispute whether memories can be repressed completely but return many years later.

Consciousness

Consciousness: It is the state of awareness of the self and the environment.

Sensorium: State of cognitive functioning of the special senses (sometimes used as a synonym for consciousness).

Confusion: Inability to think clearly.

Oneiroid state: There is dream-like imagery although the person is not asleep.

Twilight state: Prolonged oneiroid state, in which there are hallucinations.

Disorientation: Disturbance of orientation in time, place and person.

Clouding of consciousness: Disorientation in time, place and person, disturbances of perception and attention and subsequent amnesia.

Drowsiness: Further reduction in the level of consciousness, with unconsciousness if unstimulated, but can be stimulated to a wakeful state.

Somnolence: Abnormal drowsiness.

Stupor: Further loss of responsiveness. The person can only be aroused by considerable stimulation. Awareness of the environment is often maintained in depressive or catatonic stupor, but not in organic stupor.

Coma: Profound reduction of conscious level with very little or no response to stimulation.

Coma vigil (akinetic mutism): Coma in which the patient appears to be asleep but ready to be aroused.

Delirium: Acute reversible mental disorder characterised by confusion and some impairment of consciousness; generally associated with emotional lability, hallucinations or illusions, and inappropriate, impulsive, irrational, or violent behaviour.

Dream-like state: Often used as a synonym for complex partial seizure or psychomotor epilepsy.

Disturbances of Attention

Distractibility: Inability to concentrate. Occ-urs in hypomania/mania.

Selective inattention: Blocking out only those things that generate anxiety.

Hypervigilance: Excessive attention to all internal and external stimuli.

Trance: Focused attention and altered consciousness, usually seen in hypnosis, religious or spiritual experiences, and disassociative states.

Hypnosis: It is usually not encountered or done in psychiatric practice. In this controversial technique, disturbance of suggestibility results in artificial and temporary modification of consciousness.

REFERENCES

1. Sims, A. (2003). *Symptoms in the mind.* An introduction to descriptive psychopathology (3rd Edition). London: Elsevier Ltd.
2. Hamilton, M. (1985). *Fish's clinical psychopathology*. Signs and symptoms in psychiatry (2nd Edition). USA: John Wright and Sons
3. Hamilton, M. (1984). *Fish's schizophrenia* (3rd Edition). Bristol: J. Wright.
4. Jaspers, K. (1963). *General psychopathology*.

   Translated by J. Hoenig and M. Hamilton.

   Manchester: Manchester University Press.
5. B. J., Sadock and Sadock, V. A. (2007). *Kaplan and Sadock's Synopsis of Psychiatry: Behavioural sciences/ clinical psychiatry* (10th Edition). Philadelphia: Lippincott Williams and Wilkins.
6. *Essentials of Psychiatry*, Fourth Edition. Edited by Robin M. Murray Kenneth S. Kendler Peter McGuffin Simon Wessely David J. Castle, Cambridge University Press 2008. Cambridge.
7. *Psychopathology: Foundations for a Contemporary Understanding.* Edited by James E. Maddu, Barbara A. Winstead. Lawrence Erlbaum Associates, Inc. New Jersey 2005
8. *Diagnostic and Statistical Manual of Mental Disorders* Fifth edition, American Psychiatric Association, Washington 2013
9. *Adult Psychopathology and Diagnosis;* Seventh Edition Edited by Deborah C. Beidel, B. Christopher Frueh, and Michel Hersen2014 by John Wiley & Sons, Inc. New Jersey.
10. *Introductory Textbook of Psychiatry* Sixth Edition Donald W. Black and Nancy C. Andreasen 2014 American Psychiatric Publishing, Arlington, VA
11. *Lecture Notes in Psychiatry* Gautam Gulati, Mary-Ellen Lynall, Kate Saunders Eleventh Edition, 2014 John Wiley & Sons, Oxford

The Psychiatric Interview 02

It is imperative to remember that each patient is an individual and unique human being whose life has become disturbed by the mental illness. The interviewer should be keen to understand the subjective experiences and the effect they are having on the patient's life. In fact, the word psychiatry, coined by Johann Reil, a German physician and anatomist, means meeting of two minds, the mind of the patient and the mind of the doctor. It cannot be overstated that skill and proficiency in interviewing techniques is only acquired through practice and in no way should reading of books be regarded as a substitute to spending more time with the patients.

It also needs to be emphasised that interpersonal communication is a crucial skill in psychiatric assessment which should not consist of passively asking a series of questions. The rhythm and inflection of voice plays an important role, as the manner in which a question is asked is equally important as the content of the statement. It is not only essential to know what pertinent questions to ask but to be aware that these have to be asked in a sensitive, friendly and non-judgmental way. Questions should never appear to be interrogational or moralising. Patients who feel threatened or uneasy will understandably be hesitant to give full information and the whole purpose of the interview would be lost. While the interviewer must be tactful and thoughtful about what he or she says, this should not preclude behaving with natural warmth and spontaneity.

It is essential to keep in mind various factors that might influence the course and outcome of the interview. The degree of ethnic, cultural, and socioeconomic similarity between the patient and the interviewer may affect the level of rapport between patient and interviewer, the way they interpret each other's verbal and non-verbal communications (which can complement or contradict what is being said), and the meaning the interviewer attaches to the patient's statements and behaviours. The interviewer must remain open to literal and metaphorical messages from the patient, and the impact the patient is trying to make.

Transference and countertransference also play an important role in the interviewer's and patient's relationship. Transference consists of patient's attitude, beliefs and emotional responses which is brought from the past to the current situation. This is actually the quality and type of relationship which a patient had with a significant figure in the past. Similarly, countertransference is the attitude and reaction of the interviewer which is manifested unconsciously in the interaction with the patient.

The interview is the principal means of assessment in clinical psychiatry. Apart from eliciting information in a structured way, interview is used to observe, listen to, and interact with the patient. Although a psychiatric interview is similar to a general medical examination, the psychological family and social aspects of the patients have much more significance in psychiatry. The psychiatrist, moreover, attempts to build a picture of the patient's personality characteristics, especially weaknesses and strengths, as these play an important part in the prognosis of the illness.

The psychiatric interview is of paramount importance as this is the psychiatrist's primary diagnostic tool. In order to reach a diagnosis, the interviewer has to collect a substantial amount of history and conduct a thorough mental state examination. The interviewer should interpret the patient's responses correctly and appropriately and should also attempt to understand the causes and context of the mental illness. The interview, especially the first one, is not just a specialised technique for gathering information but an invaluable opportunity to establish rapport and future working relationship with the patient.

A psychiatric interview is therapeutic in its own right, and should be done in an empathetic way. Empathy is an important quality in psychiatric interviewing. While sympathy is an expression of agreement or support for another, empathy entails putting oneself in another's place and experiencing his or her state of mind. It is the ability to understand the emotional perspective of the other person, while not changing yours, and is a prerequisite for gaining the trust of the patient. As a mode of listening, empathy is an important way of understanding the patient; as a mode of response, it is important in building rapport and alliance. An example of an empathetic statement is: 'That must have been very upsetting for you. Tell me more about that'.

During the interview, it is helpful to give some reflecting comments e.g., 'you seem to be very disturbed by this'. As reflection is not the exact repetition of what the patient has stated, the patient feels assured that the interviewer is understanding the depth of the problems. Appropriate silences can be helpful as well e.g., when patient is weepy or seems to contemplate. Sometimes, however, there is a need to confront the patient with facts in a polite way especially when the patient is in denial or is not attentive to important points.

A psychiatric interview requires the clinician to ask some uncomfortable questions such as "Do you hear voices when no one is around?" or to ask about areas of life that are especially private and intimate, such as sexual preferences and practices. Questions should be asked in a tactful way, such as, 'I would like to ask about topics which are a bit more personal. Is that okay?' or 'I know these things are difficult to talk about but this information will help in understanding you better.'

Before starting the interview, it is important to ensure that structure of the room is appropriate. Patient should be sitting beside the writing desk and not across the desk as it creates a psychological barrier. Consider your safety as well. Your sitting position should be such that the patient is not able to block your exit if you want to leave the room. There should be no such objects in the room that can potentially be used by the patient in a harmful way. It is imperative that your colleagues are not only aware of the interview but are also available if you need to call them for help. On rare occasions (e.g., when there is an imminent likelihood of the patient becoming violent) it may even be preferable to terminate the interview prematurely and consult colleagues immediately. There has never been a unanimous agreement among psychiatrists about taking notes during the interview. It is generally suggested by most writers to take brief notes while at the same time maintaining appropriate eye contact with the patient.

Mentally unwell people, especially those having their first psychiatric episode, are apprehensive, upset, embarrassed and bewildered about their symptoms and morbid experiences. They feel stigmatised and struggle to make sense of their symptoms. So it is always worthwhile to make them feel at ease at the beginning of the interview. Although various campaigns and strategies have helped to reduce stigma to a significant extent, it unfortunately remains an important issue for the patients and mental health professionals. One of the commonest question patients ask is, 'what is happening to me and why?' Just as history is not simply a list of events or characters, the personal narrative of each patient is similarly more than a list of chronological events and symptoms. It is essential to take a broader and holistic look at their unique stories and not to categorise them in a homogenous way as schizophrenics or bipolars, etc.

The interview should begin with an introduction by the interviewer. While most patients would prefer to be addressed by their first names. Although calling by first may appear to be less formal or friendly, some patients may perceive it as a lack of respect. The best thing is to ask: 'What would you like me to call you?'

After introduction, patient needs to be explained the purpose and the approximate time of the interview. Also explain the necessity of taking notes and reassure the patient about confidentiality. Initially, patients should be encouraged to talk spontaneously, and open questions, which provoke variable answers (e.g.,'How can I help you?', 'What has been bothering you recently?', or 'Where shall we start?') should be asked. Closed questions and leading questions should be avoided as much as possible. Closed questions are those which restrict the answers to only yes or no (e.g.,'Do you think about ending your life?' or 'How many hours did you sleep last night?') and leading questions are ones which suggests the answers (e.g.,'You are depressed, aren't you?' or 'You must have felt angry?'). However, there is a need of asking closed or direct questions in the latter part of the interview to get specific and factual information. As majority of patients are anxious, questions should be brief and simple. Avoid multi-questions.

One of the important task of the interviewer is to control the interview in a balanced way. Interrupting prematurely or not to do it at all is equally unhelpful. Some patients repeatedly digress, indulge in unnecessary details or repeat things. They should be gently guided towards the focus of the interview without appearing to be dismissive of what they are saying. A helpful question can be: 'What you are saying is important but I need to ask you other things as well, in the given time we have. Perhaps we can come back to this again if we have time'. It is essential to ensure that the information is accurate and precise. In order to achieve this goal, one helpful question can be: 'I want to make sure that I have got the right picture. As I understand you meant that .... '. In order to clarify the information further, one helpful question can be: 'What exactly do you mean by this? Please tell me a bit more about it.'

The interviewer needs to be alert and observant of the patient's facial expressions, tone, gestures, as all of these non-verbal clues can give important and helpful information On the other hand the interviewer can utilise non-verbal means of communication (e.g., nodding, maintaining appropriate eye contact, having a relaxed posture or leaning towards the patient, etc.). To prompt and encourage the patient to continue giving information. Particular care has to be exercised when asking about childhood sexual abuse (it is not only a very sensitive area, but there is a chance of false memory syndrome as well), psychosexual history (again a delicate area to probe, and patients can feel embarrassed), substance misuse history (patients who are not using illicit substances may be surprised as to why they are being asked these questions), and forensic history (most patients are law-abiding citizens and may feel offended if the questions are not framed in a neutral way). One general helpful question for all of these areas can be: 'I hope you don't mind me asking some questions which might appear to you as odd and make you feel uneasy. We ask these from all the patients'.

Some patients pose particular difficulty for the interviewer. These include patients who are delusional, violent or agitated, hostile, confused, and seductive. Space constraints restrict elaboration on the ways for dealing with each type of these patients. However, some techniques are briefly mentioned here.

Interviews with a patient who is not in touch with reality can be quite difficult. It is recommended that the interviewer must be careful about giving reassurance and at the same time not validating the delusions. The clinician should not simply agree with a patient's bizarre belief system. He or she might instead express genuine surprise at the ideas presented. A reasonable comment could be 'it seems unlikely that ......'.

Regarding the agitated, hostile or violent patient, the interviewer must ensure a safe environment at the outset, and must take precautionary steps like having additional people nearby, and if needed measures for physical restraint or seclusion. It is important to bear in mind that responding to hostile behaviour of the patient with anger can be dangerous. At the same time ignoring the angry outbursts by the patient is not recommended, and the patient should be calmly and assertively told that behaving in that manner is not helpful. Before becoming violent, there are usually warning signals. Behavioural cues, like anger, uncooperativeness, and impulsivity are helpful in predicting violence. Physical signs like clenched jaw, flared nostrils, flushed face, clenched hands, sitting at the edge of a chair, gripping the armrest, pacing around, and loud speech can be indicative of impending violence.

Most patients who are confused (e.g., suffering from delirium or drug intoxication) will have difficulty in responding to open-ended questions. Instead, closed questions requiring yes/no or brief answers are likely to obtain most responses. These patients will also need to be frequently reminded of where they are and the purpose of being there. With confused patients, external stimuli should be at a minimum.

Regarding dishonest and deceptive patients, there can be different reasons for their behaviour. Usually these patients have a different agenda, which they feel must be kept hidden from the interviewer. The agenda is often directed toward achieving the secondary gains of illness. At times, patients may hide symptoms because of their fear of what management might be. Patients who do not trust may be reluctant or unwilling to share true and important information. Malingering is consciously lying for secondary gain(s). Those with Factitious disorder, or Munchausen syndrome, deliberately express false statements about themselves and their diseases. These are usually accompanied by hidden actions to elaborate their stories or even to induce serious symptoms. In these circumstances, there are no secondary gains, and the motivation appears to be simply to gain the patients' role and to satisfy deeper psychological needs. Malingering and factitious disorder must be distinguished from situations in which the patients are unaware that they are giving misinformation. Patients with conversion disorder experience neurological symptoms purely on a psychological basis and may be unable to speak, walk, or see with no organic defect. These patients are not being deceitful; they truly cannot function and will not until their illness is treated.

Seductive patients, especially with a personality disorder, pose another difficult scenario. The interviewer's degree of emotional openness and support can, sometimes, result in a strong desire of longing in some patients. In particular, patients who have been sexually abused as children, or those who have been unable to achieve close relationships, will sometimes find the interview an invitation to greater intimacy. These patients should be reminded of the limits of the situation, what they and the interviewer have, and the boundaries that apply. On the other hand, in some situations, the psychiatrist's own emotional reaction to the patient, including at times sexual attraction can encourage patients to respond inappropriately. This can happen more in psychotherapy as compared to initial psychiatric interviews. It should be borne in mind that the disinhibitory behaviour by some patients in the first interview may be indicative of hypomania or frontal lobe dysfunction.

Towards the end of the interview, it is always worthwhile to encourage the patient to tell anything else that he or she thinks is important and has been left out. It is recommended that patient is given truthful reassurance that everything possible to alleviate and manage the illness would be done. This will contribute in enhancing the trust.

In order to get a complete and reliable picture of the illness, it is desirable to interview a reliable relative or a close friend who knows the details of the patient's life and illness. The best way is to interview the patient and the informant separately as well as jointly. Only in exceptional circumstances should the informant be interviewed before the patient.

After determining the diagnosis, the severity of the illness needs to be ascertained. The necessary level of treatment, ranging from hospitalisation to outpatient appointments or community visits, needs to be determined. The main determinants of severity are dangerousness to self and others and impairment in the ability to care for oneself and function in social and occupational roles. It is important to determine the patient's baseline level of functioning and motivation and capacity for treatment.

It is helpful to know what environmental or psychological factors contribute to the disorder and what conditions may trigger future episodes of illness so that efforts can be made to prevent or minimise future episodes through amelioration of stressors and stressors increased social support. Assessment of baseline functioning of interpersonal relations is important as well.

All the above information has to be documented in a reliable and systematic way. The interviewer makes a summary and formulation which includes the management plan. This has to be explained to the patient to persuade them to agree with the planned interventions.

SOME USEFUL SCREENING QUESTIONS

The following lists of questions would be helpful in eliciting various psychiatric symptoms.

Symptoms of Anxiety Disorders

Generalised Anxiety Disorder

1. How do you feel about yourself usually?
2. Do you worry over trivial things most of the time?
3. Have you worried a lot over the past months?
4. What is it like when you worry?
5. Do you often feel keyed up, on edge, tense or strained?

6. Have you been so fidgety or restless that you could not keep still?
7. Have you had difficulty in relaxing during the past months?
8. Have you had times when you felt shaky and your heart pounded and you simply had to do something about it?
9. Have you been having difficulty in breathing or feeling as though you are choking?
10. What about suddenly starting to sweat?
11. Do you tend to worry about your physical health?

Panic (Anxiety) Disorder

1. Have there been times lately when these symptoms have been worse? Can you tell me about that?
2. Have you suddenly experienced episodes of increased heart rate, breathlessness, sweating, stomach pains and muscle tension?
3. Have you had the feeling that something terrible might happen?
4. How long do such episodes last?

Phobias

1. Do you get anxious in certain situations such as travelling, being alone or being in a lift or a train?
2. What about meeting people, e.g., going into a crowded room or making conversation?
3. Do you have any special fears, like some people are scared of cats, feathers, spiders or birds?
4. What difference have these symptoms made in your life?
5. Do you avoid any of these situations because you know you will feel anxious?

Obsessions

1. Do you get any distressing thoughts?
2. Do unpleasant thoughts go round and round in your mind? Can you describe them? What do you do then?
3. Are these your own thoughts or someone else's?
4. Do you try to stop them?
5. What happens then?
6. How do you feel at that time?
7. Do these thoughts keep on coming even when you try to keep them out?
8. Do you do anything (any actions) with these thoughts?
9. Do you get worried about contamination with germs?
10. Do you spend a lot of time on personal cleanliness, like washing over and over again even though you know you are clean?
11. Do you find that you have to keep on checking things that you know you have already done?
12. Do you have to count things many times or repeat the same action over and over again?
13. Do you find it difficult to make decisions about trivial things doubting yourself or your understanding of what is going on?

Somatoform Disorder

1. Do you tend to worry a lot about your physical health?
2. In what way?
3. Do you think you suffer from some physical illness?

Depersonalisation / Derealisation

1. Sometimes when people are anxious, they can have rather strange experiences. Does that happen to you? Tell me about it.
2. Some people feel as if they or their environment have changed in some way.
3. Do you ever feel as if you are detached or automatised?

Symptoms of Depressive Disorder

1. Have you been keeping reasonably cheerful or have you felt low-spirited or depressed recently?
2. Have you been feeling irritable or anxious recently?
3. Do you find any change in your mood as the day progresses?
4. Do you enjoy yourself as you used to?
5. When was the last time you enjoyed anything?
6. What about your interests? Have they changed at all?
7. Do you seem to have slowed down in your movements or have very little energy recently?
8. How is your concentration?
9. Do you find it difficult to remember things?
10. What is your sleep like?
11. Do you have difficulty in going to sleep?
12. Do you have broken sleep?
13. Are you waking earlier than usual?
14. How is your appetite?
15. What about your weight?
16. Has there been a change in your bowel habits?
17. How is your interest in sex?
18. How confident do you feel?
19. Sometimes when people are feeling rather low, they tend to dwell on their past. Does that happen to you? Is there anything you are feeling especially guilty about?
20. How is your self-esteem?

Symptoms of Suicidality

1. How do you feel about the future?
2. Sometimes when people feel low, they start to feel as though life is not worth living. Does that happen to you?
3. How often do you feel that way?
4. How strong are these feelings? Can you describe them?

5. Do you intend to harm yourself in any way?
6. Have you got plan(s) to end your life?
7. Do you intend to act on your plan(s)?
8. When do you intend to carry out your plan(s)?
9. Have you made any arrangements about your personal matters?
10. Are there factors in your life which might prevent you to kill yourself?

Symptoms of Hypomania/Mania

1. Have you felt unusually happy or irritable for no apparent reason?
2. How long does this state last?
3. Tell me about your activities during these periods.
4. Do you feel full of energy?
5. Do you spend a lot during these episodes of high mood?
6. Is there any change in your sexual libido?
7. Do you feel less need to sleep?
8. How is your concentration?
9. Do you feel as if you have got special powers?
10. Do you feel other people are jealous of your special qualities?
11. Do you think other people are conspiring against you?

Symptoms of Eating Disorders

1. Are you or anyone else worried about your eating patterns?
2. Do you fear that sometimes you might lose control of your eating?
3. Are you satisfied with your looks or are concerned about your body image?
4. Are you constantly worried that you might gain more weight?
5. What is your target weight?
6. Are you trying to lose weight by exercising, dieting or making yourself sick?
7. How much relief do these things give to you?
8. How much weight have you last in the last month?
9. When was your last menstrual period?
10. Are you able to tolerate the cold?
11. Have you noticed any changes in your body recently (skin, body hair)?

Symptoms of Schizophrenia and Related Disorders

Thought Block

Great care has to be exercised when trying to elicit this symptom as patients can be unsure of the question and may give false responses.

Delusions

Delusions are something which cannot be asked directly in the beginning but only after some rapport has been developed with the patient.

Some general starting questions about delusions:

1. Are you worried about something?
2. Has anything strange or significant happened recently?
3. Does it feel as though something strange is going on which you find hard to explain?

Persecutory Ideation/Delusions

1. How are people generally treating you?
2. Have you had trouble getting along with people?
3. Have you felt that people are against you?
4. Do you believe that people are conspiring against you or are deliberately trying to harm you?
5. Do you think your food is being poisoned?
6. What is the evidence for this?

Delusions of Reference

1. Do people seem to drop hints about you or say things with a double meaning?
2. Do you think there is some special significance for you in the objects around you?
3. Do things seem to be specially arranged to convey a message to you?
4. Do things on the TV or radio have a special meaning for you?

Delusions of Grandiosity

1. Is there something special about you?
2. Are you especially gifted?
3. Do you have unusual strength or special powers?

Nihilistic and Guilt Delusions

1. Do you believe you deserve to be punished?
2. Is there anything you feel particularly guilty about?
3. Do you think you suffer from serious physical illnesses?
4. Do you think your body is rotting?
5. Do you believe the world is coming to an end?

Hypochondriacal Delusions

1. Do you worry a lot about your physical health?
2. Do you think you suffer from any serious illness?

Delusions of Jealousy

1. What makes you believe that your wife/partner is cheating you?
2. Since when have you been suspecting this?
3. Have you confronted your wife/partner about this?
4. What does she say?

Delusions of Love

1. What makes you think that the person you mentioned is in love with you?
2. Has that person actually spoken to you or met you?

Religious Delusions

1. Do you think you are very special and holy?
2. Are you very close to God?
3. In what way does God communicate with you?

Delusions of Misidentification and Misinterpretation

1. Do you feel that people around you are not what they seem to be?
2. Do you think your relative has been replaced by an imposter?
3. Do you think these various people are actually the same person in various disguises?

Schneiderian First-Rank Symptoms

Delusion of Thought Insertion

1. Can you think clearly or is there any interference with your thoughts?
2. Do you think people are trying to put thoughts into your mind?
3. Do you believe that thoughts are coming into your head from outer space?
4. Are the thoughts in your head not your own?

Delusion of Thought Withdrawal

Do your thoughts seem to be taken out of your head as though some other person or force is removing them?

Delusion of Thought Broadcast

Are your thoughts broadcast so that other people know what you are thinking?

Delusions of Control

1. Does any outside agency or force control you?
2. Are you in control of your intentions, feelings and emotions or does it feel as though you are being controlled from the outside like a puppet or a robot?
3. Do you think your brain is being programmed by an external force?
4. Are the parts of your body under the control of someone?

Experience of Thought Echo / Thoughts Spoken Aloud

1. Do you ever experience your own thoughts being echoed?
2. Do you sometimes hear your own thoughts spoken aloud, or hear voices anticipating your thoughts?

Experience of Hearing Running Commentary

1. Do you hear voices which are commenting on your actions?
2. Have you heard voices commenting on what you are thinking?

Delusional Perception

Do you sometimes suddenly feel that certain things have special significance for you?

Hallucinations

To start with a general comment and question would be useful.

1. Some people suffering from psychiatric problems report unusual experiences. Do you have such experiences?
2. Do you ever seem to hear noise or voices when there is no one about, and nothing else to explain it?
3. Tell me about them.
4. Where do they come from?
5. How many do you hear?
6. Do they talk to you or amongst themselves about you?
7. Do they comment on what you are doing or command you to do things?
8. Do you find them pleasant or unpleasant?
9. Have you had visions or seen things which other people could not see? Tell me about them.
10. How do you explain this?
11. Did you see it with your eyes or in your mind's eye?
12. Were you fully awake or half asleep?
13. Did the vision seem to arise out of a pattern on the wall or a shadow?
14. Have you ever felt strange tastes in your mouth?
15. How do you account for this?
16. Do you sometimes notice strange smells that other people do not notice?
17. How do you explain it?
18. Have you ever felt strange sensations or felt that someone is touching you and when you look around there is no one there?
19. What was the strangest experience you ever had?

Somatic or Tactile Hallucinations

Somatic or tactile hallucinations involve experiencing peculiar physical sensations in the body. They include burning, itching sensations, or tingling sensations or the perception that the body has changed in shape or size.

Have you had burning sensations or other strange sensations in your body?

What were they?

Olfactory Hallucinations

The patient experiences unusual odours that are typically quite unpleasant. Sometimes the patient may believe that he or she smells bad. This belief should be considered a hallucination if the patient can actually smell the odour but should be considered a delusion if he or she believes that only others can smell the odour.

Have you experienced any unusual smells or smells that others do not notice?

What were they?

Visual Hallucinations

The patient sees shapes or people that are not actually present. Sometimes these are shapes or colours, but most typically they are figures of people or human-like objects. They also may be characters of a religious nature, such as the Devil or Christ. As always, visual hallucinations involving religious themes should be judged within the context of the patient's cultural background.

Have you had visions or seen things that other people cannot?

What did you see?

Insight

1. Do you think there is anything the matter with you?
2. What do you think it is?
3. Could it be a nervous or mental condition?
4. What do you think is the cause?
5. Why did you need to come to the hospital?
6. Of all the problems you have told me about, which one affects you the most?
7. What do you think might help you now?
8. Do you need treatment? What sort?
9. Do you think you need medication?

Questions Regarding Some Aspects of History Taking

Alcohol History

1. Can you tell me about your drinking habits?
2. How much do you usually drink in a day?
3. Does it vary over the weekend?
4. Do you usually drink socially or alone at home?
5. Do you sometimes feel that you really want to drink?
6. What happens if you don't get a drink then?
7. Do you get shakes and sweats when you stop drinking?
8. Have you ever heard noises or seen things that were not there while you had reduced drinking or had stopped drinking?
9. Do you have to drink to stop this from happening?
10. Have you always been drinking the same amount or has there been a change? Has there been a change in the amount of alcohol you need to be able to relax?
11. What is the longest period you've been without a drink? Why did you start drinking again?
12. Has it affected your relationships with your partner or your children?
13. Have you ever been in trouble with the law because of drinking?
14. In the past, have you ever had to go to a doctor or hospital because of drinking?
15. Have you ever had memory blackouts or had withdrawal symptoms like tremors and fits?
16. Do you tend to start drinking after a dry period?
17. When did you first start drinking?
18. Was there a time in the past when you were drinking heavily?
19. Was this the only time?
20. What was the longest period you were dry?
21. Do you find that you previously drank more but now drink in a limited way?

Screening for Alcohol Problems

The FAST Questions

1. How often do you have eight or more drinks on one occasion?
2. How often during the past year have you failed to do what was normally expected of you because of drinking?
3. How often during the past year have you been unable to remember what happened the night before because you had been drinking?

   [For these questions, score 0 for never, 1 for less than monthly, 2 for monthly, 3 for weekly and 4 for daily or almost daily.]
4. Has a relative, friend, doctor or other health worker been concerned about your drinking or suggested you cut down?

   [For this question, score 0 for never, 2 for yes but not in past year, 4 for yes in the past year.]

   The maximum score is 16, and a score of 3 or more indicates hazardous drinking.

Note that the FAST questions do not screen for alcohol dependency, which is better picked up by the CAGE questions.

The CAGE Questions

The CAGE is an alternative and widely used alcohol screening tool. Its four questions are:

1. Have you ever felt you ought to cut down on your drinking?
2. Have people annoyed you by criticising your drinking?
3. Have you ever felt guilty about your drinking?
4. Have you ever had a drink first thing in the morning (an 'Eye-opener')?

If three or more yes answers are given, the likelihood ratio for problem drinking is 250.

Drug History

1. What drugs or medications have you used recently?
2. Have you used prescribed drugs in a way that the doctor did not prescribe?
3. What street drugs have you used?
4. What about chemicals like glue or gasoline?
5. What effect did they have on you?
6. When did you first start using them?
7. What are you using now?
8. How much?
9. How often?
10. How do you take it? Where do you use it and with whom?
11. How do you take it? Do you inject? Do you share needles or water?
12. Do you get a craving for it?
13. What happens when you try to cut down or stop?
14. What is the longest period that you have been without it?
15. How has drug use affected your health?
16. Has it affected your family life?
17. What about work?
18. Have you ever been in trouble with the law because of your drug habit? Is there any case pending?
19. How do you finance your drug use?
20. Has anyone in your family also been using drugs?

Psychosexual History

First, make an empathetic initial statement such as: 'Many people find it difficult to talk about sexual matters, but, as they are important, I would like to ask you a few questions about your sexual life. Is that okay?'

1. Can you tell me a bit about your sexual experiences?
2. Do you have any particular sexual preferences?
3. Are there any special ways in which you have sexual fulfilment?
4. Did you have any unwanted sexual experiences?
5. Tell me about your past emotional relationships?
6. How long did they last?
7. How did they end?
8. Are you in a relationship at the moment?
9. Are you satisfied with your current relationship?

Forensic History

1. Have you ever been in trouble with the law?
2. Tell me a little more about it.
3. Were you ever convicted?
4. Have there been prosecutions with no convictions?

Usual Personality

1. If I ask you to describe yourself as a person, what would you tell me?
2. Can you describe what your relationships with other people, family and friends were like?
3. What do you enjoy doing in your spare time?
4. What is your mood usually like?
5. Does it fluctuate fairly rapidly?
6. How do you deal with stress?
7. When things aren't going well for you, how does that affect you? Can you give me an example?
8. Are you sensitive to criticism?
9. Are you self-conscious?
10. What is your temper like?
11. Do you fly off the handle easily?
12. Did you physically hurt anyone else?
13. Are you a religious person?
14. How do you get on with other people?
15. Do you find it easy to trust people?
16. How many friends do you have?
17. Are you a shy sort of person?
18. Do you always try to do things perfectly?
19. Are you very particular about cleanliness?
20. Do you overreact to minor things?
21. Have you been in trouble with the police?

REFERENCES

1. Aquilina, C. and Warner, J. (2004). *A guide to psychiatric examination*. Cheshire: Pastest.
2. Hill, D., Birley, J. L. T., Post, F., Cawley, R. H., Rutter, M. L., et al. (1973). *Notes on eliciting and recording clinical information*. Oxford: Oxford University Press.
3. Leff, J. P. and Isaacs, A. D. (1981). *Psychiatric examination in clinical practice* (2nd Edition). Oxford: Blackwell.
4. Poole, R. and Higgo, R. (2006). *Psychiatric interviewing and assessment*. Cambridge: Cambridge University Press.
5. Tareen, I. A. K. and Tareen I. K. (2004). *Understanding psychiatry* (2nd Edition). Lahore: Zercon Graphic.
6. *Psychiatry* Fourth edition Volume 1 The Psychiatric Interview: Settings and Techniques

   Edward K. Silberman, Kenneth Certa, Abigail Kay: Ed: Allan Tasman, Jerald Kay, Jeffrey A. Lieberman, Michael B. First, Michelle B. Riba. 2015 John Wiley & Sons, Ltd. West Sussex
7. *Introductory Textbook of Psychiatry* Sixth edition Donald W. Black and Nancy C. Andreasen 2014 American Psychiatric Publishing, Arlington, VA
8. *Lecture Notes in Psychiatry.* Gautam Gulati, Mary-Ellen Lynall, Kate Saunders. Eleventh Edition 2014 John Wiley & Sons, Oxford

History Taking and Mental State Examination

03

CHAPTER

HISTORY TAKING

The fundamental process of history taking and diagnosing is the same in psychiatry as it is in internal medicine or neurology. Obtaining a comprehensive history is a very crucial and important skill in psychiatric practice. Although the mental state examination requires an understandable background provided by history, it should not be mixed up with history and must be recorded separately. As already mentioned in the previous chapter, while interviewing and taking the history, it is important to be aware of the non-verbal communication, as emotions and attitudes are communicated through facial expressions, gestures, body position, movements of the hands, arms, legs, and feet, interpersonal distance, dress and grooming, and speech prosody.

A good clinical history is structured, goal directed and comprehensive (but not over- inclusive). All subjective and objective data should be recorded under appropriate and separate headings. Although the history should preferably be taken in the same chronological order and systematic way, in some situations it is not possible to strictly adhere to this and the interviewer would need to exhibit some flexibility. With experience, the student or trainee will learn how to adjust headings and questions depending upon the situation e.g., a slightly different style and approach might be required in interviews at A&E department (where there may be less time available and decisions regarding management might be needed quickly) as compared to a patient admitted in a psychiatric unit (where the situation may not be very urgent). Similarly, it may not be possible or even appropriate to take the history in the same order or at the same pace from a patient who is floridly psychotic as compared to one who suffers from major depressive disorder with psychomotor retardation.

A scheme of history taking is given below. All the following areas should be explored and recorded in every patient although, as mentioned above, there may variations in the order of headings, the need to prioritise certain sections in some patients, and the need for respective details.

Demographic Data

Patient's full name, age, sex, marital status, religion, address, current occupation, accommodation status, and details of other people residing with the patient should be recorded.

Informant's name, the relationship to the patient and impression about reliability should be specified

Referral

Record who referred the patient and why? What has provoked the request for an assessment now? Has the patient volunteered to come or has been forced?

Chief and Presenting Complaints

It's helpful to begin the history by determining the patient's chief complaint. Ask the patient, 'What brings you to see me/to the hospital today?' Record the answer, in his or her own words, using quotation marks (e.g., "I'm thinking of killing myself" or "The voices tell me to hurt people"). Chief complaint should be no more than one or two sentences.

Sometimes the chief complaint will be explicit (e.g., "I've been feeling very depressed," or "I've been having a pain in my head that other doctors can't explain"). At other times, the chief complaint may be relatively vague (e.g., "I don't know why I'm here—my family brought me," or "I've been having trouble at work"). When the replies are not particularly precise, the interviewer will need to follow-up his or her initial questions with others that will help determine the nature of the patient's problem (e.g.,'What kind of things have been bothering your family?', or 'What kind of trouble are you having at work?'). The initial part of the interview, devoted to eliciting the chief complaint, should take as long as is necessary to determine the patient's primary problem. When the patient is a clear, logical informant, he or she should be allowed to tell his or her story as freely as possible without interruption. When he or she is a relatively poor informant, the interviewer will need to be active and directive.

Use the chief complaint to develop a provisional differential diagnosis. As in the rest of medicine, once the patient's primary problem has been determined, the interviewer begins to construct in his or her mind, a range of explanations as to the specific diagnosis that might lead to that particular problem. For example, if the patient indicates that he or she has been hearing voices, the differential diagnosis includes a variety of disorders that produce these kinds of of psychotic symptoms, such as schizophrenia, schizoaffective disorder, mania or major depressive disorder with psychotic symptoms, substance misuse involving hallucinogens, or alcoholic hallucinosis.

After establishing the chief complaint, ask the patient about the other presenting complaints (main worries or problems). It is again very desirable to record the patient's presenting complaints in their own words rather than using technical terms.

History of Present Illness

Get a detailed and comprehensive description of the symptoms in chronological order, from the onset of the illness to the current moment. Generally speaking, the more detailed the history, the more accurate would be the diagnosis.

The mode of onset of the illness and how the illness has subsequently developed can give helpful hints as to the possible cause. Moreover, prognosis can also be based on the mode of onset, as most psychiatric disorders have a comparatively poor prognosis if they develop gradually or insidiously. Explore any precipitating events or stresses (including physical illnesses) that might have triggered the illness. Also ask about perpetuating or aggravating factors as well as anything which helps to alleviate or relieve the symptoms. Ascertain the degree of functional impairment, i.e. their effect on routines of life, work, sleep and relationships, etc. Information about the extent of distress caused by the mental symptoms can help in ascertaining the severity of the illness. Details of any medication being used or any other sort of treatment should be recorded. Additionally, note any improvement or side effects from medication.

Associated symptoms have to be probed e.g., with some depressive symptoms volunteered by the patient, other related depressive symptoms need to be asked especially suicidal ideation (which is mandatory to explore). Similarly, in patients with elevated mood, other features of hypomania/mania should be explored.

Personal History

Birth and Childhood

Date and place of birth should be recorded. Details of pregnancy (e.g., whether planned, duration, problems, etc.), and any birth complications should be noted.

Ask details about early development, achievement of milestones and any emotional, mental or physical problems, e.g., high-grade fevers, infantile convulsions or psychiatric symptoms. Questions about childhood sexual abuse can be traumatising and need to be asked in a very tactful way. There is, in addition, possibility of false memory syndrome. Get an idea about the atmosphere at home, financial difficulties and parental conflicts.

Education

Record the age of beginning and finishing school. Ask about the number of schools attended, the reasons for changing them, academic performance, and relationships with school mates and teachers. Was the patient bullied at school? Interest in sports and other extracurricular activities should also be explored. Note the details of higher education.

Sexual and Marital History

It is often not easy to gather this information in an initial interview as the patient may not be comfortable enough to confide.

Record the age of menarche along with regularity of cycles. Also, note any associated physical or psychological symptoms. What is the patient's sexual orientation? Inquire about homosexual and heterosexual experiences. Ask about sexual symptoms, e.g., lack of sexual desire, erectile or ejaculatory problems and paraphilias (sadism, fetishism, voyeurism) etc. Masturbatory fantasies are significant regarding sexual offences. Note the spouse's age, occupation, personality and compatibility. Find out the duration of acquaintance before marriage and the quality of the relationship. Enquire about any previous relationships. Ask about areas of disagreement, and issues around finances, in-laws, and children.

Children

List children chronologically, giving names, ages, personality, etc. Also ask about any miscarriages or abortions. Note the patient's attitude towards children, the physical health and psychological well-being of children.

Occupation

Note the age of starting work. List jobs held in chronological order with dates, duration and reasons for change. Details of the longest job are important. Any problems with colleagues? Describe in detail the current job and exact responsibilities. Rather than simply recording that the patient is a factory worker, it is better to know that the patient operates machinery, is a clerk or is a security guard in the factory. Is the patient satisfied with the present job? Find out about the patient's future plans and ambitions.

Premorbid Personality (Usual Personality Before the Onset of the Psychiatric Illness)

You must try to get a picture of the patient's usual self before the present illness. An independent account is important for this part of the history. Ask about the patient's usual character, interests, beliefs and habits. Some relevant good questions are, 'How would your friends describe you?' 'How do you cope in a difficult situation?' 'Would you describe yourself as a loner or as someone very sociable?' The picture of the patient's normal self can be catagorised under the following broad headings:

- **Social relations with family, friends and workmates:** Did the patient have many friends or few? Did he have any close friends who were close enough to confide in?
- **Spare time interests:** Ask about preferred books, plays or movies, and details about sport and other leisure activities.
- **Mood:** Enquire about the patient's usual mood. Get a detailed description, asking, for instance, whether the patient's mood was usually cheerful and optimistic, despondent, anxious, worrying or irritable and whether the mood usually remained stable or fluctuated.
- **Habits:** Ask about the use of tobacco, alcohol or any illicit drugs.

- **Other characteristics:** The following characteristics can be explored. Was the patient meticulous or fussy? Did he have to check things such as gas taps and locks, repeatedly? Was he inclined to be jealous or suspicious or very sensitive to criticism? Was he impulsive, selfish, timid, reserved, shy or self-conscious? How did the patient deal with stressful situations?

Family History

This should be taken in detail. Parents' ages, health, personalities and occupations should be recorded. If deceased, the age at the time of death and cause of death should be noted. Find out about the general home atmosphere. This can be done by asking an open-ended question such as, 'If I asked you to describe your family/ home, what would you tell me?' Explore the emotional relationship of the patient to parents and siblings. Find out about family history of any psychiatric disorder or general medical illness.

Medical History

In any psychiatric assessment, it is important to know about past and current medical illnesses as well as the treatment received. Previous endocrine or neurological illness is of particular relevance. Record any operations or accidents chronologically and in detail. Many medical conditions and the prescribed medications can cause psychiatric symptoms. Hypertensive medications, for example, can cause low mood. On the other hand, some psychotropic medications are not suitable for co-existing medical conditions (e.g., tricyclic antidepressants in cardiac abnormalities and lithium in a bipolar patient who has a concomitant kidney disease).

Past Psychiatric History

Get details of all psychiatric conditions, giving dates, duration and nature of treatments taken, degree of compliance, and name of the hospitals or doctors involved. It is essential to get specific details about the first episode of the illness as it can shed light on the precipitating events and the coping mechanisms used by the patient.

Forensic History

Ask about any problems with the law and any subsequent convictions; Has the patient ever been in jail? How many times? For how long? Any pending charges? A detailed risk assessment (see the chapter 'Forensic Psychiatry' for full risk assessment) is required if patient has any record of violence. Assault against whom? Were any weapons used? An extensive forensic history and patients current lack of remorse or guilt is indicative of antisocial personality disorder.

Alcohol and Drug History

Alcohol and drug misuse is quite common amongst mentally unwell people, especially in Western countries. In some patients, these could be the cause of the mental symptoms. Also ask about the abuse of benzodiazepines and over the counter medicines.

Mental State Examination (MSE)

During history taking the interviewer would have already observed and noted down some signs and symptoms of the presenting illness. Mental state examination usually confirms these observations although it is an opportunity to further explore and clarify the symptoms.

General Appearance and Behaviour

This is a very important part of MSE. Describe the patient's behaviour, both normal and abnormal, in detail and as accurately as possible.

Observe whether the attitude of the patient is cooperative, hostile, evasive, threatening, or obsequious. Does the patient displays psychomotor agitation or retardation?

Note level of consciousness (disorientated, alert, hypervigilant, somnolent, or stuporous), dress (casual, appropriate for weather, eccentric, careless, or dishevelled) grooming (style of hair, degree of makeup, shaven/ unshaven, clean), idiosyncrasies (tattoos, prominent scars), gait, and facial expressions. A strikingly unusual or inappropriate dress can provide helpful clues to diagnosis. Some patients suffering from depressive disorder wear drab colours. Patients having hypomania or mania may be dressed brightly and flamboyantly. Those suffering from schizophrenia sometimes wear strange dress combinations which have symbolic meaning for them.

Self-neglect can occur in a variety of psychiatric disorders, e.g., schizophrenia, depressive disorder and dementia. Gait and mobility of the patient can indicate certain conditions. Depressed patients usually walk slowly and hesitantly. Similarly, patients suffering from hypomania or mania may walk in an excited and brisk manner. Note whether the patient is restless or tense (anxiety disorder), has poor eye-contact and psychomotor retardation (depressive disorder), or is over-active (hypomania). Is there any eccentric behaviour? Does the patient exhibit any gestures, grimaces or mannerisms? Are there any purposeless movements like tics? Severe weight loss may be indicative of depressive disorder or anorexia nervosa.

Talk/Speech

Let the patient talk freely enough to observe how coherently his or her thoughts are connected. Most patients should be allowed to talk for at least 3 or 4 minutes without interruption in the course of any psychiatric interview. The very laconic patient, of course, will not be able to do this, but most can.

Apart from analysing a person's writing, thoughts can also be assessed by examining the speech. The form of thought (hence the term formal thought disorder), and not the content, is recorded under this heading. Thought disorder is a very significant symptom and some of the formal thought disorders are almost pathognomonic of schizophrenia.

Look for abnormalities in the organisation and form of the patient's thoughts, e.g., in loosening of associations, the patient's thoughts appear unconnected. If there are any abnormalities of thought, it is best to record a verbatim sample of the talk. Note whether the talk flows smoothly, is it spontaneous or does the patient only talk when spoken to? Is the talk excessive or little, slow or rapid and also whether it is relevant and coherent? Is the patient's talk difficult to understand or follow? Is it because of articulation problem (dysarthria)? Is there evidence for tangentiality, flight of ideas, clang associations, neologisms, paraphasias, thought block, derailment, fusion, or word salad, etc.

Mood

Mood is a pervasive and sustained emotion. At this stage the observations would have given a reasonable idea about the mood state, so the questions can be tailored and directed accordingly. Ask the patient directly about the mood as well: 'How are you feeling/How's your mood been?' Note the constancy and appropriateness of mood. Mood can be labile, blunted or flat. In mood disorders, mood is almost invariably congruent, whereas in schizophrenia it can be incongruent.

Note whether the patient is anxious, irritable, angry, frightened, perplexed, suspicious, labile, euphoric or depressed? Is the patient trying to mask the true feelings? If the mood is depressed, probe other mandatory symptoms of depressive disorder (diurnal variation of mood, self-esteem, guilt, appetite, libido, attitude about future including the extent of hopelessness, etc.). Direct questions to explore suicidal ideas and plans must not be omitted. Similarly, if the mood is elevated, related symptoms of hypomania/mania ought to be probed (excessive energy, overactivity sleep patterns, libido, and plans for future, etc.).

Thought Content

Follow-up vague or obscure replies with enough persistence to accurately determine the answer to the question. Some patients, particularly psychotic patients, have great difficulty answering questions clearly and concisely. They may say "yes" or "no" to every question asked. When a pattern of this sort is observed, the patient should be repeatedly asked to describe his or her experiences as explicitly as possible. For example, if the patient says that he or she hears voices, he or she should be asked to describe them in more detail—whether they are male or female, what they say, and how often they occur. The greater the level of detail the patient is able to provide, the more confident the clinician can feel that the symptom is truly present. Because making a diagnosis of schizophrenia or another major psychiatric disorder has important prognostic implications, the clinician should not hastily accept an answer that suggests vaguely that the patient may have a particular symptom of a disorder.

What are the patient's main preoccupations and worries? Various types of anxiety symptoms including phobias and obsessions should be explored. Record obsessional impulses, or acts.

Ask whether the patient has thoughts which are intrusive and repetitive? Ask if the patient regards them as his own thoughts and what is their appropriateness. The extent of distress caused by them. Do these obsessional thoughts have any relation to his emotional state? Does he repeat actions, such as checking and washing, unnecessarily. Does this alleviate the anxiety for a short while? Some patients (e.g., with anorexia nervosa) present with overvalued ideas.

A screening question for delusional beliefs should be followed by questions targeting common delusions, e.g., persecutory delusions, delusions of reference, delusions of grandeur, and Schneiderian first-rank symptoms of schizophrenia, etc. It is important to elaborate and specify the onset and fixity of delusional beliefs.

Perception

Perceptual abnormalities such as hallucinations and illusions can be present in relation to the self or the environment. Hallucinations are mostly auditory but could be in other four modalities (visual, olfactory, gustatory, and tactile or visceral) as well.

If hallucinations are not apparent, ask whether the patient has had any unusual experiences? Heard or seen anything unusual? For diagnostic purposes, the third person auditory hallucinations are more significant as compared to the second person hallucinations, it is, therefore, essential to specify whether the voices talk directly to the patient or do they talk about the patient or other things among themselves. If the voices address the patient in first person, ask whether the voices are commanding in nature and does the patient feel forced to comply? Ask whether the voices are pleasant, neutral or abusive? How often do these occur?

The source, vividness, reality, manner of reception, content, and all other circumstances of the experience are important and should be recorded in detail. Enquire as to whether these experiences occur at a particular time, for instance at night, when falling asleep, or when alone. Ask how does the patient respond to these experiences. Is there anything which helps to cope with these? Check for illusions.

Cognition

Orientation: Time, place, person, and situation.

Record the patient's answers to questions about his own name and address, the place where he or she is, the time of the day and the date.

Attention and Concentration

Note whether the patient's attention can easily be aroused and sustained or not? Does he or she concentrates?

Is the patient easily distracted or appears very preoccupied? To test concentration, ask the patient to tell the days of the week or the months of the year in reverse order, or to do simple arithmetical problems like subtraction of serial sevens from 100 (up to 5 answers, i.e. 93, 86, 79, 72, 65).

Abstraction: Proverb interpretation – what would someone mean by "the grass is always greener on the other side of the fence".

Similarities: How are these things alike: Apple-orange, table-chair, and eye-ear.

Computation: Number of digits successfully added or subtracted and ability to calculate change:

'If you bought fruit for forty rupees, and gave the shopkeeper a one hundred rupees note, what change would you get back?'

Memory

Record the patient's success or failure in registering, retaining, and being able to recall a number, a name, and address, or other data after 2 and 5 minutes. Give him digits to repeat forwards and backwards, and record how many he can repeat immediately after being told. In describing the state of the patient's memory, do not merely record the conclusions reached but give evidence and describe such aspects of behaviour as seem to indicate whether he was attentive, trying his hardest or being distracted by other stimuli, etc.

General Information

Tests for general information and grasp should be varied according to the patient's educational level. Useful questions here will include such things as the patient's familiarity with current affairs and political names.

Examples:

Name of the Prime Minister

Names of the capital and main cities

Recent news

Insight and Judgment

Ascertain the patient's degree of awareness and understanding of the present condition. Does the patient know that something is wrong, and that he/she is ill? Whether the patient considers the illness, as physical or psychological and is there a need of treatment? Does the patient understand the ways in which illness disrupts functions of life? Merely recording that insight is present or absent is not helpful.

Judgment should be ascertained by noting the response to standard questions (If you found a stamped letter, what would you do? If you smelled smoke in a crowded hall, what would you do?)

Ending the Interview

1. Summarise what you have been told back to the patient. This helps ensure you have gained an accurate picture, and reinforces to the patient that you have been listening carefully.
2. 'Is there anything else that I haven't asked you, that you think I should know?'
3. Give the patient an opportunity to ask questions.
4. Explain what you plan to do next.

Mini Mental State Examination

This is a brief, widely used validated clinical screening test that evaluates several dimensions of language and cognitive functioning. It is not done routinely on every psychiatric patient but may be helpful in some cases (especially elderly patients) to test attention, orientation, memory and visuospatial abilities. It is a unique test in its ability to briefly and objectively asses a patient with suspected cognitive impairment. One shortcoming of this test is its lack of sensitivity, i.e. high rate of false-negative results. Patients are asked specific questions and are also given some tasks, which are then scored. The maximum score is 30 and a score less than 24 is considered abnormal and indicative of diffuse cognitive dysfunction.

Psychological Testing

Again, psychological tests are not required in most patients but these tests can contribute very significantly to assessment and subsequent management in certain psychiatric assessments.

Aetiology

It is important to identify the contribution of various factors. These are grouped as:

Predisposing Factors

Factors that determine a person's vulnerability (genetic, and family history, etc.). This is affected by further physical, psychological and social influences. Personality is a significant contributory factor in the aetiology, because people have different coping mechanisms to deal with stressful events.

Precipitating Factors

Identify events shortly before the onset of the psychiatric illness. Physical factors include medication, tumours and medical illnesses. Personal losses and significant changes in social circumstances are psychological and social aetiological factors.

Perpetuating Factors

These would include any factors which maintain and prolong the course of the disorder. Lack of compliance and withdrawal from active life are some examples.

Cognitive Behavioural Assessment

This is one way of understanding and conceptualising the disorder. The other is from psychodynamic perspective.

Note: 24 is considered abnormal and indicative of diffuse cognitive dysfunction.

Section	Questions	Maximum points	Patient's Score
1. Orientation	a. Can you tell me today's (date)/(month)/(year)? Which day is it today? Can you tell me which season it is? b. What town/city are we in? What is the county, country? What (building) are we in and on what (floor)?	5 5	
2. Registration	I should like to test your memory. (Name three common objects: 'ball, car, man') Can you repeat the words I said? (1 point per word) (Repeat up to 6 trials until all three are remembered) Record number of trials here:	3	
3. Attention and Calculation	a. From 100 keep subtracting 7 and give each answer. Stop after 5 answers. (93_86_79_72_65) Alternatively b. Spell the word 'World' backwards. (D_L_R_O_W)	5	
4. Recall	What were the three words I asked you to say earlier? (Skip this test if all of these objects were not remembered during the registration test)	3	
5. Language Naming Repeating	Name the following objects (show a watch) and (show a pencil) Repeat the following: 'no ifs, ands or buts'	2 1	
6. Reading	(Show card or write: 'Close your Eyes') Read this sentence and do what it says.	1	
7. Writing	Now can you write a short sentence for me?	1	
8. Three stage command	(Present paper) Take this paper in your left (or right) hand, fold it in half, and place it on the floor.	3	
9. Construction	Will you copy this drawing please? 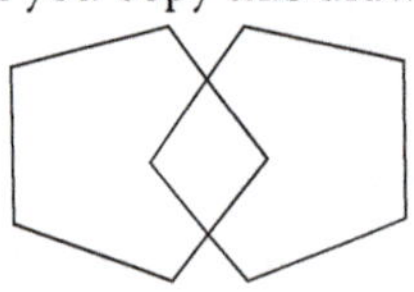	1	
Total score		**30**	

ABC model (Antecedents, Behaviours, Consequences)

1. To what extent has there been faulty early learning?
2. To what extent is the current behaviour being rewarded and therefore being reinforced?
3. To what extent avoidance is playing a part?
4. What are the cognitive distortions and the cognitive bias?

Psychodynamic Formulation

1. A psychodynamic formulation should explain how and why the patient's life has become disturbed, and how the symptoms have arisen and are being maintained. Following aspects should be considered when making this formulation.
2. Significant early experiences and their significance to the current problems.
3. What, if any, is the meaning of the symptoms? Are they providing some advantage to the patient?

4. How is the stress being handled by the patient? What are the current psychological (defences) mechanisms being used to alleviate the anxiety? Are they being excessively used so as to restrict improvement?
5. The interaction between enduring personality traits and the current symptomatology.
6. What biological and environmental influences have created the patient's vulnerability to this stress?
7. What factors in this person's life are maintaining the problems?

Physical Examination

The physical health of a psychiatric patient is important because:

- Medical conditions can present with psychological symptoms. For example, lethargy and low mood may signify anaemia, hypothyroidism or malignancy.
- Patients with psychiatric disorders have increased rates of medical illness for a number of reasons: there may be a common aetiology; the psychiatric disorder may have led them to neglect their health, or they may have medical side effects of the treatments used for psychiatric disorders.

So, in every assessment take account of the patient's physical appearance, as well as their age, symptoms, medical history, etc., and always consider what examination is required. This may include a brief examination of all systems. However, there is no pre-specified physical examination in the psychiatric assessment since it depends upon the setting, the patient, the disorder and the treatment.

A physical examination is mandatory for in-patients but it may also be required for patients in the clinics or community. The interviewer should decide what part of this examination is more relevant.

However, it is essential to palpate the thyroid gland which is crucial in postgraduate psychiatric examinations.

Neurological Examination

Like MMSE, neurological examination is also not required for most psychiatric patients. If needed, a standard neurological examination should be performed. A neurological evaluation is particularly important in psychiatric patients to rule out focal signs that might help to explain the patient's symptoms. Although it is true that the diagnosis of some neurologic disorders requires a vast experience and skill in the practice of neurology, at the same time it is not justified to neglect a general neurologic examination in those psychiatric patients in which there is any suspicion of an organic syndrome. It is beyond the scope of this book to provide a guide to neurological examination, for which the readers are suggested to consult, *Neurology for Psychiatrists* by G.S. Malhi, M.S. Matharu, and A.S. Hale.

Laboratory Investigations

Investigations should be used selectively to ensure that there is no underlying medical condition accounting for, or contributing to, the patient's psychiatric disorder, as well as baseline tests prior to commencing medication. For example:

- A urine drug screen in suspected drug-induced psychosis.
- Extensive biochemical and imageing in a patient with dementia.
- A brain scan in someone with delirium and a history of a fall.
- Thyroid function tests in a patient with anxiety, palpitations and weight loss.
- Renal function prior to commencing lithium.

For the patients presenting in out-patients' clinic, laboratory tests are not done routinely and the decision to have some done will depend on the differential diagnosis. Occasionally there is need for imageing and biochemical screening. Routine blood tests (full blood count, electrolytes, liver and thyroid function tests) are usually done at the time of admission.

Formulation / Summary

Having completed the history, the mental state examination as well as the physical examination, make a formulation/summary. Formulation has traditionally been required in psychiatric examinations. It is a concise way of summarising the psychiatric assessment. Some authors have suggested to include all the relevant information under the following headings:

1. A brief statement about the demographics of the patient
2. Main presenting problems
3. Differential diagnoses (reasons for and against each diagnosis should be given)
4. Aetiology (which should include predisposing, precipitating, and perpetuating factors)
5. Management plan (including further investigations)
6. A brief comment about prognosis

Case summaries are usually done when patient is admitted in and discharged from a psychiatric hospital or is being transferred to other psychiatric services.

Case Summary Would Include the Following Headings

1. Demographic details
2. Presenting complaints
3. Salient features of mental state examination
4. Past psychiatric history
5. Personal history
6. Family history
7. Risk assessment
8. Physical examination
9. Differential diagnosis
10. Management plan
11. Investigations
12. Prognosis

REFERENCES

For this chapter, the following articles/books were consulted:

1. Folstein, M. F., Folstein, S. E., McHugh, P. R. (1975). Mini-Mental State: A practical method for grading the cognitive state of patients for the clinician. *Journal of Psychiatry Research*, 12,189– 198.
2. Ovidio, A. de Leon. (1997). The mental status examination. In T. H. Jobe, M. Gavira and A. Kovilparambil (Eds.), *Clinical neuropsychiatry* (pp. 3–16). England: Blackwell Science.
3. *Psychiatry* The Psychiatric Interview: Settings and Techniques

   Edward K. Silberman, Kenneth Certa, Abigail Kay Fourth Edition Volume 1

   Ed: Allan Tasman, Jerald Kay, Jeffrey A. Lieberman, Michael B. First, Michelle B. Riba

   2015 John Wiley & Sons, Ltd. West Sussex
4. *Introductory Textbook of Psychiatry* Sixth edition.Donald W. Black and Nancy C. Andreasen

   2014 American Psychiatric Publishing, Arlington, VA

   Lecture Notes in Psychiatry. Gautam Gulati, Mary-Ellen Lynall, Kate Saunders, Eleventh Edition. 2014 John Wiley & Sons, Oxford

Anxiety Disorders 04

Most human problems are dimensional and not dichotomous. People's experiences vary in intensity and frequency, from having little problem to being severely incapacitated with the same problem. Most of us are anxious or worried about different things, and to a variable extent or degree. Anxiety is a common emotional experience, encountered by all of us at some time or another in our lives. Anxiety is a feeling of uneasiness, and is a normal response of an individual when exposed to a stressful or challenging situation. For example, it is natural for a student to feel anxious before going for an examination. Similarly, it is normal to feel anxious if one has to appear for a job interview. This sort of anxiety is acceptable as it serves a very useful purpose. It helps an individual to perform better and to be more efficient and more alert. Therefore, moderate levels of anxiety will improve performance and even high levels of anxiety will be desirable when they are consistent with the demands of the situation.

But then, there is another type of anxiety, which is severe, unhelpful and inappropriate. Severe anxiety can rob the capacity to plan an appropriate response and the ability to carry out the necessary action. This sort of undesirable anxiety stems out of an exaggerated and abnormal response to stress. The precipitating stress, however, differs from case to case in its nature, severity and duration. Moreover, it depends on the individual's personality and constitution as to how much stress can he or she handle effectively depending upon the coping mechanisms. There is a threshold for every individual beyond which stresses or conflicts lead to symptom formation. The person experiences the somatic manifestations of anxiety, i.e., palpitations, sweating, dizziness, tachycardia, dryness of mouth and hyperventilation, etc. Severe or persistent anxiety interferes in the normal routines of life and adversely effects work, family and social life.

Anxiety disorders are common psychiatric disorders in the general population and can be quite disabling (1). Even though a large number of patients who present at primary practice suffer with anxiety disorders, they sometimes remain undiagnosed and under-treated. In order to diagnose an anxiety disorder it is essential that dimensional information (e.g., number of panicky sensations, amount of time spent in avoidance behaviour, and extent of disability due to phobias) is gathered.

Anxiety disorders include:

- Generalised anxiety disorder
- Panic disorder with or without agoraphobia
- Specific phobias
- Social phobia
- Obsessive-compulsive disorders
- Post-traumatic stress disorder
- Acute stress disorder

Epidemiology

According to US National Comorbidity Study (NCS), one of four persons suffer from one anxiety disorder and the 12 months prevalence rate is around 17%. Findings of the same study (2)suggests the lifetime prevalence of various anxiety disorders as follows:

Generalised anxiety disorder	5.1%
Panic disorder	3.5%
Agarophobia	5.3%
Social phobia	13.3%
Specific phobia	11.3%

Although obsessive or compulsive symptoms occur in 14% of the general population, the prevalence of Obsessive-Compulsive Disorder (OCD) is 5–8%. The lifetime prevalence of post-traumatic stress disorder is about 1%. Women are more likely to have an anxiety disorder than men (2:1). The prevalence of anxiety disorders is the highest between 25–34 years (except conditions like school phobia which develops during childhood or adolescence). The prevalence of anxiety disorder decreases with higher social status.

Aetiology

Causes of anxiety can be classified under the following headings:

Psychological Theories

Four psychological theories have been put forward which provide helpful explanations about the causes of anxiety.

1. Psychoanalytic Theory

Freud has the credit of inventing the term anxiety neurosis (3). He was of the view that anxiety is a signal of the presence of danger in the unconscious. Anxiety results because of the conflict between the unconscious sexual or aggressive impulses and the superego or external reality. In response to this threat to the ego, defence mechanisms are used by the person to prevent the unacceptable feelings and thoughts from entering the conscious awareness.

2. Cognitive Theory

The proponents of this theory state that pathological anxiety derives from the misconceptions of threat and danger that are a result of cognitive distortions (the erroneous way in which the information is processed) (4).

3. Behavioural Theory

According to this theory, anxiety is a conditioned response to a specific stimulus in the environment. Social learning theory states that an individual may develop anxiety symptoms in response to the anxious behaviour of other people especially their parents.

4. Existential Theory

This school of thought is of the view that the generalised anxiety is because of the existential concerns for example, feeling that life does not have a purpose and is absurd and meaningless.

Psychosocial Causes

1. Parenting

Disturbed family relationships can play a role in the development of anxiety disorders. Anxiety can be a learnt response to stressful factors experienced in childhood. Anxious parents usually breed anxious children.

According to Bowlby, anxiety is related to separation experience in childhood. Long-term parent-child separation and disruption of bonds of affection may lead to morbid or pathological anxiety in adult life. Freud believed that anxiety is a reaction to the danger of loss of a loved object. In children, loss, through death or separation, or threat of loss of affection from parents, leads to the development of anxiety.

2. Personality Type

Some people are, by nature, more anxiety-prone than others. They are emotional, unstable, insecure and over concerned about their health. Obsessional persons, who are usually tense, rigid and over-conscientious, tend to suffer from anxiety whenever there is interference in their life pattern.

3. Life events and Trauma

Life events are important in the aetiology of Generalised Anxiety Disorder. GAD is more prevalent amongst those who have experienced a significant stress. Serious life events like loss and extreme danger have been found to be associated with mixed anxiety and depressive disorder (5).

Genetic Factors

Like other psychiatric disorders, genetics component also plays an important role in the causation of anxiety disorders. There is evidence that heredity is a predisposing factor in the development of anxiety disorders. The concordance rate in twin studies is 45% in identical twins, compared with 15% in non- identical twins. 18% of first degree relatives of patients suffering form panic disorder, have panic disorder. 60% of patients have at least one relative with the same disorder, compared with 15% of control patients. First-degree relatives of patients with specific phobias are at a higher risk of having this disorder as members of families without this. Twin studies show that similar or identical genes are responsible for generalised anxiety disorder and major depression (6).

Biological Explanations

Autonomic Nervous System (ANS)

The ANS of some patients with anxiety symptoms, not only exhibit enhanced sympathetic tone but also responds excessively to moderate stimuli.

Role of Neurotransmitters

Three major neurotransmitters play a role in anxiety symptoms: Norepinephrine (NE) (7), serotonin (8) and γ-aminobutyric acid (GABA) (9). Affected patients may have a dysfunctional regulation of noradrenergic system. Different types of stress result in increased turnover of serotonin in various parts of the brain including prefrontal cortex, nucleus acumbens, amygdala and lateral hypothalamus. The efficacy of benzodiazepines in anxiety disorders is due to their propensity to enhance the activity of GABA at the GABA type A receptors.

Hypothalamic-Pituitary-Adrenal (HPA) Axis

There is increased synthesis and release of cortisol in response to stress. In PTSD, there is evidence of alterations in HPA axis. In panic disorder, blunted Adrenocorticoid Hormone (ACTH) response to corticotropin-releasing hormone has been shown.

Corticotropin-Releasing Hormone (CRH)

Hypothalamic levels of CRH are increased in stressful states. This activates the HPA axis and increases release of cortisol.

Brain Imageing Studies

Some studies in anxiety disorders have shown increased size of cerebral ventricles. Other studies have highlighted abnormal findings in the right hemisphere, frontal cortex, occipital and temporal areas. One study in patients suffering from panic disorder discovered abnormality in the parahippocampal gyrus. In OCD and PTSD caudate nucleus and amygdala have been implicated respectively.

GENERALISED ANXIETY DISORDER (GAD)

GAD is usually a chronic disorder and results in significant disability, decreased full time employment, disruption in social and recreational activities and low satisfaction with life. It needs to be remembered that depression is almost always accompanied by anxiety. In early stages of schizophrenia, anxiety is a prominent feature. And patients in the early stages of dementia, just before insight into the illness is lost, understandably feel anxious and depressed. It is also important to rule out those medical conditions and medications that can cause anxiety (see below).

An epidemiological study (10) and a clinical study (11) suggests that the onset of GAD typically begins between the late teens and late twenties. GAD usually starts in an insidious way and has high comorbidity. Two-thirds of GAD patients also have simple phobias, social phobias, panic disorder and depressive disorder. It has more prevalence in lower social class It becomes difficult to manage with increasing age, and patients having alcohol abuse, personality disorders and family problems have comparatively poorer prognosis. In order to diagnose, the symptoms have to be present for 6 months period and before making a diagnosis, depressive episodes, phobic anxiety disorder, panic disorder and obsessive-compulsive disorder have to be excluded.

ICD-10 criteria of GAD (12)

Anxiety that is generalised and persistent but not restricted to, or even strongly predominating in any particular environmental circumstances (i.e. it is 'free-floating'). Patients may not acknowledge the excessive nature of their worries but they must be bothered by their degree of worry.

ICD-10 Criteria Guidelines

Symptoms should include elements of:

- Apprehension (worries about future misfortunes, feeling 'on edge', difficulty in concentrating, etc.)
- Motor tension (restlessness, fidgeting, tension headaches, trembling, inability to relax)
- Autonomic overactivity (light-headedness, sweating, tachycardia or tachypnoea, epigastric discomfort, dizziness, dry mouth, etc.)
    a. At least six months with prominent tension, worry and feelings of apprehension about everyday events and problems.
    b. At least four of the 22 symptoms (at least one of which must be from items 1–4)
    c. Symptoms
        1. Palpitations, pounding heart or accelerated heart rate
        2. Sweating
        3. Trembling or shaking
        4. Dry mouth
        5. Difficulty in breathing
        6. Feeling of choking
        7. Chest pain or discomfort
        8. Nausea or abdominal distress
        9. Feeling dizzy, lightheaded or faint
        10. Derealisation or depersonalisation
        11. Fear of losing control or going crazy
        12. Fear of dying
        13. Hot flushes or cold chills
        14. Numbness or tingling sensations
        15. Muscle tension or aches and pains
        16. Restlessness and inability to relax
        17. Feeling keyed-up, on edge, or mentally tense
        18. The sensation of a lump in the throat, or difficulty in swallowing
        19. Exaggerated response to minor surprises or being startled
        20. Difficulty in concentrating, or mind going blank, because of worry or anxiety
        21. Persistent irritability
        22. Difficulty in getting to sleep because of worrying

Differential Diagnosis

- Born worriers
- Panic disorder
- Phobias
- OCD
- PTSD
- Medical conditions
- Medications

Medical Conditions Associated with Anxiety Symptoms

Cardiac

Angina pectoris, arrhythmias, coronary insuffi- ciency, mitral valve prolapse, heart failure.

Endocrine

Hypercalcaemia, hyperthyroidism, pituitary disorders, Cushing's syndrome, pheochromo- cytoma, hyperparathyroidism, hypoglycaemia, carcinoid, premenstrual syndrome, menopausal symptoms.

Neurological and Other Disorders

Akathisia, temporal lobe epilepsy, vestibular nerve disease, organic brain syndrome, migraine, mass lesion, anaphylaxis, Huntington's disease, multiple sclerosis, ulcerative colitis, peptic ulcer, Wilson's disease.

Respiratory

Asthma, hypoxia, hyperventilation, chronic obstructive airway disease, pulmonary embolism.

Metabolic Disorders

Hyperkalaemia, hypoglycaemia, hypoxia, hy- ponatraemia, porphyria.

Withdrawal from CNS Depressants

Alcohol, benzodiazepines, barbiturates, narcotics.

Intoxication

Anticholinergic drugs, caffeine, theophylline, steroids, amphetamines, cocaine, hallucinogens, tobacco, sympathomimetic agents.

Miscellaneous

Systemic lupus erythematosus, pellagra, Anae- mia, vitamin B12 deficiency, collagen disease, pellagra.

Medications Causing Anxiety

Psychotropics

Antidepressants, neuroleptics, sedative-hypnotics, disulfiram.

Respiratory

Beta-adrenergic stimulants, bronchodilators.

CVS

Antiarrhythmics, antihypertensives.

Neurological

Anticonvulsants, anticholinergic agents, L-dopa.

Anaesthetic

Pre-anaesthetics, general anaesthetics.

Intoxication by Stimulants

Nicotine, caffeine, cocaine, amphetamines.

Miscellaneous

Thyroid hormone, antibiotics, non-steroidal anti-inflammatory drugs, anti-cancer drugs

Management of GAD

Most sufferers from GAD do not require hospitalisation and can be managed as outpatients. The most important aspect in the management of anxiety is a psychotherapeutic approach. A sympathetic and understanding approach in which the patient is allowed to talk freely about his problems and the doctor takes a keen interest in his patient, giving simple explanations and firm assurances about the absence of physical disease after a thorough physical examination, can have great therapeutic value in relieving anxiety. Treatment of GAD can be considered under the following headings:

Pharmacotherapy

This is mainly to provide symptomatic relief. The drugs which are used are:

a. Benzodiazepines

The efficacy of benzodiazepines in the treatment of GAD is well-established (13). Benzodiazepines are quick acting and are good for somatic symptoms. Their efficacy is maintained on long-term basis. They can, however, cause dependence, both physical and psychological, if used regularly for more than 4 weeks and it is because of this reason that their prolonged and regular use is not recommended.

b. Tricyclic Antidepressants

Tricyclic antiepressants, such as dothiepin and amitryptiline are of at least equal efficacy as benzodiazepine (14) in GAD, but full benefits may take few weeks to manifest. Their sedative properties can, however, be helpful in the meantime.

c. Selective Serotonin Reuptake Inhibitors (SSRIs)

Paroxetine and escitalopram are effective for GAD especially patients with comorbid depressive disorder.

d. SNRIs

Venlafaxine XR is also effective in treating GAD and duloxetine is also used for GAD.

e. Beta-adrenergic Blocking Agents

Their use is restricted to situational anxiety. These are more useful in patients who have predominantly autonomic symptoms of anxiety e.g., palpitation, dizziness, chest pain, etc. These are dangerous to use in people with asthma and can also cause depression (15).

f. Buspirone

This is a serotonin agonist, and is a useful anxiolytic if long-term treatment is required. In one study (16), buspirone demonstrated similar efficacy to benzodiazepines. It is more effective in reducing the cognitive symptoms of GAD than reducing the somatic symptoms. It lacks sedative and muscle relaxing properties and potentiates the effect of alcohol. One major drawback of buspirone is that it can take two to three weeks to be effective. This slow action of buspirone for transient and situational anxiety makes it less useful. However, benzodiazepine and buspirone can be initiated together and after two to three weeks benzodiazepine can be tapered off.

g. Antipsychotics

For decades, small doses of typical antipsychotics have been used as anxiolytics but there are only a few studies supporting this practice. There is also risk of akathisia. There is, however, some preliminary evidence to suggest that adding atypical antipsychotics to antianxiety or antidepressant medication to partial responders, may be helpful. The side effects of this group of antipsychotics e.g., metabolic issues, need to be borne in mind.

h. Antihistamines

These are well-established drugs for treating mild anxiety and insomnia. Although the dependence potential is low, cyclizine and diphenhydramine can be abused (17).

i. Monoamine Oxidase Inhibitors (MAOIs)

Alhough their use has not been properly evaluated, they are effective in social anxiety and panic disorder and there is reasonable assumption that they may be effective in GAD (18). Postural hypotension can be problematic and with irreversible MAOIs, dietary and drug interactions can be potentially lethal (19).

Psychological Treatments

The psychological treatments are based on the strong assumption that maladaptive and inappropriate way of dealing with stresses gives rise to pathological anxiety. These treatments help the patients to develop an insight into their problems and produce an awareness of the factors, which have led to the current symptoms. For psychotherapy to be successful, the development of a collaborative therapeutic relationship between the doctor and the patient is imperative.

Cognitive Behavioural Therapies

Evidence of the effectiveness of CBT has been found in several studies (20). Cognitive therapy is designed to help patients identify the cause of anxiety, and put their symptoms into a more accurate or logical perspective with a view to gain control over the maladaptive patterns of thoughts.

Although behavioural therapy is most effective for phobias, it is also helpful in GAD. There is some evidence of the effectiveness of exposure therapy for GAD. Cognitive therapy is, however, superior to behavioural therapy in GAD (21).

Relaxation Techniques

Patients are trained in progressive relaxation by alternating tensing and relaxing the various muscles of the body.

PANIC DISORDER

The core feature of panic disorder is the sudden attack of intense anxiety and autonomic arousal which occur out of the blue and peak within a few minutes. Although most attacks occur spontaneously they may also be provoked by an excited state or when a person is physically exhausted. The anxiety is accompanied by a sense of impending doom or a feeling that a dreadful event is about to happen. Sufferers fear a loss of control (e.g fainting, urinating, or crying out), going mad or dying from a heart attack. Between attacks, most patients experience generalised anxiety to some extent. As these attacks increase in frequency, patients become increasingly worried about future attacks and implications. Patients, moreover, start avoiding situations in which these attacks occur. This tendency, unfortunately, keeps on escalating and consequently many patients become restricted to their homes. These patients may then avoid going out altogether or may need assistance to help them going out. This is called agoraphobia. Agoraphobia is defined as a persistent and irrational fear of a specific activity or a situation that causes the patient to avoid them. Agoraphobia is almost always accompanied by panic disorder and the person fears places and situations from where escape may not be feasible. Panic disorder can be with or without agoraphobia. Approximately 65% of panic disorder patients develop agoraphobia. (22).

Panic attacks occur in other psychiatric disorders including social anxiety disorder, post-traumatic disorder, schizophrenia and depression (23). Panic disorder commonly develops between the ages of 18 and 25 years and depression can develop anytime during the course of the illness. Epidemiological studies have shown that panic disorder occurs quite frequently. Studies report a lifetime prevalence of panic disorder of 3. 5% (24). Women are more prone to develop panic disorder with female to male ratio of 2:1. The average age of onset is between 20–25 years. The clinical features of panic disorder do not appear to differ between males and females.

Evidence suggests that there is genetic vulnerability and early childhood trauma is associated with panic disorder. Medical illnesses and other life stresses can be precipitating event (25). According to a psychological model, the patients with panic disorder are caught in a vicious cycle in which they misinterpret the somatic symptoms as a warning of an impending catastrophe and severe consequences. This distorted and exaggerated thinking and worry causes further anxiety and fear (26).

Diagnosis

Diagnostic criteria of DSM- 5 (27). The criteria in 1CD-10 is similar.

A. Panic attack requires four symptoms from the following:
   - Shortness of breath
   - Choking
   - Palpitations and accelerated heart rate
   - Chest discomfort or pain
   - Sweating
   - Dizziness, unsteady feeling or faintness
   - Nausea or abdominal distress
   - Depersonalisation or derealisation
   - Numbness or tingling sensations
   - Flushes or chills
   - Trembling or shaking
   - Fear of dying
   - Fears of going crazy or doing something uncontrolled

B. At least one of the attacks has been followed by one month (no more) of one or both of the following:

- Persistent concern or worry about additional attacks or their consequences (e.g., losing control, having a heart attack, 'going crazy').
- A significant maladaptive change in behaviour related to the attacks (e.g., behaviours designed to avoid having panic attacks, such as avoidance of exercise or unfamiliar situations).

C. The disturbance is not attributable to the physiological effects of a substance (e.g., a drug of abuse, a medication) or another medical condition (e.g., hyperthyroidism, cardiopulmonary disorders).

D. The disturbance is not better explained by another mental disorder (e.g., the panic attacks do not occur only in response to feared social situations, as in social anxiety disorder: in response to circumscribed phobic objects or situations, as in specific phobia:in response to obsessions, as in obsessive-compulsive disorder: in response to reminders of traumatic events, as in post-traumatic stress disorder: or in response to separation from attachment figures, as in separation anxiety disorder).

Differential Diagnosis

Panic attacks may be seen in social phobia, simple phobia, PTSD and obsessive-compulsive disorder. In social phobia, facing the social situation may result in anxiety symptoms. Panic attacks can be distinguished from phobias as the anxiety attacks are not related to a particular stimulus or situation. In GAD, the attacks are associated with stressful situations or excessive worry. Similarly, in PTSD, the other features will predominate. About 20% of patients with major depressive disorder have panic attacks and alcohol abuse can be a consequent problem.

Hypoglycaemia may sometimes be difficult to distinguish from a panic attack. However, the symptoms of hypoglycemic attack tend to have a slower onset and last much longer and the relief of symptoms with sugar helps in diagnosis. Patients suffering from pheochromocytoma have paroxysms that resemble panic attacks. However, these patients have paroxysmal headache and hypertension is always present during the attack and also between the attacks.

Patients with simple partial seizures may have an aura, which presents as fear. However, there are usually other features, which point to the diagnosis of epilepsy. Hyperparathyroidism may also cause panic attacks but the presence of carpopedal spasm is a useful diagnostic sign. The diagnosis can be confirmed by measuring serum calcium and phosphorus.

Drugs like amphetamines may cause symptoms similar to panic attacks but their onset is usually very slow and the history of drug use confirms the diagnosis. Similarly, in benzodiazepine and alcohol withdrawal, symptoms resembling panic attacks may occur.

Excessive and acute caffeine consumption (at least 720 mg above the normal daily intake in a short period) can cause intense anxiety, whereas chronic caffeine intake may give rise to a clinical picture resembling GAD (28). Patients with panic disorder have intrinsic biological vulnerability and are extremely sensitive to caffeine. In them, even one cup of coffee (having 100 mg) can cause severe anxiety.

Management

It is now generally accepted that panic disorder is a chronic and disabling condition, and there is, therefore, a need for long-term treatment (29). Commonly used drugs are tricyclic antidepressants, selective serotonin reuptake inhibitors, monoamine oxidase inhibitors and benzodiazepines, especially clonazepam and alprazolam. Clomipramine is widely used and has a lot of evidence (30). SSRIs such as citalopram, escitalopram, fluoxetine, paroxetine and sertraline are all effective. The use of benzodiazepines is restricted because of the dependence problem.

Cognitive behaviour therapy is not only very effective treatment of panic disorder but may also have a more lasting benefit than an antidepressant like imipramine (31). If there is co-existing agoraphobia, exposure therapy is beneficial. Many people suffering from panic disorder can be helped by relaxation and breathing exercises. Patients can also be taught to control hyperventilation, which is associated with most panic attacks. Hyperventilation is a much commoner phenomenon than usually realised. Overbreathing may occur in an acute anxiety state. Rapid breathing blows off carbon dioxide producing a state of relative alkalosis. This may lead to tetany in which there is tingling in the extremities, dizziness and muscle spasms involving face and limbs. A simple remedy for this is to get the person to re-breathe into a paper bag, thus building up the carbon dioxide and hence carbonic acid in the blood, which reverses the state of alkalinity.

PHOBIC ANXIETY DISORDER

Phobic anxiety disorder has the same core symptoms as GAD, but these symptoms occur only in particular circumstances. The person tries to avoid circumstances that provoke anxiety, and experiences anticipatory anxiety when there is the prospect of encountering these circumstances. The patients remain preoccupied with the dread and despite their awareness that many other people do not have such fears about similar situations, their anxiety levels are not alleviated and they continue to perceive these situations as threatening. Phobias are persistent, intense and unrealistic fears of situations or objects. The fear is beyond voluntary control and out of proportion to the situation. It results in avoidance of the situation and, when seriously disabling or stressful, is termed as phobic disorder. The individual recognises the fear to be unreasonable and excessive but the anxiety is not relieved by the knowledge that the people do not regard the situation as dangerous.

Phobic anxiety often coexists with depression. It needs to be noted that depressive episodes can be accompanied by phobic anxiety and low mood often follows phobias. According to ICD-10, the decision to make two diagnoses or one depends on whether one disorder developed clearly before the other and if one is very clearly predominant at the time of diagnosis. If depressive disorder fulfils the criteria before the diagnosis of phobic anxiety disorder is made, than the former should have diagnostic precedence (32). Similarly, obsessional symptoms may be present along with phobic anxiety but do not dominate the clinical picture.

Agoraphobia

Unlike DSM-IV, in DSM-5 panic disorder and agoraphobia are unlinked. The former DSM-IV diagnoses of panic disorder with agoraphobia, and agoraphobia without a history of panic disorder are now replaced by two diagnoses, panic disorder and agoraphobia, each with a separate criteria. Agoraphobia affects approximately 2% of the population in one year. More than 65% of patients having agoraphobia are females and the age of onset ranges from

15 to 35 years (33). There is no significant association with social or educational status. It is, however, linked to marital and domestic discord (34). There is a strong association with panic disorder. Approximately half of people who are diagnosed as having panic disorder also have agoraphobia. Although there is some genetic basis of agoraphobia, there is often a precipitating event which can be a panic attack or any other unusual threatening situation which results in future avoidance.

Agoraphobia includes fear not only of open spaces but also of related aspects such as presence of large gatherings and the difficulty of immediate escape to their perceived safe place which is usually their own home. Agoraphobic patients are, therefore, quite anxious when they are away from home, in crowds, or in situations from where they cannot easily leave. They try their best to avoid these situations, feel anxious when anticipating them, and experience other symptoms of anxiety which are similar to those of other anxiety disorders. When they are in crowded places, they vigilantly look out for possible nearest exits which would not attract attention. They are typically worse when alone and exposed to bright light. Patients are persistently worried that help may not be readily available when needed after the anxiety attack.

The term, therefore, refers to cluster of phobias, apprehension of leaving home, fear of entering shops or other crowded public places. As agoraphobic symptoms have a strong tendency to generalize, the feared situations increase. Many patients become unable to travel alone in trains, buses or planes. They feel less anxious when accompanied by someone and even the presence of a child or their pet animal is helpful. There can also be fear of being in lifts and on bridges.

Agoraphobia is the most incapacitating of all the phobic disorders as persistence avoidance can cause significant interference in occupational and social functioning. Some sufferers become extremely disabled and completely housebound. In some cases, patients start avoiding being home alone as well. It also needs to be remembered that some people with agoraphobia experience little anxiety as they are able to consistently avoid their phobic situations.

In spite the fact that agoraphobia is included in both ICD-10 and DSM-5, some researchers have cast doubts that agoraphobia exists without panic disorder (35). Diagnostic errors have been highlighted in the initial epidemiological studies which reported large estimations of agoraphobia without panic disorder (36). Many studies have reported that panic disorder preceeds agoraphobia (37) (38) (39).

According to the ICD-10, all the following criteria should be fulfiled for a definite diagnosis.

- Psychological or autonomic symptoms must, primarily, be manifestations of anxiety and not secondary to other symptoms such as delusions or obsessional thoughts.
- Anxiety must be restricted to, or occur mainly in, at least two of the following situations: crowds, public places, traveling away from home or traveling alone.
- Avoidance of the phobic situation must have been a prominent feature.

In differential diagnosis, social phobia, delusional disorder, and Obsessive-compulsive Disorder (OCD) need to be considered.

In social phobia, patients avoid joining social gatherings and therefore may avoid leaving. In agoraphobia, however, there is fear of having a panic attack. Patients with delusional disorder may avoid public places as they are convinced that someone may harm them. Similarly, OCD patients avoid public transport because of fear of contamination.

Sometimes, severe depersonalisation can be present with agoraphobic symptoms.

Prognosis

Although there are short-lived cases, when agoraphobia persists for one year it then generally goes on for five years (40). Depressive symptoms can occur during its course. Prognosis is better for those with good marital relations and people no chronic stress.

Treatment of Agoraphobia

- Education about anxiety
- Imperative to provide these patients with information about how agoraphobia develops and how it can be overcome
- Relaxing and breathing techniques can be helpful
- Exposure therapy: In this, there is graded exposure to feared situations. Exposure therapy is more effective when combined with anxiety management (41).
- Cognitive-behavioural therapy: This is effective both in short as well as the long-term.
- Psychopharmacology
    - Benzodiazepines:

    Although there is some role of benzodiazepines, there is risk of tolerance and dependence in long-term use.

Particular caution is needed in those with a history of substance misuse.

- SSRI:

These are superior to imipramine and alprazolam (42).

- MAOIs:

Apart from the problems of dietary restrictions and interactions with other drugs, when MAOIs are stopped, most patients with agoraphobia relapse.

Social Phobic Anxiety

In social phobic anxiety (also known as social phobia) inappropriate and excessive anxiety is experienced in social situations. Patients feel very fearful, self-conscious and embarrassed. There are two clinical subtypes of social anxiety disorder, generalised social anxiety disorder and non-generalised anxiety disorder. Studies have also reported evidence for this distinction (43). The distinction between the two is on the basis of the number of feared situations. Originally thought to be a rare condition, it is now recognised as a chronic psychiatric problem with significant functional impairment.

It is the most prevalent of the anxiety disorders having a lifetime prevalence of about 13% and a 1-month prevalence rate of 4.5% (44). It is the third most frequently occurring disorder, after depression and generalised anxiety disorder (45, 46). Studies, however, report that less than 5% of people ask for professional help and treatment (47).

Secondary depression occurs in up to 40% of patients (48). People suffering from social phobia have usually been very shy during childhood, had few or no friends at school. The age of onset ranges from 15 to 35 years. It is equally common in men and women although women have a greater range of situations they are fearful of (49).

The essential feature of social phobia is fear of social interaction and being observed or scrutinised by other people in social situations such as public speaking, eating in public, using public lavatories, etc. They have a marked and persistent fear of performance as they anticipate that embarrassment or humiliation may occur. There is marked anticipatory anxiety. The most common precipitating situations, which produce social phobia, including meeting people in authority, writing in front of others, being introduced to the strangers, eating in public or at home with acquaintances, and speaking in public. Studies have reported that the most common fear is public speaking (50).

When exposed to a feared situation, they experience somatic symptoms of anxiety such as trembling, feeling shaky, increased muscular tension, palpitations, tachycardia, flushing of face or pallor, cold hands, sweating, dry mouth, twitching, difficulty in swallowing, headache and a sinking feeling in the stomach along with fear and apprehension. Avoidance of the feared situation may result in complete social isolation. Suicidal ideation and attempted suicide are quite common in social phobia. It may involve only one social situation or it may cover many social situations so that the sufferers avoid all company. It has been found that the degree of formality of the feared situation and the number of people present in that situation determines the amount of anxiety experienced by patients (51). One study has highlighted an interesting finding that in social anxiety disorder, there is little or no avoidance of shops or public transport (52). Social phobic anxiety disorder is associated with alcoholism.

Diagnosis

The ICD-10 diagnostic criteria for social phobia specifies that all of the following should be present:

- Psychological, behavioural or autonomic symptoms must primarily be manifestations of anxiety and not secondary to other symptoms such as delusions or obsessional thoughts.
- Anxiety must be restricted to or predominantly present in particular social situations.
- The phobic situation is avoided whenever possible.

The DSM-5 diagnostic criteria is similar but specifies that symptoms must have been present for at least six months.

Differential Diagnosis

In the differential diagnosis of social phobic anxiety, other disorders to consider are: inadequate social skills, normal shyness, depressive disorder, body dysmorphic disorder, generalised anxiety disorder, panic disorder with agoraphobia, avoidant personality disorder and schizophrenia.

Patients suffering from panic disorder with agoraphobia, primarily fear having a panic attack or losing control in situations from which they cannot escape. In other words, although they are very apprehensive of certain social situations, their anxiety is secondary to their fears of panic attacks and the subsequent consequences of these attacks. In social phobia, the primary fear is of scrutiny and negative evaluation of others in social situations.

In depression, a patient may avoid social contact and become socially isolated because of lack of enjoyment and energy, in contrast to social phobia where the patient withdraws from social situations as there is fear of being observed and scrutinised.

In generalised anxiety disorder, there can be apprehensions and fears of social situations but these are diffused and there is absence of significant fear of being scrutinised in a derogatory way. Patients with GAD may experience sleep problems, and headaches.

As there is high degree of comorbidity between social anxiety disorder and avoidant personality disorder, some patients meet the criteria for both disorders (53). Both the disorders are also chronic in nature. The former has a clearer onset and shorter history. People with avoidant personality disorder have a life-long history of feeling shy and lacking in confidence. Social anxiety disorder also has high comorbidity with body dysmorphic disorder (54). Patient's account regarding the imagined bodily defect is helpful to differentiate between the two.

Treatment of Social Phobia

SSRIs

These are the first choice of treatment in social phobic disorder as there is good evidence for the efficacy of SSRIs (55). Fluvoxamine, paroxetine, sertraline and fluoxetine are all helpful. In one study, escitalopram was also found to be very effective (56). The benefits are usually not visible till six weeks of treatment and SSRIs should be given for 9–12 months as many patients relapse if treatment is stopped before this period (57).

MAOIs

Although phenelzine is effective (58), its use is restricted because of dietary and drug interaction issues. Moclobemide is also helpful in some patients (59). It is important to remember that there needs to be an interval of at least two weeks between stopping an SSRI (when there is no response) and commencing an MAOI.

Benzodiazepines and Beta-Blockers

Due to the risk of dependence, benzodiazepines should preferably be used on short-term basis while patients are waiting to commence another treatment (e.g., CBT). Clonazepam (60), alprazolam (61) and bromazepam (62) are all effective. Although beta-blockers (e.g., atenolol) are helpful in the short-term for symptoms like tremors and palpitations, their overall efficacy is not established (63).

CBT

There is considerable research and evidence for CBT in the treatment of social anxiety disorder. Systematic desensitisation, imaginal flooding, muscle relaxation techniques, graduated exposure, social skills training, and cognitive restructuring are some of the behavioural and cognitive techniques that have been studied (64). CBT in groups is not as effective as individual treatment (65).

Specific Phobia

A specific phobia is a strong, persisting fear of an object or situation. Specific phobia is more common than social phobia. It is the most common psychiatric disorder among women and the second most common among men, second only to substance-related disorders (66). Specific phobia is characterised by irrational or exaggerated fear and avoidance of a particular object or situation. The range of situations that give rise to specific phobias are remarkably small. There are two groups of situations; heights, closed spaces, still water in which the danger of falling, suffocating and drowning are obvious; poisonous insects snakes and carnivorous animals from which the possibility of harm is again obvious. Everyone is wary in such situations, but people with specific phobias become anxious in anticipation of entering such a situation and when in the situation, their fear is out of proportion to the danger. Fears of blood or injury are a special case that must have a protective function. Fear of flying can be a manifestation of fears of heights, closed spaces, or agoraphobia or a conditioned fear related to previous airline trauma.

When people with specific phobias encounter their feared situation they may experience panic attacks, or complain of symptoms like:

- Accelerated heart rate/pounding heart
- Trembling
- Faintness or light-headedness
- Difficulty with breathing
- Sweating

The severity of the anxiety usually varies according to the nature and location of the stimulus (for example, the size of the animal, whether the animal is moving, distance from the animal). Generally, individuals with specific phobias will attempt to avoid the feared stimulus whenever possible, to the extent that the fear or avoidance interferes with the individual's life or causes marked distress. The feelings of anxiety are absent when the individual is not in contact with the feared stimulus or is not thinking about the stimulus. Specific phobias are usually recognised by individuals as being irrational or excessive.

Diagnosis

According to ICD-10, for a diagnosis of specific phobia the individual must display the following characteristics:

- Persistent and irrational fear of a particular object or situation (excluding fears due to panic disorder, social phobia, agoraphobia, obsessive-compulsive disorder, and PTSD).
- An immediate anxiety response when brought into contact with the stimulus.
- Avoidance of the stimulus or extreme anxiety during exposure.
- Fear, avoidance or distress interfere with the individual's normal life and social activities.
- The fear is recognised as being irrational or excessive.

The fifth edition of the Diagnostic and Statistical Manual of Mental Disorders (DSM-5) has a similar criteria but specifies that the fear, anxiety, or avoidance is persistent, typically lasting for six months or more.

Differential Diagnosis

First of all specific phobia needs to be differentiated from normal or appropriate fear. In a panic disorder, the individual experiences sudden panic attacks although the panic attacks are unpredictable and not always in response to specific stimuli. In social phobia, avoidance of social situations is due to fear of humiliation and negative evaluation by others. It is not the social situation itself that is feared but the consequences of being in that situation.

Agoraphobia involves fear and avoidance of certain places and activities. This fear and avoidance, however, stems from the possibility of having panic attacks and not being able to get help, or escape the situation.

In obsessive-compulsive disorder individuals may fear and avoid specific activities or objects so as to avoid the feared consequences (e.g., Avoiding the use of chemicals for fear of contamination, or avoiding using sharp knives in case they get the urge to stab somebody).

Similarly in post-traumatic stress disorder, the individual may avoid specific situations or objects which are associated with previous traumatic events so as to prevent the possibility of 're-living' the traumatic event.

Patients with paranoid personality disorder have generalised fear that distinguishes them from those having specific phobia. Differentiation between specific phobia and avoidant personality disorder can be difficult and may require several interviews.

Patients with hypochondriasis have fear of having a disease, whereas specific phobia patients have fear of contracting the disease. Sometimes patients with schizophrenia can also have phobic symptoms but unlike patients with specific phobia they do not have insight into the irrationality of their fears, and also have very bizarre quality to their symptoms. Specific phobia should not be diagnosed if criteria for any one of these previous differential diagnoses is met

Epidemiology

Specific phobias are very common. As many as 8% of the population have a diagnosable specific phobia although only 1% of the population will present for treatment of this phobia.

The 6-month prevalence of specific phobia is about 5 to 10 per 100 persons. Although this disorder is more common among women than among men, the ratio is closer to 1 to 1 for the fear of blood, injection, or injury. Phobias that begin during childhood generally disappear without treatment. Phobias that develop later in life, however, are usually more chronic. Most specific phobias do not usually cause enough impairment to warrant treatment since most phobic stimuli can generally be avoided without too much difficulty.

Management

The most effective treatment for specific phobias is exposure therapy and systematic desensitisation is the most frequently employed technique. In this the therapists desensitise the patients by using a series of gradual exposures to the phobic objects or situations. The anxiety provoking stimuli are graded in a hierarchy from the least to the most fearful. Patients are taught ways to cope with the anxiety e.g., relaxation and cognitive techniques. The fact that the feared or phobic situations are safe is reinforced through the cognitive-behavioural approach.

Another behavioural technique involves using sudden and intense exposure to the feared stimuli. In both imaginal flooding and flooding in vivo, patients with specific phobias are exposed to the actual phobic objects or situations and again taught to cope with the resultant anxiety. Specific phobias usually do not require any medication and it is best to avoid prescribing benzodiazepines and the like.

Acute Stress Reaction (Disorder)

Stress in one form or another is ubiquitous in everyday life. A certain level of stress is, in fact, desirable to enhance performance. However, exposure to acute or chronic stressful events, which are not tolerable and are perceived as threatening may precipitate abnormal and prolonged responses.

Acute stress reaction is a transient condition of significant severity, that develops in response to an exceptional physical or mental stress and is overwhelming to an extent so as to affect almost anyone. Examples include, natural disasters, major accidents, violence, sexual assault, and fire, etc. The traumatic events that can lead to an acute stress reaction are, therefore, of similar severity to those involved in Post-Traumatic Stress Disorder (PTSD).

Symptoms include a varying mixture of following symptoms:

- An initial state of daze
- Disorientation, reduced levels of consciousness and narrowing of attention
- Agitation and overactivity
- Social withdrawal
- Anxiety symptoms e.g., sweating, increased heart rate, flushing, etc.
- Anger and aggression
- Depression
- Amnesia

Diagnosis

According to ICD-10, there must be a temporal connection between the impact of an exceptional stressor and the onset of symptoms.

Acute stress reaction is diagnosed when:

- The individual has been exposed to a traumatic event
- Symptoms begin within few minutes (if not immediately) of the traumatic experience
- Symptoms begin to resolve within hours in those cases where the stress factor is removed. In cases where the stress factor continues, the symptoms usually begin to diminish after 24–48 hours.
- The reaction occurs in the absence of any other mental or behavioural disorder.

According to DSM-5, the essential feature of acute stress disorder is the development of characteristic symptoms lasting from 3 days to 1 month following exposure to one or more traumatic events. The clinical presentation of acute stress disorder may vary by individual but typically involves an anxiety response that includes some form of reexperiencing of or reactivity to the traumatic event.

Differential Diagnosis

Acute stress disorder has to be differentiated from adjustment disorder, panic disorder, dissociative disorder, post-traumatic stress disorder, obsessive-compulsive disorder, psychotic disorders and traumatic brain injury.

Panic disorder is diagnosed only if panic attacks are unexpected and there is anxiety about future attacks or maladaptive changes in behaviour associated with fear of dire consequences of the attacks.

Adjustment disorder involves a short-term anxiety reaction to a life stressor, however in adjustment disorder the stressor (e.g., loss of job, a relationship break-up, etc.) Is usually less traumatic than in acute stress reaction.

Acute stress reaction should not be diagnosed if the symptoms are simply an exacerbation of existing symptoms of another psychiatric disorder (with the exception of personality disorders).

Epidemiology

Various studies have come up with variable incidence but is estimated to be around 15–20% following exceptional stress. The rate of acute stress reaction reported among survivors of motor vehicle accidents is 13% (67), among victims of violent crimes (68) and among witnesses of mass shooting 33% (69).

Treatment

Pharmacological and psychological treatments given at an early stage are effective and may even be beneficial in reducing the development of PTSD (70).

The precipitating event should be dealt with through supportive therapy and healthy coping mechanisms should be reinforced.

Short-term prescription of sedatives and hypnotics may be justified, to normalise sleep and reduce overwhelming anxiety.

Adjustment Disorders

These disorders consist of psychological reactions to a stressor or life event. The clinical features of adjustment disorders include anxiety, worry, depression, irritability, anger, aggressive outbursts and disturbance of concentration. Symptoms because of autonomic arousal like palpitations, sweating and tremors may also occur. Some patients may indulge in self- harm behaviour and alcohol misuse. These disorders are distinguishable from normal adaptive responses by difficulty in psychosocial functioning and the heightened intensity of subjective distress (71).

In adjustment disorders, the disturbance and malfunctioning is gradual and more prolonged than an acute stress reaction. There is a life event which may give rise to distress and patients have difficulty in adaptation to this change. Unlike PTSD, the stressor precipitating an adjustment disorder, is not very severe. However, the severity of the stressor does not always predict the severity of these disorders. Various factors, e.g., individual predisposition or vulnerability, duration of the stressor, personal context, social support, and reversibility of the stressor, play a role in precipitating these disorders. Moreover, stressors can be single or multiple and can be recurrent as well. Significant developmental stages in an individual's life such as joining a new school, starting a career, leaving or moving home, getting married or divorced, having a child, last child leaving home (empty nest syndrome) and retiring, are all associated with adjustment disorders.

According to ICD-10, the onset of symptoms should be within one month of the stressful event or life change. The duration of the symptoms does not usually exceed 6 months, except in the case of a prolonged depressive reaction. PTSD should be considered if the symptoms persists for longer than 6 months.

ICD-10 diagnostic guidelines state that if the criteria for adjustment disorder are satisfied, the clinical form for predominant features can be classified as follows:

- Brief depressive reaction
- Prolonged depressive reaction
- Mixed anxiety and depressive reaction
- With predominant disturbance of other emotions
- With predominant disturbance of conduct
- With mixed disturbance of emotion and conduct

In brief depressive reaction, there is transient low mood, tearfulness and feelings of hopelessness. This needs to be differentiated from a major depressive disorder and uncomplicated bereavement. Prolonged depressive reaction is a mild depressive state which occurs in response to a prolonged exposure to a stressful event but its duration is not longer than two years.

Mixed features of anxiety and depressive symptoms are a hallmark of mixed anxiety and depressive reaction. These symptom, however, do not meet the criteria of an already established anxiety or depressive disorder.

In adjustment disorder with predominant disturbance of emotions, several types of emotions, such as anxiety depression, irritability, and anger, etc., are involved.

Behaviours such as truancy, vandalism, reckless driving and fighting, etc. Dominate the adjustment disorder with disturbance of conduct. Similarly, in adjustment disorder with mixed disturbance of emotion and conduct, disturbances of both emotions and conduct occur together.

Unlike ICD-10, DSM-5 criteria states a three month limit on the development of symptoms subsequent to the stressor. Both classifications require that symptoms must not persist for longer than six months after the removal of the stressor. DSM-5 lists six adjustment disorders, including an unspecified category, and this sub-classification of adjustment disorders is similar to ICD-10:

- Adjustment disorder with depressed mood
- Adjustment disorder with anxiety
- Adjustment disorder with mixed anxiety and depressed mood
- Adjustment disorder with disturbance of conduct
- Adjustment disorder with mixed disturbance of emotions and conduct
- Adjustment disorder unspecified

Epidemiology and Prognosis

The prevalence is estimated to be from 2 to 8 percent of the general population. Although adjustment disorder can occur at any age, it is more commonly diagnosed in adolescents. It is twice more common in women than in men. Most adjustment disorders last for some months and some persist for years (72). While the prognosis is good for adults, some adolescents with adjustment disorders develop psychiatric disorders in adult life (73).

Treatment

The treatment of choice for adjustment disorders is psychotherapy. Patients are helped to resolve the stressful event or situation and encouraged to adapt to stressors that are not reversible. Problem-solving techniques are provided, while maladaptive coping mechanisms are discouraged.

One study found that in patients with adjustment disorders, both brief dynamic and supportive psychotherapy were more effective than waiting list control (74). Group therapy can also be helpful for patients who had similar stresses. Individual therapy has also shown beneficial results. It explores the meaning of the stressor to the patient so as to facilitate working through the earlier traumas. A judicious use of medication on a short-term basis can help with symptomatic relief. Anxiolytic or antidepressant medication can be used depending on the type of adjustment reaction.

Post-Traumatic Stress Disorder (PTSD)

PTSD is characterised by the development of a long-lasting anxiety response following a traumatic or catastrophic event. Typically, the individual experiences or witnesses a traumatic event such as actual or threatened death, serious injury to oneself of another person, or a threat to the personal integrity of oneself or others. The individual's response involves helplessness, intense fear, or horror. Typical traumatic events include: violent assaults (e.g., sexual or physical assault or mugging); torture, being taken hostage, kidnapped, or held as a prisoner of war; terrorist attacks; severe car accidents; being victims of natural or man-made disasters; being diagnosed (or having a loved one diagnosed) with a life-threatening illness; witnessing or learning about the unexpected death or injury of another person. The nature and severity of the trauma is of fundamental importance. Traumas caused by humans generally cause more lasting damage than the stress caused by natural disasters (75). Some researchers suggest that trauma should be sudden (so there is no time for mental preparedness), dangerous (life-threatening) and overwhelming (so that the victim feels helpless) (76). Trauma may be physical or emotional, isolated or repeated. After the trauma, the patient undergoes a period of confusion and disbelief and tries to make sense of what has actually happened. Later, the anxiety symptoms like tachycardia, sweating, hyper alertness, sleep disturbance, aggression, rage, helplessness and guilt feelings appear. The patient usually feels numb and detached from the surroundings, and is unable to perform day-to-day work. The onset of post-traumatic stress disorder is usually delayed for weeks or months after the stressful event. Symptoms can fluctuate over time, being especially worse during periods of stress. The patient persistently re- experiences the trauma through nightmares or in the form of intrusive or unwanted thoughts or memories. This is the central feature of PTSD and is essential for the diagnosis of PTSD. Symptoms of PTSD usually develop within 3–6 months of the traumatic event (although sometimes longer) and involves:

- Images, dreams or flashbacks of the traumatic event
- Avoidance of cues that act as reminders of the traumatic event
- Amnesia about important aspects of the traumatic event
- Intense arousal and anxiety on exposure to traumatic cues
- Depressed or irritable mood
- Social withdrawal
- Concentration and memory difficulties
- Nightmares and disturbed sleep
- Being easily startled

Diagnosis

For decades the very entity and diagnosis of PTSD has been a matter of controversy. One reason being that there is considerable litigation and compensation involved in PTSD cases. Clinically there is also a debate about whether PTSD is an anxiety or a mood disorder.

There are substantial differences between DSM-5 and DSM-IV in the diagnostic criteria for PTSD. The stressor criterion is more explicit with regards to events that qualify as 'traumatic' experiences. Moreover, another criterion, the subjective reaction to the traumatic event has been removed. There are four symptom clusters in DSM-5 instead of three given in DSM-IV (re-experiencing, avoidance/numbness and arousal). The avoidance/numbness cluster has been divided into two distinct clusters: avoidance and persistent negative alterations in cognition and mood. The cluster of persistent negative alterations in cognitions and mood contains new or reconceptualised symptoms, such as persistent negative emotional states. The final cluster (arousal), also includes irritable behaviour or angry outbursts and reckless or self-destructive behaviour.

According to ICD-10, PTSD should not generally be diagnosed unless there is evidence that it arose within six months of a trauma which should be of an exceptionally threatening or catastrophic nature and is likely to cause pervasive distress in almost anyone. This definition of ICD-10 is included to differentiate PTSD from other psychiatric disorders by implying that is an understandable reaction and also that severe trauma is necessary to precipitate the disorder. It should be borne in mind, however, that majority of people who experience similar traumatic events do not develop PTSD. Those patients in whom the PTSD symptoms occur after 6 months should be given a diagnosis of probable PTSD provided the symptoms are typical. The more chronic cases should be classified under the category of enduring personality change (77).

Comorbidity

Over half of PTSD patients have a comorbid psychiatric disorder (78). According to another study, most people who have PTSD also meet the criteria for at least one other psychiatric disorder (79). Depression is the most common comorbidity. Alcohol and drug misuse is quite common among men while women suffer more from depression and anxiety disorders. Those with PTSD also have a higher rate of OCD (80). There can also be conspicuous and persistent changes in personality after the trauma.

Differential Diagnosis

the unpleasant experience (s) as they do in PTSD. PTSD is usually distinguished from acute stress disorder in terms of the time frame in which symptoms are experienced. Acute stress disorder should resolve within four weeks whereas symptoms of PTSD are prolonged. In OCD, there are recurrent intrusive thoughts but unlike PTSD, the content of the thoughts does not represent the trauma (in case there is a precipitating life event). Flashbacks can also occur in dissociative disorders, but can be differentiated by other features.

Epidemiology

The prevalence of PTSD varies across different parts of the world depending upon the prevalence of traumatic events in particular communities. In those parts of the world where there are wars and other significant conflicts, the rates of PTSD would be higher.

The lifetime incidence of PTSD is estimated to be 9% to 15%, and the lifetime prevalence is about 8% of the general population. One study in USA found prevalence among adult population to be 8%, with women (10%) twice as likely as men (5%) to have PTSD at some point in their lives (81). In another study among community populations affected by war and forced migration, the prevalence of PTSD was found to be between 14% and 37% (82). Although PTSD can appear at any age, it is most prevalent in young adults. This is probably because of their comparatively more exposure to traumatic events. PTSD is more likely to occur in those who are single, divorced, widowed, socially isolated and who belong to a low socioeconomic class.

Aetiology

As many people who have experienced similar traumatic events do not develop PTSD, it seems plausible that PTSD is the result of the interaction between vulnerability and resilience factors. Vulnerability is the predisposition of an individual to be adversely affected. Resilience has been defined as the ability to maintain a state of normal equilibrium in the face of extremely unfavourable circumstances (83).

According to one study, three factors predict the onset of PTSD: the scale of the trauma, the patient's previous experience of trauma and the level of social support available (84). Other predisposing factors include childhood abuse, female gender, past psychiatric history, family history, psychiatric disorders, personality disorders, previous experience of trauma (especially during childhood), previous acute stress reaction, feelings of helplessness and lack of control during and after the traumatic event.

Perceived lack of social support after the trauma and disassociation at the time of trauma (85) (86) have been highlighted as significant contributory factors in the development of PTSD. Although the significance of intensity and extent of trauma has been highlighted by some researchers, other studies have come up with opposite findings. In two studies involving fire fighters, no association was found (87) (88). Another study also failed to link the severity of the stressor and the subsequent development of PTSD (89).

The role of genetic factors has also been highlighted by some robust studies. It has been put forward by one researcher that people who develop PTSD are more likely to have first degree relatives with psychiatric disorders than those who do not have PTSD (90). In another study involving monozygotic and dyzygotic twins, genetic factors accounted for about 34% of PTSD symptoms (91).

There is substantial evidence that neurobiological abnormalities are present in patients with PTSD. Neurobiological findings like altered hypothalamic-pituitary-adrenal feedback mechanisms, with low urinary cortisol, have been demonstrated in PTSD (92). Abnormality in the opioid system is suggested by low plasma B-endorphin concentrations in people with PTSD. Studies found increased urine epinephrine and catecholamine concentrations in veterans and sexually abused girls respectively (93).

People with PTSD show morphological and functional abnormalities of the brain and areas implicated include amygdala, hippocampus and prefrontal cortex

(94). Studies have shown decreased activity in medial prefrontal and anterior cingulated areas to be correlated with increased activity in the amygdala (95).

Course of PTSD

PTSD is often a chronic disorder associated with significant disability and handicap, affecting relationships, work and physical health. Half recover within five years, the speed of recovery being greater for individuals who have received professional treatment. More than one-third continue to have PTSD symptoms after many years (96). Symptoms can have troublesome effect on work and family, etc. Social support, being widowed or divorced, having low education and low income, and low psychosocial functioning play a role in chronically maintaining symptoms of PTSD (97).

Management

Trauma-focused psychological treatments, e.g., Trauma-focused cognitive-behavioural therapy and eye movement desensitisation and reprocessing) should be first-line of treatment, and medication should be tried afterward (98). Trauma focused cognitive-behavioural interventions have lot of evidence for efficacy (99) (100) (101). Research has now shown that psychological debriefing is not very effective (102).

Cognitive-Behavioural Therapy

Cognitive and behavioural approaches are successful, especially in reducing the intrusive symptom (103). CBT includes exposure techniques, cognitive restructuring procedures, and anxiety management programmes. Exposure therapy has the strongest evidence. Both exposure in imagination and exposure in real-life to trauma-related events appear to be therapeutic (104).

Eye Movement Desensitisation and Reprocessing (EMDR)

EMDR became popular following a randomised control trial with a group of individuals suffering from post-traumatic stress disorder (105). Since then there have been at least twenty RCT's on EMDR and PTSD.

EMDR can usefully be understood in terms of Adaptive Information Processing systems (106). EMDR seems to directly influence the way that the brain functions in processing new information, via its protocol based structure and the specific technique of bilateral stimulation. It helps to restore normal ways of dealing with problems (i.e. information processing). Following successful EMDR treatment, memories of the event are no longer emotionally painful when brought to mind. What happened can still be recalled, but it is less upsetting. EMDR appears to mimic what the brain does naturally on a daily basis during dreaming, or REM sleep, and therefore EMDR can be thought of as an inherently natural therapy, which assists the brain in working through distressing material.

The AIP model suggests that remembered information is stored in memory networks of related thoughts, images, sounds, smells, tastes and emotions, being organised around the earliest related events. It is suggested that traumatic experiences, at any point in a person's life, or persistent unmet needs, during crucial periods in development, may produce problems in the normal functioning of the adaptive information processing system in attempting to resolve this material.

Pharmacological Treatment

NICE guidelines recommend that treatment for PTSD should be continued for at least one year. SSRIs such as paroxetine and sertraline, are the first-line of drug therapy as they have been researched extensively for the treatment of PTSD. Paroxetine has a lot of evidence (107) (108), and is also recommended by NICE. One study showed no benefit from using 40 mg of paroxetine instead of 20 mg (109). Because of the potential problems, e.g., Withdrawal syndrome, some researchers have advocated that it should be used cautiously (110).

Sertraline is also recommended as an effective treatment (111) (112), but for fluoxetine the data is not impressive, as one study did not show any statistical difference (113).

Among tricyclics, the efficacy of imipramine and amitriptyline is supported by a number of well-controlled trials. Amitriptyline, however, has more evidence for efficacy than imipramine (114). Dosage of both these tricylics should be the same as those used to treat depressive disorder.

Regarding MAOIs, one study has shown that phenelzine is effective for PTSD (115). Studies have also shown improvement with Reversible Monoamine Oxidase Inhibitors (RIMAS). Trazadone, valproate and carbamazepine may be helpful.

Mirtazapine has also shown promising results in one study (116), and is also recommended by NICE guidelines. Venlafaxine has also been tried but one randomised controlled study (117) failed to show significant efficacy.

Because of noradrenergic hyperactivity in patients with PTSD, the use of antiadrenergic agents such as clonidine and propranolol has also been advocated.

Atypicals antipsychotics have been used as an add on therapy with SSRIs. Some researchers have recommended to augment SSRIs with olanzapine (118) if there is no substantial improvement. Olanzapine on its own, however, as a first-line treatment for PTSD, does not have much evidence (119). In another study, risperidone was unsuccessfully tried as an adjunctive therapy (120).

Obsessive-Compulsive Disorder

DSM-5 does not include Obsessive- Com-pulsive Disorder (OCD) under anxiety disorders, and has a new separate chapter 'Obsessive-Compulsive and Related Disorders'.

Obsessive-Compulsive Disorder (OCD) is characterised by persistent and intrusive thoughts or impulses that increase anxiety, and ritualistic behaviours or mental acts, that serve to alleviate the anxiety. The unwanted thoughts that recur are called obsessions or obsessional ruminations, and the unwanted repetitive acts that the patient realises as absurd or ridiculous (but is unable to resist) are called compulsions or compulsive rituals. Obsessional thoughts can be words, ideas and beliefs that enter the patients mind forcibly and repeatedly. Obsessional impulses are repetitive urges to perform socially embarrassing or violent acts e.g., shouting blasphemies or injuring someone. In some patients obsessional phobias can occur when they start avoiding certain situations in which their distress is increased, e.g., when they have urges to harm others in the presence of items that can potentially be used in a dangerous way.

One very important aspect of OCD is that the symptoms are egodystonic and patients recognise these irrational thoughts as products of their own minds. Obsessions may also take the form of doubts, ruminations and obsessional hesitancy. Most patients have a mixture of both obsessions and compulsions and it is uncommon for someone to have only one of these. The thoughts and behaviour do not give any pleasure but, as mentioned above, help in decreasing the discomfort and worry. In fact, the obsessions and compulsions not only cause significant distress, but also consume a lot of the time of the patient and interfere with the social and occupational functioning. Many patients become so preoccupied with the obsessional behaviours that their life comes to a standstill as they are unable to perform the routine requirements of their lives. That is why OCD is a serious and frequently disabling illness which results in causing high cost to the individuals and the society. OCD is detrimental to the educational pursuits and considerably effects the work performance of the sufferers. Many patients have to consequently lower their job or career responsibilities and aspirations. Some cease to work at all and there are, therefore, significant economic implications.

Patients also try to enlist the help of friends or relatives. The effect on their families can be devastating as the relatives not only find it very difficult to deal with them but also find their own lives being restricted because of their involvement with the tiresome obsessional behaviours. The relationships are understandably affected very adversely.

There is a higher rate of suicide attempts in people with OCD as compared to general population and there are even higher rates when comorbid depression exists. Two-thirds of OCD patients have depressive symptoms (121). Commonly, OCD patients suffer with these symptoms in isolation for years before seeking professional help. One possible explanation is they do not appreciate medical treatment can help with these problems. The other being that they are worried about being labelled as crazy or insane.

Although many patients with OCD have a combination of symptoms, the predominant symptoms can be broadly classified into clusters. The most common obsession is of contamination and it is accompanied by washing compulsion. These patients spend a considerable time washing parts of their body and are also very vigilant in avoiding objects from which they think they can get contaminated, e.g., door handles, switches, and other people's hands etc. The other group of patients are predominantly concerned with checking, and are unfortunately not satisfied by repeated checking. Sometimes, while driving, patients drive back to check to ensure they have not caused an accident or have injured someone.

Other patients are preoccupied with intrusive thoughts which have aggressive or sexual themes. As the aggressive thoughts usually involve hurting the dear ones, patients suffering from these symptoms are understandably very distressed. Similarly, some patients have inappropriate and perversive sexual thoughts, images and impulses about children, animals and holy figures.

In obsessional slowness, patients take hours trying to lay things in perfect order. Another symptom cluster consists of hoarding behaviour. Patients suffering from this symptom are extremely reluctant to throw even unwanted and trivial things as they fear they might lose something important.

Risks Associated with OCD

Some authors have distinguished the consequent risks of OCD into primary and secondary. The primary risks arise directly because of OCD symptoms and are not only apparent but also more easily managed. These include the chance of acting on an obsession aggressive or sexual impulses). Fortunately, there is minimal risk of this happening. Secondary risks are more serious as they are not routinely appreciated by clinicians as well as carers. Patients with contamination, for example, may start avoiding food and drinks to the extent of malnourishment or dehydration. The growth of children suffering from OCD may be adversely affected. There may be harms due to over exposure to disinfectants when patients repeatedly and incessantly clean their bodies.

Diagnosis

As mentioned above, the hallmark of OCD are obsessions and compulsions. Common obsessions and compulsions e.g., contamination, hand-washing, thoughts about harming others and checking, give diagnostic clues to the interviewer. Sometimes, however, patients may not readily complain of these problems, as they may regard these as personality traits or may feel very embarrassed to disclose them. There may, therefore, be a need to probe about these symptoms routinely and directly. This is especially important when seeing children as they are more likely not to disclose about them spontaneously. Occasionally, compulsions may be entirely mental, e.g., mental checking, and pose diagnostic difficulty as they are less obvious and hard to describe. Similarly, patients with obsessional slowness (where patients suffer with extreme slowness that is out of proportion to other symptoms), are not easily recognised as having OCD.

According to the ICD-10, for a definite diagnosis, obsessional symptoms or compulsive acts or both must be present on most days for at least two successive weeks and be a source of distress or interference with activities. The obsessional symptoms should have the following characteristics:

- They must be recognised as the individual's own thoughts or impulses.
- There must be at least one thought or act that is still resisted unsuccessfully, even though others may be present which the sufferer no longer resists.
- The thought of carrying out the act must not, in itself, be pleasurable. (Simple relief of tension or anxiety is not regarded as pleasure in this sense).
- The thoughts, images, or impulses must be unpleasantly repetitive.

Differential Diagnosis

Some patients who do not have OCD may be misdiagnosed. These include misdiagnosis of ruminations in depressive disorder, worries in generalised anxiety disorder (GAD), and intrusive symptoms in post-traumatic stress disorder (122). Depressive episodes are often accompanied by obsessional symptoms and about 15% of patients report a lifetime history of depression have also suffered with OCD (123).

A careful history and a thorough mental state examination would differentiate between OCD and GAD. In post-traumatic stress disorder there would be a clear and distinctive onset after a trauma. The features of OCD, being bizarre, may resemble schizophrenia. In psychotic illness, there is a lack of resistance and lack of insight, whereas OCD patients recognise their obsessional thoughts and acts as senseless and inappropriate. They also realise these originate from their own minds rather than from other people or external agencies. However, many patients with schizophrenia have OCD symptoms in the early and prodromal stages and 15% of patients with schizophrenia meet the diagnostic criteria of OCD. In these cases, the prognosis is relatively poor for both conditions (124). Some patients suffering from schizophrenia have stereotyped symptoms which mimic compulsions.

Some people have perfectionist traits which are more conspicuous and problematic in obsessive-compulsive personality disorder (also called anankastic personality disorder). Patients with body dysmorphic disorder have obsessive and compulsive symptoms about their imagined or perceived physical ugliness. Similarly, in hypochondriasis there are obsessions and compulsions about their imagined illness.

Obsessions and compulsions are also present in medical disorders such as Sydenham's chorea, Huntington's disease, temporal lobe epilepsy and encephalitis lethargica. As OCD frequently develops before the age of 30, OCD symptoms in older patients should raise the possibility of neurological disorders. About 90 percent of patients with Tourette's disorder have compulsive symptoms and as many as two-thirds fulfil the diagnostic criteria for OCD (125).

Epidemiology

Obsessive-compulsive disorder is far more common than used to be thought, the lifetime prevalence in the general population being 2–3%. The Epidemiological Catchment Area (ECA) study reported one month prevalence of 1.1% in males and 1.5% in females (126).

OCD occurs most frequently in late adolescence or early adulthood. The mean age of onset is about 20 years, although men have a slightly earlier age of onset than women. Single persons are affected more than married ones although it is likely that this finding is compounded by the fact that the sufferers have difficulty in maintaining relationships. About 25% of OCD patients have premorbid obsessional traits.

Aetiology

Genetics

There is evidence for genetic influence (127) and (128) and another study has provided support for familial involvement (129).

Serotonergic Function

Clinical drug trials have supported the hypothesis that in OCD there is dysregulation of serotonin. There is less support for the involvement of noradrenergic system.

Brain-Imageing Studies

There is evidence of abnormal metabolism in the orbito-frontal cortex, in the anterior cingulate and in the basal ganglia. Studies show hypermetabolism in these areas.

Learning and Cognitive Theories

According to this theory, abnormal learning causes symptoms of OCD. Obsessional rituals, for example, are a form of avoidance response.

Cognitive theory states that the root cause is the patient's inability to control the intrusive thoughts. Patients with OCD, somehow hold themselves responsible for their possible consequences (130). This attitude then leads to further futile attempts to avoid such thoughts by indulging in compulsive and avoidance behaviour.

Prognosis

About 20 to 30 percent of patients have significant improvement and 40 to 50 percent have moderate improvement (131). When there is a precipitating event and good social or occupational adjustment, the prognosis is much better. Interestingly, the content of the obsessions do not have any bearing on the prognosis. Some OCD patients have comorbid psychopathology with schizophrenia and it has also been noted that clozapine may initiate or exacerbate OCD symptoms in patients with schizophrenia (132). Prognosis is worse when OCD symptoms start in childhood and there is a personality disorder.(133)Patients having schizotypical personality disorder respond poorly to both behaviour therapy and pharmacotherapy (134) (135). Male patients may have a poor prognosis. Males also have more obsessions with symmetry and consequently have more obsessional slowness, whereas checking and cleaning rituals are more common in females (136).

Management

Clomipramine

Although clomipramine is very effective in OCD, the full benefit may not be seen until six weeks of treatment. Moreover, the anticholinergic side effects of clomipramine may be quite troublesome. Many patients taking this medication relapse within few weeks of stopping the drug (136) but if exposure therapy is combined with this tricyclic antidepressant, then relapse rate is reduced (137).

SSRIs

SSRIs including fluoxetine, fluvoxamine, paroxetine and sertraline, are effective in OCD (138) (139), but are less effective than clomipramine (140). Many patients respond to an adequate dose and duration, both the dose and duration being higher than depression (141). If a patient fails to respond adequately to an SSRI, the first step is to change the SSRI to an another SSRI, as there is evidence for this strategy (142). The second strategy is to augment the first SSRI with another one. However, it is important to carefully monitor patients when they are being treated with combination of these medications (143).

Other Pharmacological Strategies

Augmentation of SSRIs by neuroleptics in small doses may prove useful in the treatment of both obsessions and compulsions. Similarly, adding lithium, fenfluramine, buspirone and tryptophan to an SSRI may be helpful. Anxiolytic drugs have a role in the magement of OCD but should be prescribed on short-term basis.

Behaviour Therapy

Behaviour therapy is as effective as pharmaco-therapy in OCD and there is also evidence that the effects of behaviour therapy last longer (144). The main approaches are exposure and response prevention but desensitisation, thought stopping, flooding, implosion therapy and aversive conditioning have also been suc- cessfully used.

Other Therapies

There is only anecdotal evidence for long-term individual therapy (145). Family therapy can help reduce the relationships conflicts and some patients with OCD find group therapy helpful.

ECT

Although the evidence for the efficacy of ECT in OCD is reported in some studies (146), it is not compelling as the beneficial effect of ECT may have been on the depressive symptoms which are present in 40% of the patients with OCD. ECT should, therefore, be reserved for severely depressed and suicidal patients.

Neurosurgery

Neurosurgery is now rarely done. Types of operations include anterior cingulotomy, anterior capsulotomy, subcaudate tractotomy, and limbic leucotomy. The most common complication of neurosurgery is the development of seizures.

REFERENCES

1. Lader, M. H. and Uhde, T. H. (2006). *Fast facts: anxiety, panic and phobias* (2nd Edition). Oxford: Health Press.
2. Kessler, R. C., McGonagle, K. A., Zhao, S., Nelson, C. B., Hughes, M., Eshleman, S., Wittchen, H. U. and Kendler, K. S. (1994). Lifetime and 12 month prevalence of DSM III-R psychiatric disorders in the United States. Results from the National Comorbidity Survey. *Archives of General Psychiatry*, 51, 8–19.
3. Freud, S. (1894). The justification for detaching from neurasthenia a particular syndrome: the anxiety neurosis. *Collected Papers*, 1, 76–106.
4. Wells, A. and Butler, G. (1997). *Generalised anxiety disorder*. In D. M. Clark and C. G. Fairburn (Eds.), Science and practice of cognitive behaviour therapy. University Press: Oxford.
5. Finlay-Jones, R. and Brown, G. W. (1981). Types of stressful life event and the onset of depressive and depressive disorders. *Psychological Medicine*, 11, 803–815.
6. Kendler, K. S. (1996). Major depression and generalised anxiety disorder: same genes, (partly) different environments-revisited. *British Journal of Psychiatry*, 168, 68–75.
7. Nutt, D. J. (1992). Pharmacoendocrine studies in anxiety. *Clinical Neuropharmacology*, 15, 214–215.
8. Deaken, J. F. (1998). The role of serotonin in panic, anxiety and depression. *International Clinical Pharmacology*, 13, 1–5.
9. Nutt, D. J. and Malizia, A. L. (2001). New insight into the role of the GABA-A benzodiazepines receptor in psychiatric disorder. *British Journal of Psychiatry*, 179, 390–396.
10. World Health Organisation. (1992). *ICD-10 Classifications of mental and behavioural Disorder*: Clinical descriptions and diagnostic guidelines. Geneva: World Health Organisation.
11. Burke, K. C., Burke, J. D. Jr, Rae, D. S. and Reigier, D. A. (1991). Comparing age at onset of major depression and other psychiatric disorders by birth cohorts in five US community populations. *Archives of General Psychiatry*, 48, 789–795.
12. Rogers, M. P., Warshaw, M. G., Goisman, R. M., Goldenberg, I., Rodriguez-Villa, F., Mallya, G., Freeman, S. A. and Keller, M. B. (1999). Comparing primary and secondary generalised anxiety disorder in a long-term naturalistic study of anxiety disorders. *Depression and Anxiety*, 10(1), 1–7.
13. Davidson, J. R. T. (2001). Pharmacology of generalised anxiety disorder. *Journal of Clinical Psychiatry*, 62(11), 46–50.
14. Davidson, J. R. T. (2001). Pharmacology of generalised anxiety disorder. *Journal of Clinical Psychiatry*, 62(11), 46–50.
15. Nutt, D., Asgyropoulos, D. S. and Forsall, S. (1998). *Generalised anxiety disorder*. London: Martin Dunitz.
16. Enkelmann, R. (1991). Alprazolam versus buspirone in the treatment of outpatients with generalised anxiety disorder. *Psychopharmacology*, 105, 428–432.
17. Johnstone, E. C., Owens, D. G. C., Lawrie, S. M., Sharpe, M. and Freeman, C. P. L (2004). *Companion to psychiatric studies* (7th Edition). London: Elsevier.
18. Nutt, D., Asgyropoulos, D. S. and Forsall, S. (1998). *Generalised anxiety disorder*. London: Martin Dunitz.
19. Lader, M. H. and Uhde, T. H. (2006). *Fast facts: Anxiety, panic and phobias* (2nd Edition). Oxford: Health Press.
20. Butler, G., Cullington, A., Hibbert, G., Klimes, I.and Gelder, M. (1987). Anxiety management for persistent generalised anxiety disorder. *British Journal of Psychiatry*, 151, 535–542.
21. Butler, G., Fennell, M., Robson, P. and Gelder, M. (1991). Comparison of behaviour therapy and cognitive behaviour therapy in the treatment of generalised anxiety disorder. *Journal of Consulting and Clinical Psychology*, 59, 167–175.
22. Lader, M. H. and Uhde, T. H. (2006). *Fast facts: Anxiety, panic and phobias* (2nd Edition). Oxford: Health Press.
23. Nutt, D., Asgyropoulos, D. S. and Forsall, S. (1998). *Generalised anxiety disorder*. London: Martin Dunitz
24. Kessler, R. C., McGonagle, K. A., Zhao, S., Nelson, C. B., Hughes, M., Eshleman, S., Wittchen, H. U. and Kendler, K. S. (1994). Lifetime and 12 month prevalence of DSM III-R psychiatric disorders in the United States. Results from the National Comorbidity Survey. *Archives of General Psychiatry*, 51, 8–19.
25. Johnstone, E. C., Owens, D. G. C., Lawrie, S. M., Sharpe, M. and Freeman, C. P. L (2004). *Companion to psychiatric studies* (7th Edition). London: Elsevier.
26. Clark, D. M. (1986). A cognitive approach to panic disorder. *Behaviour Research and Therapy*, 24, 461–470.
27. American Psychiatric Association.(2013). *Diagnostic and statistical manual of mental disorders* (5th Edition). Arlington, VA: American Psychiatric Publishing.
28. Lader, M. H. and Uhde, T. H. (2006). *Fast facts: Anxiety, panic and phobias* (2nd Edition). Oxford: Health Press.
29. David, J. R. T. (1998). The long-term treatment of panic disorder. *Journal of Clinical Psychiatry*, 59, 17–21.
30. Fahy, T. J., O'Rourke, D. O., Brophy, J., et al. (1999). The Galaway study of panic disorder. Clomipramine and lofepramine in DSM-III-R panic disorder: a placebo controlled trial. *Journal of Affective Disorders*, 25, 63–76.
31. Barlow, D. H. (1997). Cognitive-behavioural therapy for panic disorder: current status. *Journal of Clinical Psychiatry*, 58, 32–36.
32. World Health Organisation. (1992). *ICD-10 Classifications of mental and behavioural disorder*: Clinical descriptions and diagnostic guidelines. Geneva: World Health Organisation.
33. Buckley, P., Prewette, D., Bird, J. and Harrison G. (2005). *Examination notes in psychiatry*. New York: Holder Education.
34. Wright, P., Stern, J. and Phelan, M. (2005). *Core psychiatry* (2nd Edition). London: Elsevier Saunders.
35. Lader, M. H. and Uhde, T. H. (2006). *Fast facts: Anxiety, panic and phobias* (2nd Edition). Oxford: Health Press.
36. Nutt, D. and Ballinger, J. (2005). *Anxiety disorders panic disorder and social anxiety disorder*. Oxford: Blackwell Publishing.
37. Garvey, M. J. and Tuason, V. B. (1984). The relationship of panic disorder to agoraphobia. *Comprehensive Psychiatry*, 25, 529–531.
38. Thyer, B. and Himle, J. (1985). Temporal relationship between panic attack onset and phobic avoidance in agoraphobia. *Behaviour Research and Therapy*, 23, 607–608.
39. Uhde, T., Boulenger, J., Geraci, H., Vittone, B. and Post, R. (1985). Longitudinal course of panic disorder. *Progress in Neuro-psychopharmacology and Biological Psychiatry*, 9, 39–51.
40. Marks, I. M. (1969). *Fears and Phobias*. London: Heinemann.
41. Cohen, S. D., Monteiro, W. and Marks, I. M. (1984). Two year follow-up of agoraphobics after exposure and imipramine. *British Journal of Psychiatry*, 144, 276–281.
42. Boyer, W. (1995). Serotonin uptake inhibitors are superior to imipramine and alprazolam in alleviating panic attacks: a meta-analysis. *International Clinical Pharmacology*, 10, 45–49.
43. Turner, S. M., Beidel, D. C. and Townsley, R.M. (1992). Social phobia: a comparision of specific and generalised

subtypes and avoidant personality disorder. *Journal of Abnormal Psychology*, 101, 326–331.

44. Magee, W. J., Eaton, W. W., Witchen, H. U., mcgonagle, K. A. and Kessler, R. C. (1996). Agoraphobia, simple phobia and social phobia in the National Comorbidity Survey. *Archives of General Psychiatry*, 43, 519–522.
45. Kessler, R. C., Stang, P., Wittchen, H. U., Stein, M. and Walters, E. E. (1999). Lifetime comorbidities between social phobia and disorders in the US National Comorbidity Survey. *Psychological Medicine*, 29, 555–567.
46. Goldberg, D. P. and Lecrubier, Y. (1995). Form and frequency of mental disorders across centres. In T. B. Ustan and N. Sartorious (Eds.), *Mental illness in general healthcare: an international study*. New York: John Wiley and Sons.
47. Schneier, F. R., Spitzer, R. L., Gibbon, M., Fyer, A. J., Liebowitz, M. R. and Weissman, M. M. (1992). Social phobia: Comorbidity in an epidemiological sample. *Archives of General Psychiatry*, 49, 282–288.
48. Wright, P., Stern, J. and Phelan, M. (2005).*Core psychiatry* (2nd Edition). London. Elsevier Saunders.
49. Turk, C. L., Heimberg, R. G. and Orsillo, S. M. (1998). An investigation of gender differences in social phobia. *Journal of Anxiety Disorders*, 12, 209–223.
50. Holt, C. S., Heimberg, R. G. and Hope, D. A. (1992), Avoidant personality disorder and the generalised subtype of social phobia. *Journal of Abnormal Psychology*, 101, 318–325.
51. Rapee, R. M. (1991). Descriptive psychopathology of social phobia. In R. G. Heimberg, M. R. Leibowitz, D. A. Hope and F. R. Scheiner (Eds.), *Social phobia: diagnosis, assessment and treatment*. New York: The Guildford Press.
52. Wright, P., Stern, J. and Phelan, M. (2005).*Core psychiatry*, 2nd Edition. London: Elsevier Saunders.
53. Schneier, F. R., Spitzer, R. L., Gibbon, M., Fyer, A. J., Liebowitz, M. R. and Weissman, M. M. (1992). Social phobia. Comorbidity in an epidemiological sample. *Archives of General Psychiatry*, 49, 282–288.
54. Zimmerman, M. and Matia, J. I. (1998). Body dysmorphic disorder in psychiatric outpatients: recognition, prevalence, comorbidity, demographic, and clinical correlates. *Comprehensive Psychiatry*, 39, 265–70.
55. Ballenger, J. C., Davidson, J. R. T., Lecrubier, Y., et al. (1998). Consensus statement on social anxiety disorder from the International Consensus Group on Depression and Anxiety. *Journal of Clinical Psychiatry*, 59(17), 54–60.
56. Seigfried, K. (2005). Escitalopram in the treatment of social anxiety disorderrandomised, placebo-controlled, flexible-dosage study. *The British Journal of Psychiatry*, 186, 222–226.
57. Haug, T. T., Blomhoff, S., Hellstorm, K., et al. (2003). Exposure therapy and sertraline in social phobia: 1-year follow-up of a randomised controlled trial. *British Journal of Psychiatry*, 182, 312–318.
58. Liebowitz, M. R., Gorman, J. M. and Fyer, A. J. (1988). Pharmacotherapy of social phobia: an interim report of placebo controlled comparison. *Journal of Clinical Psychiatry*, 49, 252–257.
59. Schneier, F. R., Goetz, D., Campeas, R., et al. (1998). Placebo controlled trial of moclobemide in social phobia. *British Journal of Psychiatry*, 172, 70–77.
60. Jefferson, J. W. (2001). Benzodiazepines and anticonvulsants for social phobia. *Journal of Clinical Psychiatry*, 62, 50–53.
61. Jefferson, J. W. (2001). Benzodiazepines and anticonvulsants for social phobia. *Journal of Clinical Psychiatry*, 62, 50–53.
62. Versiani, M., Nardi, A. E., Figueira, I., Mendlowicz, M. and Marques, C. (1997). Double blind placebo controlled trial with bromazepam in social phobia. Jornal Brasileiro de Psiquiatria, 46, 167–171.
63. Turner, S. M., Beidel, D. C. and Jacob, R. G. (1994). Social phobia: comparison of behaviour therapy and atenolol. *Journal of Consulting and Clinical Psychology*, 62, 350–358.
64. Schneier, F. R. (1991). *Social phobia. Psychiatry Annals*, 21, 349–353.
65. Stangier, U., Heidenreich, T., Peitz, M., et al. (2003). Cognitive therapy for social phobia: individual versus group treatment. *Behaviour Research and Therapy*, 41, 991–1007.
66. Sadock, B. and Sadock, V. (2007). *Kaplan's and Sadock's synopsis of psychiatry* (10th Edition). Philadelphia: Lippincott Williams and Wilkins.
67. Harvey, A. G. and Byrant, R. A. (1998). The relationship between acute stress disorder and post-traumatic disorder: a prospective evaluation of motor vehicle accident survivors. *Journal of Consulting and Clinical Psychology*, 66, 507–512.
68. Brewin, C. R., Andrews, B. and Rose, S. (1999). Acute stress disorder and post-traumatic stress disorder in victims of violent crimes. *American Journal of Psychiatry*, 156, 360–366.
69. Classen, C., Koopman, C., Hales, R., et al. (1998). Acute Stress Disorder as a predictor of post-traumatic stress symptoms. *American Journal of Psychiatry*, 155, 620–624.
70. Bisson, J. (2002). Post-traumatic stress disorder. *Clinical Evidence*, 7, 913–919.
71. Casey, P., Dowrick, C. and Wilkinson, G. (2001). Adjustment Disorders. *British Journal of Psychiatry*, 179, 479–481.
72. Gelder, M., Harrison, P. and Cowen, P. (2006). *Shorter Oxford Textbook of Psychiatry* (5th Edition). Oxford: Oxford University Press.
73. Andreason, N. C. and Hoenck, P. R. (1982). The predictive value of adjustment disorders: a follow-up study. *American Journal of Psychiatry*, 139, 584–590.
74. Maina, G., Forner, F. and Bogetto, F. (2005).Randomised controlled trial comparing brief dynamic and supportive therapy with waiting list condition in minor depressive disorders. *Psychotherapy and Psychosomatics*, 74, 43–50.
75. Argyropoulos, S., Campbell, A. and Stein, G. (2007). In G. Stein and G. W. Gaskell (Eds.), *Anxiety disorders in seminars in general adult psychiatry*. London: The Royal College of Psychiatrists.
76. Figley, C. R. (1985). Traumatic stress: the role of the family and social support system. In C. R. Figley (Ed.), *Trauma and its wake*. The study of Post-traumatic Stress Disorder. New York: Brunner/Mazel.
77. Figley, C. R. (1985). Traumatic stress: the role of the family and social support system. In C.R. Figley (Ed.), *Trauma and its wake*. The study of Post-traumatic Stress Disorder. New York: Brunner/Mazel.
78. Kessler, R. C., Sonnega, A., Bromet, E., et al. (1995). Post-traumatic stress disorder in the National Comorbidity Survey. Archives of General Psychiatry, 52, 1048–1060.
79. Fairbank, J. A., Ebert, L. and Costello, E. J. (2000). Epidemiology of traumatic events and post-traumatic stress disorder. In D. J. Nutt, J. R. Davidson and J. Zohar (Eds.), *Post-traumatic Stress Disorder*: Diagnosis, management and treatment. London: Martin Dunitz.
80. Helzer, J., Robins, L. N. and McEvoy, L. (1987). Post-traumatic stress disorder in the general population. Findings from the Epidemiological Catchment Area Survey. *The New England Journal of Medicine*, 317, 1630–1634.

81. Kessler, R. C., Sonnega, A., Bromet, E., et al. (1995). Post-traumatic stress disorder in the National Comorbidity Survey. *Archives of General Psychiatry*, 52, 1048–1060.

82. Karunaka, U. K., Neuner, F., Schauer, M., et al. (2004). Traumatic events and symptoms of post- traumatic stress disorder amongst Sudanese nationals, refugees and Uganfians in the West Nile. *African Health Sciences*, 4, 83–93.

83. Bonanno, G. A. (2004). Loss, trauma and human resilience: have we underestimated the human capacity to thrive after extremely aversive events? *American Journal of Psychology*, 59, 20–28.

84. Van der Kolk, B. (1996). The body keeps the score: the evolving psychobiology of post- traumatic stress. In H. G. M. Westenberg, J. A. Den Boer and D. L. Murphy (Eds.), *Advances in the neurobiology of anxiety disorders*. Chichester: Wiley.

85. Brewin, C. R., Andrews, B. and Valentine, J. D. (2000). Meta-analysis of risk factors for post- traumatic stress disorder in trauma-exposed adults. *Journal of Consulting and Clinical Psychology*, 68, 748–766.

86. Ozer, E. J., Best, S. R., Lipsey, T. L., et al. (2003).Predictors of post-traumatic stress disorder and symptoms in adults: a meta-analysis. *Psychological Bulletin*, 129, 52–73.

87. McFarlane, A. (1998a). Relationship between psychiatric impairment and a natural disaster: the role of distress. *Psychological Medicine*, 18, 129–139.

88. MacFarlane, A. (1998b). The aetiology of post- traumatic stress disorders following a natural disaster. *British Journal of Psychiatry*, 152, 116–121.

89. Feinstein, A. and Dolan, R. (1991). Predictors of post-traumatic stress disorder following physical trauma: an examination of the stressor criterion. *Psychological Medicine*, 21, 85–91.

90. Davidson, J., Swartz, M. and Storck, M. (1985).A diagnostic and family study of post-traumatic stress disorder. *American Journal of Psychiatry*, 142, 90–93.

91. True, W. R., Rice, J., Eisen, S. A., et al. (1993). A twin study of genetic and environmental contributions to liability for post-traumatic stress symptoms. *Archives of General Psychiatry*, 50, 257– 264.

92. Yehuda, R., Giller, E., Southwick, S. Et al. (1991). Hypothalamic-pituitary-adrenal dysfunction in post-traumatic stress disorder. *Biological Psychiatry*, 30, 1031–1048.

93. Sadock, B. and Sadock, V. (2007). *Kaplan's and Sadock's synopsis of psychiatry* (10th Edition). Philadelphia: Lippincott Williams and Wilkins.

94. Ahmed, A. S. (2007). Post-traumatic stress disorder, resilience and vulnerability. *Advances in Psychiatric Treatment*, 13, 369–375.

95. Bremner, J. D. (1999). Does stress damage the brain? *Biological Psychiatry*, 45, 797–805.

96. Kessler, R. C., Sonnega, A., Bromet, E., et al. (1995). Post-traumatic stress disorder in the National Comorbidity Survey. *Archives of General Psychiatry*, 52, 1048–1060.

97. Zlotnick, C., Rodriguez, B. F., Weisberg, R. B., et al. (2004). Chronicity in post-traumatic stress disorder and predictors of the course of post-traumatic stress disorder among primary care patients. *Journal of Nervous and Mental Disease*, 192, 153–159.

98. National Collaborating Centre for Mental Health. (2005). Post-traumatic Stress Disorder: The management of PTSD in adults and children in primary and secondary care. *National clinical practice guideline number 26*. Leicester: Gaskell and British Psychological Society.

99. Byrant, R. A., Harvey, A. G., Dang, S. T., et al. (1998). Treatment of acute stress disorder: a comparison of cognitive-behavioural therapy and supportive counselling. *Journal of Consulting and Clinical Psychology*, 66, 862–886.

100. Ehlers, A., Clark, D. M., Hackmann, A., et al. (2003). A randomised control trial of cognitive therapy, a self-help booklet, and repeated assessments as early interventions for post-traumatic stress disorder. *Archives of General Psychiatry*, 60, 1024–1032.

101. Bisson, J. I., Shepherd, J. P., Joy, D., et al (2004). Early cognitive-behavioural therapy for post- traumatic stress symptoms after physical injury. Randomised controlled trial. *British Journal of Psychiatry*, 184, 63–69.

102. Rose, S., Bisson, J. and Churchill, R. (2002).Psychological debriefing for preventing PTSD. *Cochrane Database of Systematic Reviews*, 2, CD000560.

103. Solomon, S., Gerrity, E. and Muff, A. (1992). Efficacy of treatments for post-traumatic disorder: an empirical review. *The Journal of the American Medical Association*, 268, 633–638.

104. Rothbaum, B. O. (2000). Psychosocial treatment of post-traumatic stress disorder. In D. Nutt, J. Davidson and J. Zohar (Eds.), *Post-Traumatic Stress Disorder* diagnosis, management and treatment. London: Martin Dunitz.

105. Shapiro, F. (1989). Efficacy of the eye movement desensitisation procedure in the treatment of traumatic memories, *Journal of Traumatic Stress Studies*, 2, 199–223.

106. Dworkin, M. (2005). *EMDR and the relational imperative*. New York: Routledge.

107. Marshall, R. D., Beebe, K. L., Oldham, M., et al. (2001). Efficacy and safety of paroxetine treatment for chronic PTSD: a fixed-dose, placebo-controlled study. *American Journal of Psychiatry*, 158, 1982–1988.

108. Stein, D. J. (2000). *Improving treatment options– new clinical data on paroxetine*. CINP.

109. Marshall, R. D., Beebe, K. L., Oldham, M., et al. (2001). Efficacy and safety of paroxetine treatment for chronic PTSD: a fixed-dose, placebo-controlled study. *American Journal of Psychiatry*, 158, 1982–1988.

110. Duff, G. (2004) Safety of Selective Serotonin Reuptake Inhibitor Anti-depressants. Retrieved from http:// www. Info. Doh. Gov. Uk/doh/ embroadcast. Nsf/ vwdiscussionall/9AA9EC56B07B3B4F80256F61004BAA88

111. Friedman, M. J., Davidson, J. R. T. and Mellman, T. A. (2000). Pharmacotherapy. In E. B.Foa, T. M. Keane and M. J. Freidman (Eds.), Effective treatments for PTSD: *Practice guidelines from the International* Society *for Traumatic Stress Studies*. New York: Guilford Press.

112. Stein, D. J., Zungu-Dirwayi, N., Van der Linden, G. J. H., et al. (2004). Pharmacotherapy for post-traumatic stress disorder (PTSD). *Cochrane Library*, 2. Wiley Interscience.

113. Martenyi, F., Brown, E. B., Zhang, H., et al. (2002). Fluoxetine versus placebo in post-traumatic stress disorder. *Journal of Clinical Psychiatry*, 63, 199–205.

114. Kosten, T. R., Frank, J. B., Dan, E., et al. (1991). Pharmacotherapy for post-traumatic stress disorder using phenelzine or imipramine. *Journal of Nervous and Mental Disease*, 179, 366–370.

115. Kosten, T. R., Frank, J. B., Dan, E., et al. (1991). Pharmacotherapy for post-traumatic stress disorder using phenelzine or imipramine. *Journal of Nervous and Mental Disease*, 179, 366–370.

116. Davidson, J. R. T., Weisler, R. H., Butterfield, C.D. C., et al. (2003). Mirtazapine vs placebo in post-traumatic stress

disorder: a pilot trial. *Society of Biological Psychiatry*, 53, 188–191.

117. Davidson, J., Baldwin, D., Stein, D. J., et al. (2006). Treatment of post-traumatic stress disorder with venlafaxine extended release: a 6-month randomised controlled trial. *Archives of General Psychiatry*, 63, 1158–1165.

118. Butterfield, M. I., Becker, M. E., Connor, K. M., et al. (2001). Olanzapine in the treatment of post-traumatic stress disorder: a pilot study. *International Clinical Psychopharmacology*, 16, 197–203.

119. Stein, M. B., Kline, N. A. and Matloff, J. L. (2002). Adjunctive olanzapine for SSRI-resistant combat-related PTSD: a double-blind, placebo- controlled study. *American Journal of Psychiatry*, 159, 1777–1779.

120. Hamner, M. B., Faldowski, R. A., Ulmer,H. G., et al. (2003). Adjunctive risperidone treatment in post-traumatic stress disorder: A preliminary controlled trial of effects on comorbid psychotic symptoms. *International Clinical Psychopharmacology*, 18, 1–8.

121. Montgomery, S. and Zohar, J. (1999). *Obsessive-compulsive Disorder*. London: Martin Dunitz.

122. Stein, D. and Emsley, R. (1999). Treatment of the difficult obsessive–compulsive disorder patient. In M. Lader and D. Naber (Eds.), *Difficult problems in psychiatry*. London: Martin Dunitz.

123. Harrison-Read, P., Tyrer, P. and Sharpe, M. (2004). In E. Johnstone, D. C. Owens, S. Lawrie,M. Sharpe and C. P. Freeman (Eds.), *Companion to psychiatric studies* (7th Edition). Edinburgh: Churchill Livingstone.

124. Berman, I., Kalinowski, A., Berman, S. M., et al. (1995). Obsessive and compulsive symptoms in chronic schizophrenia. *Comprehensive Psychiatry*, 36, 6–10.

125. Sadock, B. and Sadock, V. (2007). *Kaplan's and Sadock's synopsis of psychiatry* (10th Edition). Philadelphia: Lippincott Williams and Wilkins.

126. Regier, D., Narrow, W. and Rae, D. (1990). The epidemiology of anxiety disorders: the epidemiological catchment area (ECA) experience. *Journal of Psychiatry*, 24(2), 3–14.

127. Carey, G. and Gottesman, I. I. (1981). Twin and family studies of anxiety, phobic and obsessive disorders. In D. F. Klein, J. Rabin (Eds.), *Anxiety: New research and changing concepts*. New York: Raven Press.

128. Rasmussen, S. A. and Tsuang, M. T. (1986). Clinical characteristics and family history in DSM–III obsessive-compulsive disorder. *American Journal of Psychiatry*, 143, 317–322.

129. Pauls, D. L., Towbin, K. E., Leckerman, J. F., et al. (1995). A family study of obsessive-compulsive disorder *American Journal of Psychiatry*, 152, 76– 84.

130. Salkovskis, P. (1997). Obsessive-compulsive disorder. In D. M. Clark and C. G. Fairburn (Eds.), *Science and practice of cognitive behaviour therapy*. Oxford: Oxford University Press.

131. Sadock, B. and Sadock, V. (2007). *Kaplan's and Sadock's synopsis of psychiatry* (10th Edition). Philadelphia: Lippincott Williams and Wilkins.

132. Baker, R. W., Bermanzohn, P. C., Wirshing, D.A., et al. (1997). Obsessions, compulsions, clozapine and risperidone. *CNS Spectrums*, 2, 26–36.

133. Iancu, I., Dannon, P. N. and Zohar, J. (2000). Obsessive-compulsive disorder. In M. G. Gelder andJ. J. Lopez-Ibor Jr (Eds.), *The New Oxford textbook of psychiatry*. Oxford: Oxford University Press.

134. Jeneke, M. A., Baer, L., Minichiello, W. E., Schwartz, C. E. and Carey, R. J. (1986). Concomitant obsessive-compulsive disorder and schizotypal personality disorder. *American Journal of Psychiatry*, 143, 530–532.

135. Minichiello, W. E., Baer, L. and Jenike, M. A. (1987). Schizotypal personality disorder: a poor prognostic indicator for behaviour therapy in the treatment of obsessive-compulsive disorder. *Journal of Anxiety Disorders*, 1, 273–276.

136. Pato, M. T., Zohar-Kadouch, R., Zohar, J., et al. (1988). Return of symptoms after discontinuation of clomipramine in patients with obsessive-compulsive disorder. *American Journal of Psychiatry*, 145, 1521–1525.

137. Pato, M. T., Zohar-Kadouch, R., Zohar, J., et al. (1988). Return of symptoms after discontinuation of clomipramine in patients with obsessive-compulsive disorder. *American Journal of Psychiatry*, 145, 1521–1525.

138. Goodman, W. K., Price, L. H., Rasmussen,S. A., et al. (1989). Efficacy of fluvoxamine in obsessive–compulsive disorder. *Archives of General Psychiatry*, 46, 36–44.

139. Jenike, M. A., Hyman, S., Baer, L., et al. (1990). A controlled trial of fluvoxamine in obsessive-compulsive disorder: implications for serotonergic theory. *American Journal of Psychiatry*, 147, 1209–1215.

140. Ackerman, D. and Greenland, S. (2002). Multivariate meta-analysis of controlled drug studies for obsessive-compulsive disorder. *Journal of Clinical Psychopharmacology*, 22, 309–317.

141. Tollefson, G. D., Birket, M., Koran, L., et al. (1994). Continuation treatment of OCD: double blind and open-label experience with fluoxetine. *Journal of Clinical Psychiatry*, 55, 69–76.

142. Piggot, T. A., Pato, M. T., Bernstein, S. E., et al. (1990). Controlled comparisons of clomipramine and fluoxetine in the treatment of obsessive –compulsive disorder. *Archives of General Psychiatry*, 47, 926–932.

143. Szegedi, A., Wetzel, H., Leal, M., et al. (1996).Combination treatment with clomipramine and fluvoxamine: drug monitoring, safety, and tolerability data. *Journal of Clinical Psychiatry*, 57, 257–264.

144. Sadock, B. and Sadock, V. (2007). *Kaplan's and Sadock's synopsis of psychiatry* (10th Edition). Philadelphia: Lippincott Williams and Wilkins.

145. Sadock, B. and Sadock, V. (2007). *Kaplan's and Sadock's synopsis of psychiatry* (10th Edition). Philadelphia: Lippincott Williams and Wilkins.

146. Maletzky, B., McFarland, B., Bart, A. (1994). Refractory obsessive-compulsive disorder and ECT. *Convulsive Therapy*, 10, 34–42.

CHAPTER

05 Mood (Affective) Disorders

Mood disorders are illnesses in which the predominant abnormality is of the mood. Since mood is also used synonymously with affect, affective disorders is another term for these disorders. Mood disorders can be conceptualized as falling into two main categories: unipolar and bipolar disorders. These disorders include depression and hypomania or mania (according to the degree of severity of the illness). When only episodes of depression occur in isolation without hypomania or mania, it is termed as unipolar depressive disorder. This is further classified into mild, moderate or severe, depending upon the number of symptoms and hence the severity of the condition. The repeated episodes of depression are called recurrent depressive disorder.

When episodes of depression and mania or hypomania occur in the same patient, it is called bipolar affective disorder (previously called manic-depressive illness or psychosis). In some patients manic and depressive symptoms may be intermingled together. This condition is called mixed affective disorder or state.

Unipolar Depressive Disorder

In unipolar depression, a patient suffers from one or more depressive episodes. As already mentioned above, a depressive episode can be mild, moderate or major (also called severe). A depressive episode is defined as persisting for a period of at least two weeks, with at least one of two cardinal features, depressed mood and anhedonia. In anhedonia, there is loss of pleasure in activities that are usually enjoyable. In unipolar depressive episodes, five of the following nine symptoms are present: depressed mood, anhedonia, appetite or weight changes, insomnia or hypersomnia, psychomotor agitation or retardation, loss of energy, feelings of worthlessness or guilt, diminished ability to concentrate or indecision, or suicide ideation. Because of the depressed mood there is change in the person's normal functioning. In addition, symptoms and altered functioning must be associated with significant distress or impairment. A depressive episode, on average, lasts for six months but about 25 percent of patients have longer episodes. About 10–20 percent of patients have a chronic and unremitting course (1).

Depressive disorder is a common and serious human affliction. Up to 50% of patients with major depression have comorbid medical or psychiatric disorder (2). Presence of co-morbid mental and physical disorders worsens prognosis as compared to depression alone.

Severe or Major Depressive Disorder (MDD) is very debilitating, and is increasingly seen as a chronic and relapsing illness. Much of the burden of Major Depressive Disorder (MDD) is linked to the recurrent nature of the disorder. 75–90% of patients with MDD have multiple episodes. With each new episode, the next episode occurs sooner and is comparatively more treatment-resistant. The importance of stress in precipitating subsequent depressive episodes also diminishes. This phenomenon has been called kindling effect (3).

Symptoms of a major depressive episode often begin with a mild form but can later escalate into a full-blown episode. Most patients completely recover from their symptoms, although approximately 20% to 30% of individuals recover only partially from the episode and in these cases the symptoms remain in a low-grade depressive state.

Typically, the number of previous episodes is a good predictor of the probability of future episodes. Periods of remission usually tend to shorten with each passing episode and more than 80% of people experience recurrent episodes. Those who achieve partial remission are more likely to develop another episode. Studies have shown that one year after being diagnosed with a major depressive episode, 40% of individuals still met the criteria for the major depressive episode, 20% of individuals were in partial remission, and the remaining 40% evidenced no symptoms of depression.

Depression shows a strong association with many chronic medical disorders, like arthritis, multiple sclerosis, and chronic obstructive pulmonary disease. Sustained depression has systematic consequences and may have increased morbidity with stroke and diabetes. Major depressive disorder has a close and adverse relationship with cardiovascular disease (4). There is significant economic burden, psychological distress, reduced quality of life, increased propensity to accidents, delayed development of children (because of depressed mothers inability to look after them adequately), continued impairment in work and relationships and ongoing risk of suicide.

A recent study highlights the significance of painful physical symptoms in depression and the decreased chances of recovery (5). Unipolar depression is the second highest cause of worldwide disability after heart disease (6).

Clinical Features

Sadness or low mood is a universal and common life experience as many people feel gloomy, run-down or low in spirits in response to demands and stresses of everyday life. In depression, however, the mood is significantly lowered, there is a loss of interest and pleasure in activities that were previously a source of enjoyment (anhedonia), and one is unable to cope adequately with the everyday functioning of life. This pathological low mood, which is usually worse in the morning (diurnal variation) is also distinguishable by its severity, persistence and duration. The mood in depression does not improve significantly in response to pleasant situations (e.g., after hearing some good news) where normally people would feel happy.

Other characteristic disturbances in depression (called biological features) include decreased sleep with early morning awakening, decreased appetite, loss of weight, and loss of libido, etc. Lack of interest and enjoyment in activities that were previously a source of pleasure (anhedonia) is a frequent complaint. Lack of reactivity to external events, irritability, constipation and amenorrhea may also be present.

Sometimes reversed biological features like increased sleep (hypersomnia), increased appetite and weight gain may be present. They are usually present in what is called Atypical depression. These patients also have pronounced anxiety and a persistent tendency to react to real or perceived rejection (rejection sensitivity)(7).

Frequently presented complaints include apathy, lack of interest, insomnia, loss of appetite, loss of weight, loss of interest, tiredness, loss of energy, inability to concentrate, loss of libido, generalised aches and pains (usually pain in the back). Complaints of poor memory are quite common and memory disturbance can be severe in some cases so as to mimic dementia (called depressive pseudodementia).

Speech in depression is usually slow, monotonous and retarded. Thought content predominantly consists of negative and pessimistic views of self, the world and the future. Patients tend to have selective recall of unpleasant experiences.

Mood congruent delusions, auditory and other hallucinations may also occur. The common themes of delusions in severe depression are of worthlessness, guilt, poverty and physical health. Hypochondriacal concern, especially with bowels, is also seen in some patients and patients with hypochondriacal delusions are convinced that they have serious illnesses.

Cognitive distortions, feelings of worthlessness, guilt, hopelessness, lack of confidence and loss of self-esteem may increase to the extent of making patients suicidal. Rates of suicide in mood disorders are at least 12 times greater than those of the general population (8). Risk is higher in patients with major depression who have been inpatients as compared to those in the community. Anxiety is frequently associated with moderate depression and is very common in severe depression. Other features like depersonalisation, obsessional symptoms, panic attacks and disassociative symptoms can occur and occasionally dominate the whole clinical presentation.

In Eastern cultures, it is socially more acceptable, to present with physical symptoms on account of stigma attached to mental disorders. Common complaints presented by these patients are flatulence or gas in stomach, abdominal pain, indigestion and headache. Anxiety is commonly seen in many of these patients and they may present with palpitations, dizziness and headache, which is usually described as a feeling of constriction or a tight band around the head.

Diagnosis and Classification of Depressive Disorder

The historical distinction between depression caused by external factors or stresses, such as financial loss, failure in examination or break- up of a relationship (reactive, neurotic or psychogenic depression) and one which arises out of the blue independently, without any apparent external reason (endogenous depression), is not given much consideration now. Both DSM-5 and ICD-10 do not recommend these terms. The reason is that such distinction is not always clear-cut, and in clinical practice it sometimes becomes difficult to differentiate between the two. Other terms like agitated depression, and melancholic depression are also no longer used in current classifications like ICD- 10. Similarly the term retarded depression (where psychomotor retardation is prominent) is no longer considered a separate entity. For psychotic depression, the currently preferred term is a severe depressive episode with psychotic symptoms.

ICD-10 Diagnostic Criteria

Symptoms required for diagnostic criteria for a depressive episode are as follows:

A

- Depressed mood
- Loss of interest and enjoyment
- Reduced energy and decreased activity

B

- Reduced concentration
- Reduced self-esteem and confidence
- Ideas of guilt and unworthiness
- Pessimistic thoughts
- Ideas of self-harm
- Disturbed sleep
- Diminished appetite

ICD-10 requires a duration of two weeks for all grades of depressive disorder but accepts shorter periods if symptoms are unusually severe and have rapidity of onset. The differentiation between the three grades of depressive disorder depends on the number, type and severity of symptoms present. The extent of disruption in social and occupational life is a reasonable guide to ascertain the severity of symptoms.

The ICD-10 subdivides depressive episodes as follows:

- Mild depressive episode (with or without somatic symptoms)
- Moderate depressive disorder (with or without somatic symptoms)

- Severe depressive disorder (with or without psychotic symptoms)

For diagnosis of the mild depressive episode:, at least two symptoms from group A and at least two from group B are required. Moderate depressive episode requires at least two symptoms from group A and three from group B, for its diagnosis. For a severe depressive episode, all three symptoms from group A and at least four from group B are required.

In mild depressive disorder, the symptoms are more like an exaggeration of ordinary unhappiness with marked tearfulness. Mood varies, depending on external circumstances and fluctuates from day-to-day. There is also marked anxiety and patients tend to be irritable. They brood over their problems and have difficulty in getting to sleep. There are no delusions or hallucinations and somatic symptoms are not prominent. Mild depression responds best to psychological treatment rather than physical methods of treatment.

In moderate depressive disorder, depressed mood, loss of interest and enjoyment and increased fatigability are usually present along with symptoms of reduced self-esteem, ideas of guilt and unworthiness and a disturbance of sleep and appetite. The low mood varies little from day-to-day and is often unresponsive to circumstances, yet may show a characteristic diurnal variation as the day goes on. An individual with moderately severe depression will usually have considerable difficulty in continuing with domestic, social or work activities.

Severe depressive disorder (with or without psychosis) is characterised by a pervasive sadness of mood. Biological symptoms, e.g., early morning awakening, diurnal variation of mood, anorexia and weight loss are often prominent, and psychotic symptoms such as delusions and hallucinations may be present. Severe depression usually responds best to physical methods of treatment rather than psychological treatment alone.

Persistent Affective Disorders

ICD-10 has a category of persistent affective disorders, which include cyclothymia and dysthymia.

Cyclothymia

This is a persistent instability of mood involving periods of mild depression and mild elation, which are not significant enough to fulfil the criteria for bipolar affective disorder or recurrent depressive disorder. In DSM-5, the diagnosis of cyclothymic disorder is given to adults who experience at least two years (for children, a full year) of both hypomanic and depressive periods without ever fulfiling the criteria for an episode of mania, hypomania, or major depression (9).

This disorder has early onset in adult life and takes on a chronic course. It is often difficult to diagnose as the individuals enjoy the periods of mild elation and may not think it warrants medical help. Only by prolonged and consistent observation, cyclothymia may be diagnosed. Cyclothymia is common in relatives of bipolar disorder patients and there are cases when some of these patients have eventually developed bipolar disorder.

Dysthymia

Dysthymic disorder is a chronic, low-grade depression that lasts for at least two years. The symptoms are the same as in a major depressive episode, but they are fewer and less severe. Because of the chronicity of dysthymic disorder, the depressed mood and associated symptoms often become integrated into a person's normal functioning. After the first two years of depressed mood, if a major depressive episode also occurs, the combination is referred to as a double depression. On the other hand some patients suffering from major depression may subside into dysthymia (10).

DSM-5 requires that the depressed mood is present for most of the day, for more days than not, as indicated by either subjective account or observation by others, for at least two years. In children and adolescents, however, the mood can be irritable and the duration must be at least one year. As dysthymia responds to antidepressant treatment, it seems plausable that its pathophysiology overlaps with that of major depression (11).

Recurrent Brief Depression

In this disorder, there are short episodes of severe depression which last for a few days or a week. Some patients may develop major depression and similarly others with major depression may show conversion to recurrent brief depression (12).

Seasonal Variation

Some patients experience depressive symptoms during a particular time of the year, most commonly in winter. This is known as Seasonal Affective Disorder (SAD). These patients usually have atypical symptoms of depression like hypersomnia, hyperphagia, but not rejection sensitivity (13). Some of these patients may respond well to light therapy but the evidence for this treatment is not strong. Some studies have shown no advantage in SAD of bright light over dim light (14). The status of SAD and light therapy, therefore, is currently unclear and controversial.

Mixed Anxiety and Depressive Disorder

Although ICD-10 classifies this order under anxiety disorders, it is mentioned here for the sake of convenience. In this symptoms of both anxiety and depression are present, but neither group of symptoms are severe enough to justify a diagnosis.

Depressive Disorder and Suicide

Severely depressed patients frequently have suicidal ideation which can lead to suicide. This risk should always be kept in mind. Suicidal ideation should be inquired in all depressed patients, as there is no evidence that asking about suicide increases the risk of suicide.

Unfortunately, there are no current psychological or biological measures that can help to exactly estimate the risk of suicide in depressed patients. However, there are certain risk factors which can assist in identifying those with high risk. Risk factors for suicide in depression include, greater severity of illness, previous suicidal attempt, male sex, self-neglect, impaired concentration/memory, hopelessness, living al-one or being unmarried, bereavement, alcohol and drug problem, early loss of a parent,coexisting medical illness, recent stress, e.g., loss of job, breakdown of relationship, family history of suicide and recent discharge from psychiatric hospital.

Epidemiology and Aetiology

Gender

Depression is more common in females than males, with lifetime prevalences of 20% and 10%, respectively (15). Not only do at least twice as many women suffer from the disorder as compared to men, but they have an increased rate of both physical and emotional disorders associated with depression (16). This excess rate in women is a source of controversy as some authors have stated that men may be less likely to acknowledge depression and are more likely to forget previous symptoms experienced by them (17). Although the precise reasons for female preponderance are not established, many reviews have confirmed that the difference is real (18). This difference in the incidence of depression is less marked after menopause. Women also have more complex and severe clinical features in the course of the depressive disorder. Studies have reported that depressed women complain more of fatigue, excessive sleep and psychomotor retardation, whereas insomnia and irritability is more conspicuous in men (19). About 10% of women have depression after childbirth (postnatal depression) and 30% of these women have further episodes after future pregnancies. The hormonal levels of women suffering from postnatal depression are not different from those not having this disorder and it is felt that psychosocial factors are perhaps more important (20).

Age and Marital Status

Peak onset of depression is between 20 to 45 years of age. Severe depression is less common in elderly population, although they have higher incidence of dysthymia and mild depression. There is evidence of increasing incidence of depression in young people. The point prevalence (measure of the proportion of people in a population who have a condition at a particular time), of major depression in children is in the range of 0.5–2.5%. Depression is higher in single and divorced people. This risk is somewhat higher in men.

Social and Personality Factors

Early childhood experiences seem to play a part in the genesis of depression in later life. Bowlby, in his famous hypothesis of 'maternal deprivation', stressed that motherless children have a greater risk of developing depression later in life (21). Link between parental loss and depression is quite well-established now.

Depression occurs in all social classes. Studies in UK which have mainly been on females, have found a higher association of depression with lower social class (22). This association has not been confirmed by ECA study in USA. Patients from lower social class, nevertheless, have poor prognosis. Social isolation, and unemployment are other risk factors for depression. It has been highlighted that the social bonds of depressed patients are week and provide less support (23). There is a lack of consistent data for the commonly held view that depression has a higher association with urban than with rural population (24).

Stressful life situations invariably predispose an individual to affective disorders. There is increasing evidence that stressful life events precede the onset of affective disorder in about 80% of cases. Brown and Harris, in their famous study, found that depression is more common in women who are not working outside their homes. They described 'vulnerability factors' which predispose women to depression. These factors are loss of mother before the age of 11, having three or more children under the age of 15 at home and lack of a confiding relationship with husband (25).

Certain personality traits may predispose individuals to affective disorder. People who have low self-esteem, are sensitive, have obsessional traits, and have an excessive tendency to depend upon others for support are more vulnerable to develop depression.

Genetic Factors

Twin studies show concordance of 40–50% in monozygotic twins and 25% in dizygotic twins (26). The prevalence of unipolar affective disorders in the first degree relatives of patients is 10–15% respectively, which is much greater in comparison to the prevalence of 1–3% in general population. Adoption studies have confirmed that there are increased rates of depressive disorder in biological relatives compared with adopted relatives of probands. The inheritance is polygenic/multifactorial and not in Mendelian fashion. It seems that the depressed people inherit the propensity to develop depression in response to life events.

Biological Factors

Biogenic Amines

There is consistent data that dysregulation of norepinephrine and serotonin is implicated in the pathogenesis of mood disorders. One strong evidence for this is the correlation between the down-regulation of β-adrenergic receptors and clinical antidepressant responses. Another support for this theory comes from the finding that activation of alpha-2 adrenergic receptors results in a decrease in the amount of norepinephrine released.

The effectiveness of Serotonin-Specific Reuptake Inhibitors (SSRIs) in depression suggests that serotonin is involved in the pathophysiology of depression. Depletion of serotonin may precipitate depression, and low concentrations of serotonin metabolites and low concentrations of serotonin uptake sites on platelets are found in some suicidal patients (27). Dopamine is also thought to play a role as there is some data to suggest that dopamine activity may be reduced in depression.

Other Neurochemical Factors

GABA, vasopressin and endogenous opiates, adenylate cyclase, phosphatidylinositol, and calcium regulation, have been implicated in the pathophysiology of mood disorders (28). Some investigators have suggested that increased intracellular sodium levels are of casual relevance (29).

Endocrinological Causes

A variety of neuroendocrine dysregulations have been observed in patients with mood disorders. The relationship between myxo-oedema and depressed mood, the prominent mood changes in Cushing's syndrome and the persistence of depressed mood in patients with hypothyroidism, prompted researchers to look into hormonal disturbances in affective disorders.

The Hypothalamic-Pituitary- Adrenocortic (HPA) system

HPA overactivity in depressive disorders has been established. Cortisol is the main hormone involving stress. Depressed patients have increased cortisol levels (30). Lowering cortisol levels by administration of cortisol synthesis inhibitors results in improvement of depressive symptoms.

Dexamethasone Suppression Test (DST) is based on the fact that normal people show decreased cortisol levels throughout the following day after being administered a dose of 1–2 mg of dexamethasone. Many depressed patients, in contrast to this, continue to produce cortisol either at normal levels or even slightly raised levels. The DST, however, has modest sensitivity (it fails to identify 20–30 percent of depressed patients). Moreover, in recurrent depressive episodes, DST may not be abnormal in all episodes (31).

The Hypothalamic-Pituitary-Thyroid System

Clinical disorders of thyroid function are known to cause mood changes. Thyrotropin Releasing Hormone (TRH) allows secretion of Thyroid Stimulating Hormone (TSH) which stimulates release of thyroxin (T4) and triiodothyronine (T3). Studies have demonstrated reduced TSH response to TRH and increased TRH production in depressed subject (32). Antithyroid antibodies are present in about 9–20 percent of depression. Moreover, T3 or T4 augmentation enhances the efficacy of antidepressant medication.

Sleep Changes

One consistent abnormality in depressed subjects is reduction of the time between onset of sleep and commencement of Rapid Eye Movement (REM) sleep. This finding is more conspicuous in major depression and in elderly people (33). This reduced REM latency may persist even when people recover and indicate a vulnerability to relapse. Another finding is that many antidepressants decrease REM sleep time and increase the latency to its onset. Moreover, total sleep deprivation and selective REM sleep deprivation can temporarily result in mood enhancement (34).

Brain Changes

A number of structural brain abnormalities have been found in subjects suffering from major depression, by Computerised Tomography (CT) and Magnetic Resonance Imageing (MRI). These include enlarged brain ventricles, decreased hippocampal volume, decreased volume of basal ganglia, and decreased grey matter volume of the subgenual prefrontal cortex.

According to the neurotrophic hypothesis of depression, stress causes atrophy and death of neurons and down-regulation of adult neurogenesis especially in the hippocampus (35). Studies have also reported a reduction in cerebral blood flow in frontal regions of depressed subjects (36). Reduced metabolic rate of glucose in the caudate nucleus of depressd people has also been reported (37).

Psychological Theories

Wolpe explained depression as a form of behavioural conditioning in which the person is conditioned to become depressed by a loss because of the association of repeated losses and depression in the past. Seligman suggested that depression occurs in a situation in which the rewards and punishments are not in control of the person and he or she learns to behave as if helpless, a condition called learned helplessness.

The cognitive theory, first proposed by Beck and currently much respected, states that depressed mood may result from a habit of negative thinking, interpreting all events in their worst possible light and drawing generalised pessimistic conclusions from an isolated minor incident.

Freud suggested that in depression, the patient regresses to an emotional stage where aggressive impulses are directed inwards and the self is bitterly criticised. Other psychoanalysts regard the loss of self-esteem as a crucial factor in depression. They view mania as a defence reaction against intolerable unhappiness and depression, which they call 'manic defence' and 'flight into mania'.

Differential Diagnosis of Depression

Depression is often associated with a number of other illnesses and, at times, it becomes difficult and rather confusing to make the correct diagnosis.

Anxiety

Although anxiety as a symptom is quite common in depression, mild depressive disorder is sometimes difficult to differentiate from anxiety disorders. The precise order and severity of symptoms of both these disorders can help with the primary diagnosis.

Patients suffering from a primary anxiety disorder feel anxious rather than sad and less helpless in contrast to hopelessness expressed by depressed people. Speech and motor activity are reduced in depression and there is usually guilt and apathy as well. Insomnia in depression can be early, middle or late but in anxiety, insomnia is usually early.

Grief

In grief there is a low mood without diurnal variation. There is, moreover, no loss of self- esteem and self-confidence.

Dementia

Sometimes patients with severe depression present with considerable memory problems and differentiating it from dementia may pose a diagnostic difficulty. The presence of biological features of depression will help clarify the diagnosis.

In dementia, there is apparently no role of life events, duration of illness is longer, intellectual deterioration starts before the onset of depression, the effect is labile and superficial, symptoms are worse at night, patients minimise cognitive disturbances and unlike depressed patients, there may be confabulation. Moreover dysphasia, apraxia, and agnosia may be present and there is no decrease in REM latency.

Somatoform Disorders

In these patients, symptoms appear after a minor event and biological features are usually less prominent. There is usually no past history of depression, physical symptoms usually worsen at the end of the day.

Patients are preoccupied with physical symptoms, exaggerate their distress, and they are unwilling to accept psychological explanations about the origin of the symptoms. They endlessly shop around for medical help, and are very keen to discuss their symptoms with other people. The response to antidepressants is usually inadequate.

Schizophrenia

Sometimes difficulty arises when severely depressed patients have psychotic symptoms. In schizophrenia, features like poor premorbid adjustment, personality deterioration, formal thought disorder and bizarre thought content differentiate it from depression. Moreover, in schizophrenia, delusions and hallucinations are not mood congruent. It should, however, be remembered that many schizophrenia patients secondarily develop significant depressive symptoms which may warrant further and different management.

Organic

a. Infections such as influenza, glandular fever and infective hepatitis may precipitate depression.
b. Endocrine changes likely to cause depression are those associated with hypothyroidism, Cushing's disease, menopause, puerperium and hyperparathyroidism.
c. Surgical procedures, such as hysterectomy, may precipitate depression.
d. Anaemias due to iron or B12 deficiency may mimic depression.
e. Neurological diseases such as Parkinsonism, disseminated sclerosis, intracranial tumours, SLE, syphilis and epilepsy may present as or precipitate depression.
f. Certain drugs like reserpine, methyldopa, steroids, barbiturates, L-Dopa, and chronic amphetamine use may precipitate depression.

Rating Scales for Depression

Following are some of the rating scales used in measuring depression:

- Hamilton Rating Scale for Depression
- Montgomery-Asberg Depression Rating Scale
- Beck Depression Inventory
- Hospital Anxiety and Depression Scale
- Visual Analogue Scale

Treatment

Regarding depressive disorder it is imperative that achieving remission should be the target, as depressed patients with residual symptoms are three times more likely to relapse than those without residual symptoms (38). Lack of remission adversely affects physical, social, occupational and marital functioning. Well-being of the offsprings of depressed mothers, is also compromised and there remains an increased risk of suicide. Depression is treated by one of the following methods or in some cases by a combination of them:

1. Chemotherapy
2. Psychotherapy
3. ECT and other physical methods of treatment

Chemotherapy

The following are antidepressant drugs commonly used these days:

a. Specific Serotonin Reuptake Inhibitors (SSRIs)

Fluvoxamine, sertraline, fluoxetine, citalopram, escitalopram, and paroxetine, are now considered to be the treatment of first choice because they are as effective as tricyclics antidepressants and they have fewer side effects (39). They are also comparatively safe in overdoses.

Side effects include, nausea, vomiting, diarrhoea, headache, sexual dysfunction, and sleep disturbance. Restlessness and anxiety can also occur in the first week but does not persist in most cases. There is no strong evidence that SSRIs cause higher rates of aggression and suicide. It is recommended that SSRIs are not stopped abruptly as this results in withdrawal side effects.

b. Serotonin Noradrenaline Reuptake Inhibitors (SNRIs)

Venlafaxine and duloxetine

These have a dual action of blocking re-uptake of both noradrenaline and serotonin. They have less histaminergic, alpha adrenergic and cholinergic effects than tricyclic antidepressants. They should be used carefully in people with hypertension. Venlafaxine appears to be a little more effective than SSRIs in severely depressed patients (40).

c. Tricyclic Antidepressants

Tricyclics can be broadly divided into sedative TCAs (amitriptyline, dothiepin and clomipramine) and the less sedative one (imipramine, nortriptyline and lofepramine). TCAs are very effective drugs for the treatment of severe depression but are less often prescribed as they are comparatively less safe than SSRIs in over dosages. Moreover, autonomic side effects like dry mouth, increased sweating, blurring of vision, constipation, urinary hesitancy and postural hypotension, can be troublesome. These effects are mostly related to higher dosage and can be minimised by adjusting the optimal dose. Lofepramine is less cardiotoxic but amitriptyline is contraindicated in patients with a recent history of myocardial infarction or heart failure.

d. Monoamine Oxidase Inhibitors (MAOIs)

MAOIs are very rarely considered as the first-line of treatment. Patients who fail to respond to a tricyclic antidepressant or SSRI may respond dramatically to MAOIs. Phenelzine and tranylcypromine are, however, less often prescribed because of the adverse reactions (e.g., Phenelzine causes hypotension even in low doses) and dietary restrictions. Reversible MAOIs like moclobemide do not have problems with diet. MAOIs have an important role in treatment of atypical depression.

The combination of MAOIs and SSRIs (and clomipramine) is contraindicated as this can result in toxic effects even at therapeutic doses.

e. Miscellaneous Other Antidepressants

Maprotiline, mianserin, mirtazepine, reboxetine, trazodone, are also used. Mirtazepine has got robust evidence for efficacy (41).

f. Lithium

Although lithium is used primarily in bipolar affective disorder, it can also be used to reduce the frequency of depressive episodes in recurrent depressive disorder. Lithium carbonate is also used to potentiate the effects of tricyclic antidepressants when they have not produced the desired improvement. But lithium is a drug that should be used with caution because of its narrow therapeutic window and various side effects. Nausea, slight tremor in hands, fatigue, muscle weakness, polyuria and polydipsia are common side effects. There may also be some weight gain. Severe adverse reactions like vomiting, diarrhoea, dizziness, stiffness of muscles and coarse tremors of hands can be very troublesome and the drug has to be discontinued. It is important to monitor the level of lithium in blood, and the serum lithium level should ideally be maintained between 0.6–1.2 mEq/L.

g. Quetiapine

Quetiapine is used as an adjunctive treatment for depression which has not responded to an antidepressant.

h. Aripiprazole

This is licensed in the USA as an adjunctive antidepressant, but not in the UK.

Psychotherapy

Psychotherapy, in combination with antidepressants, is more effective in the management of depression than either treatment alone.

a. Cognitive Therapy

This therapy focuses on the cognitive distortions thought to be present in depressive illness and is specifically designed to challenge and modify patterns of habitual negative thinking, in particular the cognitive triad; feelings of helplessness about oneself, one's future, and one's past. Selective attention to the negative aspects of the circumstances, and unrealistic and pathological inferences about what might happen in future, are examples of cognitive distortions.

Cognitive therapy aims to improve depressive mood and to prevent its occurrences by assisting the patients in identifying and testing the negative thoughts. The patient is encouraged to have a flexible and positive style of thinking. Effectiveness of cognitive therapy for the treatment of depressive episodes of all grades is well-established.

b. Behaviour Therapy

Based on the theories of learning, behaviour therapy operates on the assumption that by addressing maladaptive behaviour patterns, depressed patients would behave in such a positive way that they will receive positive reinforcement from the people in their lives. The operant conditioning technique of positive reinforcement can be very effective in the treatment of depression especially if combined with antidepressants.

c. Interpersonal Therapy

Interpersonal therapy is also effective in depression (42) although there is less data on its efficacy in major depression. It is a systematic approach to relationship difficulties and life problems. It focuses on the patient's current interpersonal issues. The assumptions behind this approach are that the current interpersonal difficulties are likely to be the result of early dysfunctional relationships and that the current interpersonal difficulties are responsible for precipitating or maintaining the present depressive symptoms. This therapy usually consists of 12 to 16 weekly sessions.

d. Supportive Psychotherapy

The primary aim of supportive therapy is to provide emotional support with a view to help solve emotional problems. One important aspect to be kept in mind is that the patients must be encouraged to make all decisions by themselves.

e. Family Therapy

Family therapy is not considered to be the primary psychological treatment for depression. It is particularly indicated when patient's depression is disrupting family life and when the depressive illness is thought to be related to, or caused by family events.

ECT and Other Physical Methods of Treatment

ECT is an important treatment for major depression especially in patients who have psychotic features and are not eating or drinking because of severe retardation. It is also indicated for treatment-resistant depression. The effectiveness of ECT is supported by clinical trials (43).

Factors associated with good response to ECT in depression include absence of precipitating factors, diurnal variation of mood, early morning awakening, family history of depression,self blame and guilt feelings and psychomotor retardation.

Other physical methods to treat depression include Repetitive Transcranial Magnetic Stimulation (RTMS), Vagus Nerve Stimulation (VNS), Deep Brain Stimulation (DBS) and psychosurgery (anterior cingulotomy and anterior capsulotomy). There are no large scale studies for all these methods but some modest evidence is there.

Treatment-Resistant Depression (TRD)

About one-third of patients do not respond to the first course of antidepressant therapy. A further 10–15% are helped by another antidepressant from a different class of antidepressants or ECT. There remains a residual group of patients (about 5–10%) for whom multiple interventions are unhelpful. These patients remain depressed and are not able to achieve a reasonable level of functioning (44). This group of patients are referred to as treatment-resistant, refractory depression or intractable depression.

Different researchers have put forward different criteria for this group of patients. One generally accepted definition is when a patient has failed to respond to two successive courses of pharmacologically different antidepressants given in adequate doses and for a sufficient time period (45).

Strategies for TRD Include

Combination of Antidepressants

Combination of TCA and SSRI can be helpful. It should be noted that combination of TCA and an MAOI is contraindicated.

Lithium Augmentation

When lithium is added to TCAs, SSRIs or MAOIs, there is response in about 50% of patients who were previously resistant to improvement. Enhanced response to a TCA- Lithium combination has been confirmed in studies (46). Addition of lithium to the monoamine oxidase inhibitors like isocarboxazid and tranylcypromine has shown to be effective as well.

Augmentation of lithium to SSRIs has also been recommended. The possibility of serotonin syndrome, when combining lithium to TCAs or SSRIs, should be kept in mind. Lithium augmentation therapy requires regular monitoring as symptoms of lithium toxicity can occur within the therapeutic lithium serum levels (47).

Esketamine Nasal Spray

This has recently been licensed for use in combination with a selective serotonin reuptake inhibitor (SSRI) or serotonin and norepinephrine reuptake inhibitor (SNRI), for adults with treatment-resistant major depressive disorder (TRD).

Thyroid Hormone Augmentation

There is evidence for the efficacy of this strategy (48). Studies have suggested that T3 augmentation to TCAs is helpful in more than 50% of cases which were unresponsive to TCA alone. It has also been observed that in these patients, augmentation with T3 gave a higher response than augmentation with T4. Thyroid function status of patients may also play a role in the response.

Addition of an Atypical Antipsychotic

This strategy can be effective as well. Some atypical antipsychotics, when added to an SSRI or SNRI, have shown improvement in depressive symptoms. The best evidence is for aripiprazole (49).

Miscellaneous Augmentations

Augmentations with pindolol (with an MAOI or SSRI), bupropion (with an SSRI), and tryptophan (with MAOI) have also been tried successfully in some depressed patients Adding mood stabilisers like carbamazepine, valproate and lamotrigine to various antidepressants can also be helpful sometimes.

ECT

ECT remains an important choice in TRD.

Psychosurgery

It is now very rarely done.

BIPOLAR AFFECTIVE DISORDER

Bipolar affective disorder is characterised by episodes of mania/hypomania and depression. Because of its devastating psychosocial consequences, the World Health Organisation has labelled bipolar disorder to be the sixth leading cause of disability worldwide (50). It ought to be noted that episodes of depression are associated with greater impairment in work, family and social life than are episodes of mania (51). For the diagnosis of bipolar disorder, the mood disturbance has not to be caused by substance abuse or a general medical condition.

According to the diagnostic criteria of DSM-5, the presence of a single episode of hypomania or mania qualifies the disorder to be termed bipolar disorder. DSM-5 also separates bipolar disorder into two main types bipolar I and bipolar II. For a diagnosis of bipolar I disorder, it is necessary to meet the criteria for a manic episode. The presence of psychoses or an episode of major depression is not a requirement for the diagnosis of bipolar I disorder. The manic episode may have been preceded by and may be followed by hypomanic or major depressive episodes. Although hypomanic episodes are common in bipolar I disorder they are not required for the diagnosis of bipolar I disorder.

Bipolar II disorder requires the lifetime experience of at least one episode of major depression and at least one hypomanic episode.

Bipolar disorder II is no longer considered a milder condition than bipolar I, primarily because of the amount of time individuals with this condition spend in depression. Moreover, there is serious impairment in work and social functioning. DSM-5 also contains cyclothymic disorder in which patients have two years (for children, a full year) history of both hypomanic and depressive periods without ever fulfiling the criteria for an episode of mania, hypomania, or major depression.

In bipolar disorder not otherwise specified (NOS), there are manic symptoms but criteria is not met for bipolar I disorder, bipolar II disorder, or cyclothymia. Depressive symptoms are not required. For the diagnosis of bipolar disorder, ICD-10 requires at least two episodes of mood disturbances, which should consist of mania or hypomania and depression. Unlike DSM-5, there is no distinction between bipolar I and bipolar II disorders.

There is a lot of evidence that bipolar affective disorder may be under-diagnosed or misdiagnosed as depression or personality disorder (52). Approximately 35–45% of patients with bipolar I disorder are misdiagnosed with unipolar depression. One possible explanation for this is that patients more often seek help for depressive symptoms than manic symptoms. Moreover, some patients may regard the elevated mood and associated symptoms as normal or desirable.

Anxiety disorder and schizophrenia are other disorders with which bipolar disorder is misdiagnosed. Delay in diagnosis and subsequent lack of appropriate treatment understandably results in more instability, increased psychosocial impairment, more complications and comorbidities, and adverse prognosis. There is evidence that treatments, both psychopharmacological and psychosocial, may be less helpful in patients whose initial episodes have not been appropriately treated (53).

Mania

In mania, there is significant disinhibition of psychomotor function. Symptoms of mania include elated or irritable mood, overactivity, pressure of speech, flight of ideas, decreased sleep, and increased libido. Patients may exhibit various type of reckless behaviours such as, sexual promiscuity, dangerous driving and over spending, etc. Psychotic symptoms are relatively common in mania and according to some studies, are seen in 50% of cases at any one time and approximately 70% of cases on a lifetime basis. Delusions are usually mood congruent and have grandiosity as the central theme. It is imperative to appreciate that some patients with mania, may have mood-incongruent psychotic features (including Schneiderian first-rank symptoms) just like those in schizophrenia. The presence of psychotic symptoms, however, do not necessarily reflect the severity in mania. Presence of psychosis has an adverse bearing on the prognosis as it is associated with increased relapse (54). Unipolar recurrent mania is rare.

In mania, the mean rate of occurrence of irritability is 80%, of euphoria 71%, flight of ideas 71%, poor concentration 71%, delusions 48%, and hallucinations 15% (55). Apart from the increasing clinical observation that bipolar disorder is misdiagnosed, about 10 percent of patients presenting with unipolar depression will eventually have a manic relapse. Young patients having major depression with psychoses are especially likely to be misdiagnosed. According to another study, as many as 50% of unipolar depression, who are hospitalised are eventually diagnosed with bipolar disorder (56). Moreover, the risk of mania in a patient with repeated depressive episodes, remains throughout the life. The diagnostic criteria for mania in ICD-10 and DSM-5 are similar.

DSM-5 Diagnostic Criteria for a Manic Episode

a. A distinct period of abnormally and persistently elevated, expansive, or irritable mood and abnormally and persistently increased goal-directed activity or energy, lasting at least one week and present most of the day, nearly every day (or any duration if hospitalisation is necessary).

b. During the period of mood disturbance and increased energy or activity, three (or more) of the following symptoms (four if the mood is only irritable) are present to a significant degree and represent a noticeable change from usual behaviour:

   i. Inflated self-esteem or grandiosity

   ii. Decreased need for sleep (e.g., feels rested after only three hours of sleep)

   iii. More talkative than usual or pressure to keep talking

iv. Flight of ideas or subjective experience that thoughts are racing
v. Distractibility (i.e. attention too easily drawn to unimportant or irrelevant external stimuli) as reported or observed
vi. Increase in goal-directed activity (either socially, at work or school, or sexually) or psychomotor agitation (i.e. purposeless non-goal-directed activity)
vii. Excessive involvement in activities that have a high potential for painful consequence (e.g., engageing in unrestrained buying sprees, sexual indiscretions, or foolish business investments)

c. The mood disturbance is sufficiently severe to cause marked impairment in social or occupational functioning or to necessitate hospitalisation to prevent harm to self or others, or there are psychotic features.
d. The episode is not attributable to the physiological effects of a substance (e.g., a drug of abuse, a medication, other treatment) or to another medical condition.

Note: A full manic episode that emerges during antidepressant treatment (e.g., medication, electroconvulsive therapy) but persists at a fully syndromal level beyond the physiological effect of that treatment is sufficient evidence for a manic episode and, therefore, a bipolar I diagnosis.

Hypomania

Hypomania is the term used to describe a mild degree of mania. The extent of functional impairment is an important distinction between mania and hypomania. Hypomanic symptoms are less severe than those in mania, and states of euphoria and overactivity are not as marked. Although patients with hypomania have serious problems at work or in their social circle, they are not as severe as those present in a manic episode. Some patients may, in fact, view it as positively desirable. They report pleasant periods of increased productivity and sense of humour. However, these phases can still be very problematic for most patients and their families. A hypomanic phase may also result in a full-blown manic episode. Like mania, hypomania is also associated with depressive episodes.

DSM-5 Diagnostic Criteria for a Hypomanic Episode

a. A distinct period of abnormally and persistently elevated, expansive, or irritable mood and abnormally and persistently increased activity or energy, lasting at least four consecutive days and present most of the day, nearly every day.
b. During the period of mood disturbance and increased energy and activity, three (or more) of the following symptoms (four if the mood is only irritable) have persisted, represent a noticeable change from usual behaviour, and have been present to a significant degree:
i. Inflated self-esteem or grandiosity
ii. Decreased need for sleep (e.g., feels rested after only three hours of sleep)
iii. More talkative than usual or under pressure to keep talking.
iv. Flight of ideas or subjective experience that thoughts are racing.
v. Distractibility (i.e. attention too easily drawn to unimportant or irrelevant external stimuli), as reported or observed
vi. Increase in goal-directed activity (either socially, at work or school, or sexually) or psychomotor agitation
vii. Excessive involvement in activities that have a high potential for painful consequence (e.g., engageing in unrestrained buying sprees, sexual indiscretions, or foolish business investments)

c. The episode is associated with an unequivocal change in functioning that is uncharacteristic of the individual when not symptomatic.
d. The disturbance in mood and the change in functioning are observable by others.
e. The episode is not severe enough to cause marked impairment in social or occupational functioning or to necessitate hospitalisation. If there are psychotic features, the episode is, by definition, manic.
f. The episode is not attributable to the physiological effects of a substance (e.g., a drug of abuse, a medication, other treatment).

Note: A full hypomanic episode that emerges during antidepressant treatment (e.g., medication, electroconvulsive therapy) but persists at a fully syndromal level beyond the physiological effect of that treatment is sufficient evidence for a hypomanic episode diagnosis. However, caution is indicated so that one or two symptoms (particularly increased irritability, edginess, or agitation following antidepressant use) are not taken as sufficient for diagnosis of a hypomanic episode, nor necessarily indicative of a bipolar disorder.

Mixed Affective States

Mixed affective states are difficult to diagnose. These are states where there is a mixture of both manic and depressive symptoms. In mania there can be transient low mood, a mixed affective state is diagnosed when symptoms of both mania and depression are consistently present.

DSM-5 criteria requires the occurrence of an episode with sufficient associated features to fulfil the criteria for mania and depression over a one week period. The two most common presentations are rapidly alternating mania and depression, and severe depression with complete absence of euphoria but showing irritability, hostility and paranoia.

Rapid Cycling

Patients who have four or more episodes of mania, hypomania, mixed state or depression in one year, are described as having rapid cycling. Rapid cycling can occur at the onset of the illness but is usually present in the later course of bipolar disorder. It is the most malignant type of bipolar illness and is characterised by severe morbidity and a refractory clinical course. It is commoner in females as compared to males.

Some patients exhibit periods of remission in between the episodes while others continuously switch from one episode to another. Although there is no robust evidence for a causal relationship, rapid cycling may result after exposure to antidepressants or becoming worse with antidepressants. It occurs in 10–15% of bipolar patients with equal frequency in bipolar I and bipolar II patients. These patients are usually unresponsive to lithium and may respond better to carbamazepine. In ultra rapid cycling there are four or more episodes in a month. These are very rare cases in which manic and depressive episodes occur every 48 hours.

Delirious Mania

Sometimes patients having severe mania develop confusional state, in which they become disorientated and have visual hallucinations. There is usually severe neglect and physical exhaustion preceding the confusional state.

Dysphoric Mania

In some patients, manic symptoms are accompanied by significant anxiety, anger or depression. This is called dysphoric mania.

Secondary Mania

A mania-like state sometimes develops following a disturbance by certain medications or medical conditions. This is called secondary mania. Levodopa, corticosteroids in high doses, amphetamines, anabolic steroids, benzhexol, procyclidine, thyroid disease lesions, right- sided cerebral vascular lesions and head injury can produce a mania-like picture. According to DSM-5, mania/hypomania which is induced by antidepressants is not regarded as diagnostic of bipolar disorder.

Comorbidity

Bipolar disorder is associated with a high rate of psychiatric comorbidity. Anxiety disorders are common. Alcohol and substance misuse occurs in 60% of cases. Attention-deficit disorder and personality disorders are also frequently encountered.

There is an association with eating disorders and more than 10% of bipolar patients have eating disorders. Lifetime prevalence of bipolar disorder among individuals with anorexia or bulimia nervosa is 4–6%. Among non-psychiatric comorbidities, obesity and overweight are conspicuous. Obesity is present in about 21–32% of patients with bipolar affective disorder, and about 58% of patients are overweight (57). In obese bipolar patients there are more depressive and manic episodes, longer duration of acute episodes, more suicide attempts and shorter time of recurrence. There is also association of bipolar disorder with diabetes, thyroid disease, hypercholesterolaemia, heart disease and hypertension (58).

Suicide

Approximately 25–50% of bipolar patients attempt suicide at least once during their lifetime. One in five suicide attempts are completed because of higher occurrence of severe recurrent depressive episodes in bipolar I patients, the risk of suicide is greater than bipolar II patients. Rates of attempted suicide are similar in bipolar I and bipolar II patients. After depressive episodes in bipolar disorder, mixed states and the presence of psychotic symptoms have the next higher risk. Manic episodes have the lowest risk (59). The overall rate of suicide in bipolar patients is 0.40% per year (60). Some of the factors which increase suicides in bipolar disorder are increased comorbidities (e.g., anxiety, and substance misuse, etc.), earlier onset, mixed states, less psychomotor retardation, more impulsivity, more psychosocial stress-related to longer periods of depression and rapid cycling.

Aetiology

Bipolar disorder has a strong hereditary basis. Although it runs in families, the mode of inheritance is not Mendelian. It seems that multiple genes play a role. First degree relative of bipolar patients have higher rates of bipolar I, bipolar II disorder and major depression than the general population.

Hypothalamo-pituitary-adrenal axis abnormalities, thyroid abnormalities, neurotrans- mitter/receptor imbalances, second messenger abnormalities, and mitochondrial dysfunction have been implicated in the pathogenesis of bipolar disorder (61). Dysfunctions in the prefrontal cortex, amygdala, and hippocampus have been implicated through neuroimageing and postmortem histopathology studies (62).

There is role of environmental factors as well. Studies have highlighted the role of recent negative or stressful events in the onset as well as recurrence of episodes. The negative life events precede both mania/hypomanic episodes as well as depressive episodes. Deprivation of sleep and disruption of daily social rhythms is postulated to be the final common pathway that leads to mania (63).

Epidemiology and Course of Illness

For bipolar I disorder, the lifetime prevalence is 1% (range 0.5–1.6%) (64) with an equal male to female ratio. The age of onset is earlier than major depression. Just like schizophrenia, the age of onset in males is earlier as compared to females. Females have less manic episodes but have a higher risk of rapid cycling (65). They also have more and longer depressive episode (66). Lifetime prevalence of bipolar II disorder is around 1. 5–2.5% (67). It is more common in females (68).

The first episode onset is usually during second or third decade (peak age of onset being 15–25 years). The initial episode is followed by a longer remission than the subsequent episodes (4.5 years median). Over the first ten years, there are about four major episodes. Over a longer term, episodes of mood elevation will be fewer and briefer than the depressed episodes. If untreated, bipolar patients are likely to have about ten episodes during their lifetime (69). Although the course of bipolar disorder includes periods of remission, without treatment, patients will always relapse (70). In majority of patients there are more depressive episodes than manic episodes, the duration of depressive phases being longer (median: 6 months) than the manic episodes (median: 4 months).

Rapid cycling patients suffer more from depressive symptomatology and at a very high risk of attempting suicide. Chronic subsyndromal states cause significant disability because of the substantial amount of impairment experienced by patients.

Almost 50% of patients experience a recurrence despite adequate treatment for bipolar disorder. Few patients (26%) achieve full symptom resolution. Residual symptoms increase the risk of a recurrence and contribute to earlier relapse. They cause psychosocial and cognitive impairment (poor work performance). Remission should, therefore, be the goal of treatment. Many patients who show signs of improvement, continue to experience psychosocial and vocational impairments that affect normal daily living. Over a 1-year period, functional recovery occurred in only 24% of patients.

Screening Tools

Although a number of screening tools can be used for bipolar disorder, it needs to be emphasised that no screening tool is a gold standard and there is no substitute for taking a careful and comprehensive history from the patients as well as the carers. Some of the tools for depression have been mentioned in the earlier part of this chapter. The following tools are helpful in diagnosing and monitoring bipolar disorder:

- Mood disorder questionnaire
- Bipolar spectrum diagnostic scale
- Clinician administered rating scale for mania
- Young mania rating scale
- Hypomania checklist

Acute Treatment of Mania/ Hypomania

As a good clinical practice, it is essential to ascertain the severity of symptoms, the presence of psychotic symptoms, response to previous medication in case this is not the first episode, and presence of any psychiatric as well as non-psychiatric comorbid conditions. The aim of the treatment is safe and rapid control of manic symptoms. Antimanic treatment has to be continued at least until full remission is achieved as residual symptoms are associated with a substantial risk of relapse.

Lithium

Lithium has the largest pool of studies regarding its anti-manic efficacy. Lithium has been the drug of choice for decades for the treatment of acute manic attacks (it is also used as an established prophylactic agent). It has proven efficacy in the treatment of 'classical mania' and is reported to have specific anti suicidal effect (71). Mixed states and rapid cycling disorders do not respond adequately to lithium. Moreover, lithium's effect in treating psychoses is debatable, and antipsychotics are indicated as part of the treatment package.

In spite of the narrow therapeutic window and risk of toxicity, poor tolerability, unsuitability in certain medical conditions (e.g., renal disease and thyroid dysfunction, etc.), contraindications, and serious risk of rebound mania when it is abruptly stopped, lithium remains a fairly popular drug. Early side effects of lithium are nausea, vomiting, abdominal discomfort, diarrhoea, fine tremor, polyuria and thirst. If vomiting and diarrhoea are severe and persistent,then toxicity should be suspected.

Late side effects are weight gain, nephrogenic diabetes insipidus, thyroid enlargement (goitre) and hypothyroidism in 5–10%. Lithium can cause benign reversible T-wave flattening or inversion. It can also produce or exacerbate acne and psoriasis. Other late side effects are teratogenic effects, and toxicity. It is essential to do regular serum lithiums levels, thyroid function tests and kidney function tests. The therapeutic lithium serum levels are in the range of 0.6–1.0 mmol/l.

Carbamazepine

Some studies have shown that carbamazepine efficacy is equal to lithium (72), whereas others have demonstrated that lithium is superior in efficacy (73). There is role for carbamazepine in mixed affective states and rapid cycling (74). It has reportedly slower onset as compared to neuroleptics and valproate but a slightly faster response than lithium. Its main shortcomings are its interactions with other psychotropic drugs e.g., several antipsychotics, antidepressants and anticonvulsants (75). This limits the use of carbamazepine.

Valproate

The efficacy of valproate in the treatment of mania has been well-established (76). Compared to carbamazepine, valproate is superior in efficacy (77). Although valproate is efficacious in treating classical mania, it is probably less efficacious than lithium. It is, however, superior to lithium in treating rapid cycling disorder.

Other Anticonvulsants

There is lack of large randomised controlled trials regarding efficacy of other anticonvulsants. Gabapentin, topiramate, levetiracetam, zonisamide, pregabaline, and tiagabine have some anti-manic efficacy. Similarly, evidence for oxycarbamazepine is not substantial. Phenytoin has shown antimanic efficacy but its side effect profile is not encourageing. Lamotrigine has less antimanic potential and is more efficacious in bipolar depression and rapid cycling.

Antipsychotics

Typical antipsychotics, like haloperidol, are very effective in the treatment of acute mania. Their onset is probably faster than lithium. Extrapyramidal side effects are not only quite troublesome but occur commonly. More importantly, their propensity to cause tardive dyskinesia limits their use. Atypical antipsychotics like aripiprazole, quetiapine, olanzapine, risperidone, and ziprasidone are all effective in treating manic episodes. Clozapine is usually reserved for refractory cases. Aripiprazole has demonstrated superiority in efficacy as compared to lithium and valproate (78). Discontinuation in aripiprazole is quite low (79). It is also very effective in preventing relapses of manic episodes (80). The long-term side effect profile of aripiprazole is also superior to other atypicals. It has, therefore, been given the highest overall ranking regarding both efficacy and comparatively better side effect profile, by the World Federation of Societies of Biological Psychiatry (81). As aripiprazole is not a sedating drug, and may cause restlessness and agitation on initation, it is advisable to add small doses of benzodiazepines or antihistamines on a short-term basis.

Benzodiazepines

Clonazepam and lorazepam are commonly used in the management of acute mania but they are not used as primary antimanic agents but only as adjunctive medications. They have an important role to play.

Other Miscellaneous Drugs

Tamoxifen and nimodipine (calcium antagonist) have shown some benefits in acute mania.

Combination Strategies

Combination of lithium and carbamazepine can have a useful synergistic action. Combining mood stabilisers, like lithium, carbamazepine as well as new anticonvulsants e.g., semi-sodium valproate, lamotrigine, etc., with atypical antipsychotics is also a useful option. Although monotherapy remains the first preferred option, a greater efficacy of combination treatment is supported by a meta-analysis (82).

ECT

Although there is a lack of randomised controlled studies, some authors state that ECT has some beneficial role in mania, especially with psychotic features. ECT may be considered for treating mania that is associated with life-threatening physical exhaustion or for mania which has not responded to drug treatment. It is also a valuable last resource in severe delirious mania (83).

Bipolar Depression

Bipolar depression typically emerges before the age of 25 years. Suicide is a significant risk factor during bipolar depression. Episodes of bipolar depression are shorter than unipolar depression and may be abrupt in onset. The diagnostic criteria for a major depressive episode in bipolar disorder is essentially the same as those of major unipolar depression. A diagnosis of bipolar depression requires that five or more of the key symptoms are present for more than two weeks.

Some features of bipolar depression like more psychomotor retardation, fewer anxiety symptoms, less somatic complaints and hypersomnia, can help differentiate it from unipolar depression. Bipolar depression may be less responsive to medication.

Monotherapy with antidepressants is not recommended for bipolar I disorder as there is an increased risk of switching to mania. They should also be used with caution in bipolar II disorder. Tricyclics and venlafaxine carry a greater risk of precipitating a manic episode as compared to SSRIs. However, tricyclics have a role in treatment-resistant depression. SSRIs have a modest efficacy in bipolar depression. Combination of an SSRI and a mood stabiliser like lithium and valproate can be tried. Similarly, SSRI can be added to an antipsychotic agent.

ECT should be considered for patients with high suicide risk and psychoses. Quetiapine XL has been licensed in the UK for bipolar depression.

Long-Term Management of Bipolar Disorder

Prophylactic treatment should be considered after a second major episode of bipolar disorder, especially if the interval between the episodes is only a few years. As already mentioned, the interval between the first and second episode tends to be longer than between subsequent episodes. For this reason, maintenance treatment is justified only if there is no precipitating event, episode is very severe, there is high suicide risk, or if there is a significant occupational or social repercussion for the person.

Patients with typical bipolar disorder who have complete recovery in between the episodes are most likely to benefit from lithium prophylaxis (84). Patients whose first episode was manic also do better on lithium. The long-term treatment with lithium reduces suicidal behaviour and suicide.

In patients where lithium prophylaxis is not indicated, alternative treatments are with valproate, carbamazepine and lamotrigine. Similarly, apart from their efficacy in acute mania, antipsychotics both typical and atypical have a role in the maintenance treatment of bipolar disorder. They are more effective in preventing manic episodes than depressive one. Those patients who have compliance issues can benefit from depot antipsychotic formulations.

Psychotherapy

No psychological intervention has shown efficacy in controlled studies in comparison to a placebo intervention in the management of bipolar disorder. Psychoeducation has long-standing prophylactic effects in bipolar disorders and helps to reduce the number of hospitalisations. The main objective of psychoeducation is to empower patients to manage their illness effectively. Patients are helped to understand their symptoms, course of the illness, early warning signs of relapse, and rationale for the acute and long-term treatment. They are made aware of how to avoid potential triggers such as substance abuse and encouraged to have regular sleep patterns.

REFERENCES

1. Angst, J. (2000). Course and prognosis of mood disorders. In M. G. Gelder, J. J. Lopez-Ibr Jr andN. C. Andreasen (Eds), *The New Oxford textbook of psychiatry*. Oxford: Oxford University Press.
2. Keane Veronica, O. (2000). In M. Steiner, K. A. Yonkers andE. Eriksson (Eds.), *Mood disorders in women*. London: Martin Dunitz.
3. Kendler, K. S., Thornton, L. M. and Gardner, C. O. (2000). Stressful life events and previous episodes in the aetiology of major depression in women: an evaluation of the 'kindling' hypothesis. *American Journal of Psychiatry*, 157(8), 1243–1251.
4. Musselman, D. L., Evans, D. L. and Nemeroff, C. B. (1998). The relationship to cardiovascular disease: epidemiology, biology, and treatment. *Archives of General Psychiatry*, 55, 580–592.
5. Bahk, W. M., Park, S., Jon, D. I., Doon, B. H., Min, K. J. and Hong, J. P. (2011). Relationship between painful physical symptoms and severity of depressive symptomatology and suicidality. *Psychiatry Research*, 189(3), 357–361.
6. Angst, J. (2000). Course and prognosis of mood disorders. In M. G. Gelder, J. J. Lopez-Ibr Jr and N. C. Andreasen (Eds.), *The New Oxford textbook of psychiatry*, Oxford: Oxford University Press.
7. Gelder, M., Harrison, P. and Cowen, P. (2007). *Shorter Oxford textbook of psychiatry*. Oxford: Oxford University Press.
8. Harris, E. C. and Barraclough, B. M. (1995). Suicide as an outcome for medical disorders. *Medicine*, 73, 281–96.
9. American Psychiatric Association.(2013). *Diagnostic and statistical manual of mental disorders* (5th Edition). Arlington, VA: American Psychiatric Publishing
10. Gelder, M., Harrison, P. and Cowen, P. (2007). *Shorter Oxford textbook of psychiatry*. Oxford: Oxford University Press.
11. Lima, M. S. and Moncrieff, J. (2000). A comparison of drugs versus placebo for the treatment of dysthymia. *Cochraine Database of Systematic Reviews*, 2, CD001130.
12. Angst, J. (1996). Cormobidity of mood disorders: a longitudinal prospective study. *British Journal of Clinical Psychiatry*, 55, 31–37.
13. Rosenthal, N. E., Sack, D. A., Gillin, G. C., Lewy, A.J., Goodwin, F. K., Davenport, Y., Mueller, P. S., Newsome, D. A. and Wehr, T. A. (1984). Seasonal affective disorder. A description of the syndrome and the preliminary findings with light therapy. *Archives of General Psychiatry*, 41(1), 72–80.
14. Wilman, S. M., Eagles, J. M., Andrew, J. E., et al. (2001). Light therapy for seasonal affective disorder in primary care. Randomised controlled trial. *British Journal of Psychiatry*, 178, 311–316.
15. Sadock, B. J. and Sadock, V. A. (2000). *Kaplan and Saddock's comprehensive textbook of psychiatry* (7th Edition). Philadelphia: Lippincott Williams and Wilkin.
16. Merikangas, K. R. (2000). In M. Steiner, K. A. Yonkers and E. Eriksson (Eds.), *Mood disorders in women*. London: Martin Dunitz.
17. Angold, A. and Worthman, C. W. (1993). Puberty onset of gender differences in rates of depression: a developmental, epidemiologic and neuroendocrine perspective. *Journal of Affective Disorders*, 29, 145–158.
18. Steiner, M., Yonkers, K. A. and Eriksson, E. (2000), *Mood disorders in women*. London: Martin Dunitz.
19. Khan, A. A., Gardner, C. O., Prescott, C. A. and Kendler, K. S. (2002). Gender differences in the symptoms of major depression in opposite-sex dizygotic twin pairs. *American Journal of Psychiatry*, 159, 1427–1429.
20. Baldwin, D. S. and Hirschfield, R. (2005) *Fast facts: Depression* (2nd Edition). Oxford: HealthPsychiatric Publishing.
21. Bowlby, J. (1969). Attachment. *Attachment and loss*: Vol. 1. Loss. New York: Basic Books.
22. Brown, G. W. and Harris, T. O. (1978). *Social origins of depression*. London: Tavistock.
23. Wessely, S. and Cleare, A. (2001). In L. Appleby, D. M. Forshaw, T. Amos and H. Barker (Eds.), *Postgraduate psychiatry clinical and scientific foundations* (2nd Edition). London: Arnold.
24. Murray, R. M., Hill, P. and McGuffin, P. (1997). *The essentials of postgraduate psychiatry* (3rd Edition). Cambridge: Cambridge University Press.
25. Brown, G. W. and Harris,T. (1978). *Social origins of depression*. London: Tavistock.
26. McGuffin, P., Katz, R. and Rutherford, J. (1991). Nature, nurture and depression; a twin study. *Psychological Medicine*, 21(2), 329–335.
27. Kaplan, H. I. and Daddock, B. J. (1996). *Concise textbook of clinical psychiatry* (7th Edition). Baltimore: Lippincott Williams and Wilkin.
28. Kaplan, H. I. and Daddock, B. J. (1996). *Concise textbook of clinical psychiatry* (7th Edition). Baltimore: Lippincott Williams and Wilkin.
29. Wessely, S. and Cleare, A. (2001). In L. Appleby, D. M. Forshaw, T. Amos and H. Barker (Eds.), *Postgraduate psychiatry clinical and scientific foundations* (2nd Edition). London: Arnold.
30. Kelly, W. F., Checkley, S. A. and Bender, D. A (1989). Cushing's syndrome, tryptophan and depression. *British Journal of Psychiatry*, 142, 16– 19.
31. Coryll, W., Keller, M., Lavori, P. and Endicott, J. (1990). Affcetive syndromes, psychotic features and prognosis. I. Depression. *Archives of General Psychiatry*, 47,651–657.
32. Checkley, S. A. (1992). Neuroendocrine mechanisms and the precipitation of depression by life events. *British Journal of Psychiatry*, 160, 7–17.
33. Kupfer, D. J., Spiker, D. G., Rossi, A., et al. (1983). Recent diagnostic and treatment advances in REM sleep and depression. In P. Clayton and J. Barrett (Eds.), *Treatment of depression: old controversies and new approaches*. New York: Raven Press.
34. Nishino, S. (2004). Sleep And Biological Rhythms,http://onlinelibrary. Wiley. Com/doi/10. 1111/sbr. 2004. 2. Issue-s1/issuetoc 1(2), 11–12.
35. Dunman, R. S. (2004). Role of neurotrophic factors in the aetiology and treatment of mood disorders. *Neuromolecular Medicine*, 5(1), 11–25.
36. Baxter, L. R. Jr, Schwartz, J. M., Phelps, M. E., et al. (1989). Reduction of prefrontal cortex glucose metabolism common to three types of depression. *Archives of General Psychiatry*, 46, 243–250.
37. Buchsbaum, M., Wu, J., Delisi, L., et al. (1986). Frontal cortex and basal ganglia metabolic rates assessed by positron emission tomography with 2–dexyglucose in affective illness. *Journal of Affective Disorders*, 10, 137–152.
38. Judd, L. L., et al. (1998). Major depressive disorder: a prospective study of residual subthreshold depressive symptoms as predictor of rapid relapse. *Journal of Affective Disorders*, 50, 97–108.
39. Song, F., Freemantle, N. and Sheldon, T. A. (1993). Selective serotonin reuptake inhibitors: meta-analysis of efficacy and acceptability. *British Medical Journal*, 306, 683–687.

40. Smith, D., Dempster, C., Glanville, J., et al. (2002). Efficacy and tolerability of venlafaxine compared with selective serotonin reuptake inhibitors and other antidepressants: a meta- analysis. *British Journal of Psychiatry*, 180, 396–404.

41. Cipriani, A., Furukawa, T. A., Salanti, G., Geddes, J. R., Higgins, J. P. T., et al. (2009). Comparative efficacy and acceptability of 12 new-generation antidepressants: A multiple- treatments meta-analysis. *The Lancet*, 373(9665), 746–758.

42. Elkin, I., Shea, T. and Watkins, J. T. (1989). National Institute of Mental Health Treatment of Depression Collaborative Research Programme: general effectiveness of treatments. *Archives of General Psychiatry*, 46, 971–982.

43. UK ECT Review Group (2003).Electroconvulsive Therapy-systematic review and meta-analysis of efficacy and safety in depressive disorders. *The Lancet*, 36, 799–808.

44. Fava, M. and Davidson, K. G. (1996). Definition and epidemiology of treatment-resistant depression. *The Psychiatric Clinics of North America*, 19, 179–200.

45. Helmchen, H. (1991). Therapy resistance in depression. In M. Gaspar and P. Kielholz (Eds.), *Problems in psychiatry in general practice*. Lewiston, New York: Hogrefe and Huber.

46. Stein, G. and Bernadt, M. (1993). Lithium augmentation therapy in tricyclic-resistant depression. A controlled trial using lithium in low and normal doses. *British Journal of Psychiatry*, 162, 634–640.

47. Bernadt, M. (2007). Drug treatment of depression. In G. Stein and G. Wilkinson (Eds.), *Seminars in general adult psychiatry* (2nd Edition). London: Royal College of Psychiatrists.

48. Joffe, R. T., Singer, W., Levitt, A. J., Macdonald, C. and Brierer, A. (1993). A placebo-controlled comparison of lithium and triiodothyronine augmentation of tricyclic antidepressants in unipolar refractory depression. *Archives of General Psychiatry*, 50(5), 387–393.

49. Shelton, R. C. and Papakostas, G. I. (2008). Augmentation of antidepressants with atypical antipsychotics for treatment-resistant major depressive disorder. *Acta Psychiatrica Scandinavia*, 117, 253–259.

50. Murray, C. J., Lopez, A. and Jamison, D. T. (1994). The global burden of disease in 1990: summary results, sensitivity analysis and future directions. *Bull World Health Organisation*, 72, 495–509.

51. Calabrese, J., Hirschfield, R., Reed, M., et al. (2003). Impact of bipolar disorder on a US community sample. *Journal of Clinical Psychiatry*, 64, 425–432.

52. Hirschfield, R. M. (2001). Bipolar spectrum disorder: improving its recognition and diagnosis. *Journal of Clinical Psychiatry*, 62(14), 5–9.

53. Swann, A. C., Bowden, C. L., Morris, D., et al. (1997). Depression during mania. Treatment response to lithium or divalproex. *Archives of General Psychiatry*, 54, 37–42.

54. Tohen, M., Waternaux, C. M. and Tsuang, M. T. (1990). Outcome in mania. A four year prospective follow-up of 75 patients utilizing survival analysis. *Archives of General Psychiatry*, 47, 1106–1111.

55. Goodwin, F. K. and Jamison, K. R. (1990). *Manic-Depressive illness*. New York: Oxford University Press.

56. Goldberg, J. F., Harrow, M. and Whiteside, J. E. (2001). Risk for bipolar illness in patients initially hospitalised for unipolar depression. *American Journal of Psychiatry*, 158, 1265–1270.

57. Elmslie, J. L., Silverstone, J. T., Mann, J. I., et al. (2000). Prevalence of overweight and obesity in bipolar patients. *Journal of Clinical Psychiatry*, 61, 179–184.

58. Bayer, J., Kuchibhatla, M., Gersing, K., et al. (2005). Medical cormobidity in a bipolar outpatient clinical population. *Neuropsychopharmacology*, 30, 401–404.

59. Tondo, L. and Baldessarini, R. J. (2000). Reduced suicide risk during lithium maintenance treatment. *Journal of Clinical Psychiatry*, 61(9), 97–104.

60. Tondo, L., Isacsson, G. and Baldessarini, R. (2003). Suicidal behaviour in bipolar disorder: risk and prevention. *CNS Drugs*, 17, 491–511.

61. Vieta, E. (2007). *Manageing mania in clinical practice*. London: Current Medicine Group.

62. Sachs, G. (2004). *Manageing bipolar affective disorder*. London: Science Press.

63. Wehr, T. A. (1991). Sleep loss as a possible mediator of diverse causes of mania. *British Journal of Psychiatry*, 159, 576–578.

64. Kessler, R. C., Berglund, P., Demler, O., et al. (2005). Lifetime prevalence and age of onset distributions of DSM-IV disorders in the National Comorbidity Survey Replication. *Archives of General Psychiatry*, 5, 63–68.

65. Arnold, L. M. (2003). Gender differences in bipolar disorder. *The Psychiatric Clinics of North America*, 26, 595–620.

66. Angst, J. (1986). The course of affective disorders. *Psychopathology*, 19(2), 47–52.

67. Hantouche, E.G. Adiskal, H. S., Lancrenon, S., et al. (1998). Systematic clinical methodology for validating bipolar II disorder: Data in mid stream from a French national multi-site study (EPIDEP). *Journal of Affective Disorders*, 50, 163–173.

68. Hantouche, E.G. Adiskal, H. S., Lancrenon, S., et al. (1998). Systematic clinical methodology for validating bipolar II disorder: data in mid stream from a French national multi-site study (EPIDEP). *Journal of Affective Disorders*, 50, 163–173.

69. Hirschfeld, R. M. A., Bowden, C. L., Perlis, R. H., et al. (2002). American Psychiatric Association. Practice guideline for the treatment of patients with bipolar disorder. *American Journal of Psychiatry*, 159(4), 1–50.

70. Vieta, E. (2007). *Manageing mania in clinical practice*. London: Current Medicine Group.

71. Thies-Flechtner, K., Muller-Oerlinghausen, B., Seibert, W., et al. (1996). Effect of prophylactic treatment on suicide risk in patients with major effective disorders. Data from a randomised prospective trial. *Pharmacopsychiatry*, 29, 103–107.

72. Small, J. G., Klapper, M. H., Milstein, V., et al. (1991). Carbamazepine compared with lithium in the treatment of mania. *Archives of General Psychiatry*, 48, 915–921.

73. Lere, B., Moore, N., Meyendorff, F., et al. (1987). Carbamazepine versus lithium in mania: a double blind study. *Journal of Clinical Psychiatry*, 48, 89–93.

74. Post, R. M., Udhe, T. W., Roy-Bryne, P. P., et al. (1987). Correlates of antimanic response to carbamazepine. *Psychiatry Research*, 21, 71–83.

75. Spina, E., Pisani, F. and Perucca, E. (1996). Clinically significant pharmacokinetics drug interactions with carbamazepine. *Clinical Pharmacokinetics*, 31, 198–214.

76. Macritchie, K. A. N., Geddes, J. R., Scott, J., et al. (2003). Valproate for acute mood episodes in bipolar disorder. *Cochrane Database of Systematic Reviews* (Online), 1, CD004052.

77. Vasudev, K., Goswami, U. and Kohli, K. (2000). Carbamazepine and valproate monotherapy: feasibility, relative safety and efficacy, and therapeutic drug monitoring in manic disorder. *Psychopharmacology*, 150, 15–23.

78. Vieta, E., Owen, R., Baudelet, C., Sanchez, R. D. M. R. and Marcus, R. N. (2010). Assessment of safety, tolerability and effectiveness of adjunctive aripiprazole to lithium/valporate in bipolar mania: a 46-week, open label extension following a 6-week double-blind study. *Current Medical Research and Opinion*, 26(6), 1485–1496.

79. Rana, T. A. (2010). Clinical trials to clinical practice: Retrospective analysis of 25 patients with bipolar mania treated with aripiprazole (Poster). Amsterdam: ECNP.

80. Rana, T. A. and Malik, T. (2010). Clinical trials to clinical practice: Retrospective analysis of 25 patients with bipolar mania treated with aripiprazole. *Progress in Neurology and Psychiatry Case Notes*, 14(5), 1–8.

81. Grunze, H., et al. (2009). The World Federation of Societies of Biological Psychiatry Guidelines for the Biological Treatment of Bipolar Disorders: Update 2009 on the Treatment of Acute Mania. *The World Journal of Biological Psychiatry*, 1092, 85–116.

82. Smith, L. A., Cornelius, V., Warnock, A., Tacchi, M. J. and Taylor, D. (2007). Acute bipolar mania: a systematic review and meta-analysis of co-therapy vs monotherapy. *Acta Psychiatrica Scandinavia*, 115, 12–20.

83. Karmacharya, R., England, M. L. and Ongur,D. (2008). Delirious mania: clinical features and treatment response. *Journal of Affective Disorders*, 109, 312–316.

84. Grof, P., Alda, M., Grof, E., et al. (1993). The challenge of predicting response to stabilising lithium treatment. The importance of patient selection. *British Journal of Psychiatry*, 163(21), 16–19.

CHAPTER

06 Schizophrenia and Related Disorders

Although schizophrenia was described more than a century ago, it remains one of the most challenging, disabling and destructive mental illnesses. Despite trends toward community-oriented treatment, about 25% of all psychiatric hospital beds are occupied by persons with schizophrenia. The costs of treating schizophrenia are significant in terms of both financial and personal costs. Despite the economic costs, the impact on the person's social and occupational functioning over a lifetime may be even more devastating. In fact, the largest indirect cost associated with schizophrenia is the loss of productivity over the lifetime. The burden of schizophrenia places the disorder as one of the top 10 most disabling conditions in the world in terms of illness-adjusted life years. Even when persons with schizophrenia receive optimal treatments, many continue to experience substantial impairments throughout most of their lives.

The outcome in many cases remains fragmented and unsatisfactory. Schizophrenia is a very complex condition that profoundly affects not only the life of the patient but also of the family members and other carers as well. It exists in all cultures and in all countries and the symptoms are more or less similar around the world. However, there is variability in symptoms and the course of the illness among individuals. The clinical presentation can, moreover, vary within the same individual at different stages of the illness. Schizophrenia accounts for a large proportion of patients who need long-term psychiatric care in hospitals and even outside them, on a supportive basis, in the community.

As there is no specific test and pathology, there has been an ongoing controversy as to whether it can be classified as a disease. It is, therefore, preferable to regard schizophrenia as a syndrome (that can be identified by a characteristic cluster of symptoms). The illness is usually associated with deterioration of personality, and the patient's thought processes, perception, behaviour and emotions are all adversely affected. There is a tendency of withdrawal from social contact and retreat from reality. A disturbance of the development and maintenance of adequate ego-boundaries is a central feature of the schizophrenic process.

The onset of the first episode of schizophrenia may be sudden or gradual. It is usually preceded by escalating adjustment problems, a period referred to as the prodromal phase. There is some evidence that longer untreated psychotic episodes may be harmful for schizophrenia patients and may result in a worse course of illness. However, this conclusion is controversial, and some researchers suggest that the relation between a longer duration of untreated psychosis and worse prognosis may be a product of poorer premorbid functioning and an insidious onset.

Kraepelin, in 1896, was the first to group these disturbances of thoughts, feelings and volition under the term dementia praecox (1). He mentioned that this illness started at an early age and invariably led to a complete deterioration of personality and ultimately to dementia. Bleuler, who introduced the term schizophrenia, in 1911, believed that the disorder was due to a loosening of association between thought processes and between different psychic functions which, although, often left the personality scarred, was likely to remit in several cases (2).

Bleuler's fundamental symptoms ('the four As')

- Loosening of associations (thought disorder)
- Blunted or incongruous affect
- Autism (social withdrawal)
- Ambivalence (apathy)

Clinical Features

Many different clinical pictures may occur in schizophrenia and the onset of illness may be acute or insidious, leading to a gradual and significant deterioration of personality in many cases. Schizophrenia is usually characterised by delusions, hallucinations, formal thought disorder and negative symptoms.

Hallucinations

Hallucinations are perception-like experiences in the absence of external stimuli. They are not under voluntary control. Although they occur in any modality, auditory hallucinations are quite common in schizophrenia. They may be voices talking directly to the patient (second person hallucinations) and/or talking about the patient in third person (third person hallucinations). Some patients also hear voices commenting on their actions, or giving commands.

Delusions

Delusions are fixed beliefs that are not amenable to change in light of conflicting or contradictory evidence. Their content may include a variety of themes (e.g., persecutory, referential, somatic, religious, grandiose). Persecutory delusions and delusions of reference are very common in schizophrenia although any type of delusion may exist.

Delusions are considered to be bizarre if they are clearly implausible and not understandable and do not derive from ordinary life experiences. It is important to rule out any cultural belief.

A primary delusion or a bizarre delusion (e.g., Aliens have landed and taken control of the patient) is very important from a diagnostic point of view. It arises suddenly without any prior morbid experiences. A secondary delusion develops subsequent to a previous symptom patient having nihilistic delusion after low mood) and is of less diagnostic significance. Delusions of thought control and passivity phenomena are again important for diagnostic purposes. These may take the form of thought insertion, thought withdrawal, thought broadcasting, made feelings, made impulses and made actions.

Formal Thought Disorder

Formal thought disorder does not imply delusional ideation, but is disorder of the formation of thought. It is a very important and characteristic feature of schizophrenia. The patient complains of having confused or muddled thoughts. The normal association of ideas becomes disconnected and it may be difficult to follow the patient's flow of talk which is more often vague and unclear. Derailment or loosening of associations, poverty of content of thought, word salad, thought block and neologism are some examples.

Disorders of Emotion

There is a characteristic reduction in the intensity of emotional expression (blunting or flattening of affect) and in addition patient's affective response is not appropriate or compatible with the ideas being discussed (inappropriate or incongruous affect).

Disorders of Volition

The patients shows lack of drive or initiative especially in the chronic stages of the illness and find it difficult to go through the day-to-day routines of life. They become more and more withdrawn and asocial with diminished interest in the outside world. Personal hygiene and appearance also gets increasingly neglected and there is often a significant decline in social and occupational spheres.

Disorganised or Abnormal Motor Behaviour

This may manifest itself in a variety of ways including catatonic behaviour (marked decrease in reactivity to the external events), mutism and stupor (complete lack of verbal and motor rsponses), catatonic excitement (purposeless and excessive motor activity). It is important to remember that catatonic symptoms can also occur in bipolar disorder and depressive disorder as well as in medical conditions.

Cognitive and Emotional Deficits

Among the most well-established aspects of schizophrenia are the cognitive deficits that accompany the illness. Schizophrenia patients manifest performance deficits on a broad range of cognitive tasks, from simple to complex. One of the most basic is the deficit in the very earliest stages of visual information processing. Schizophrenia patients are slower in the initial processing of stimuli. Among the higher-level cognitive functions, schizophrenia patients show deficits in verbal and spatial memory, abstract reasoning, psychomotor speed, and planning.

Lack of Insight

Most patients either do not have awareness of their mental condition or their insight is very limited. This has implications for compliance with medications and other treatments, relapses and hospital admissions.

Positive and Negative Symptoms

Patients usually represent an increase or distortion of normal functioning, i.e. formal thought disorder, inappropriate affect, disorganised behaviour, delusions and hallucinations. However, patients (usually in chronic stage) also have decreased or loss of normal functioning which includes blunting of affect, poverty of thought and speech, impaired volition and social withdrawal. This group constitutes negative symptoms and they account for a substantial portion of burden associated with schizophrenia. Relatives and carers of patients with schizophrenia often find it more difficult to cope with the negative symptoms.

Crow's Type I Syndrome (3)

This is characterised by positive symptoms (delusions, hallucinations, and thought disorder). It has acute onset.

Crow's Type II Syndrome

This is characterised by negative symptoms (affective flattening, apathy and poverty of speech).

Liddle's Classification (4)

- Psychomotor poverty (poverty of speech, flat effect, decreased spontaneous movement)
- Disorganisation (disorder of form of thought and inappropriate affect)
- Reality distortion (delusions and hallucinations)

SUBTYPES OF SCHIZOPHRENIA

In DSM-5 as well as ICD 11, subtypes of schizophrenia have been eliminated because of their limited diagnostic validity, low reliability and poor validity. Clinically this sub-division is of a limited value as many patients may present with different types at different stages and there may be considerable overlapping of symptoms.

ICD-10 Has the Following Subtypes

1. Paranoid schizophrenia
2. Hebephrenic schizophrenia
3. Catatonic schizophrenia
4. Simple schizophrenia
5. Residual schizophrenia
6. Undifferentiated schizophrenia
7. Post-schizophrenic depression

Paranoid Schizophrenia

Persecutory delusions and auditory hallucinations are prominent in this type. Personality is often well preserved for a number of years before declining. Disturbances of affect, volition and speech and catatonic symptoms are not prominent.

Hebephrenic Schizophrenia

The onset is insidious and the patient often presents with prominent affective changes. Mood is inappropriate and speech is incoherent. There is a marked volitional disorder and disorganisation of personality. Hallucinations may be fleeting and fragmentary.

Catatonic Schizophrenia

This usually has an acute onset and is characterised by motor abnormalities accompanied by hallucinations and delusions. The patient's behaviour is withdrawn and negativistic. Bizarre mannerisms, posturing and grimacing occur and a particular posture may be maintained over a prolonged period of time.

Simple Schizophrenia

The onset of this type of schizophrenia is also insidious but there is progressive development of oddities of conduct, inability to meet the demands of society and a decline in total performance. Delusions and hallucinations are not evident. There is loss of interest in routines of life e.g., studies. These patients show extreme apathy and a total lack of ambition or plans for the future.

Undifferentiated Schizophrenia

This includes those clinical pictures which do not seem to fit in any of the above described types or which exhibit the features of more than one of them, without a clear predominance of one or the other. This type should only be diagnosed after an attempt has been made to classify the condition into one of the above four types.

Post-Schizophrenic Depression

In this disorder, the depressive symptoms are prolonged, arising in the aftermath of a schizophrenic illness. ICD-10 diagnostic criteria empathises that some schizophrenic symptoms must still be present but no longer dominate the picture. The depressive symptoms are rarely sufficiently severe or extensive to meet criteria for a severe depressive episode.

Diagnosis of Schizophrenia

As no laboratory tests are available, detailed psychiatric history and mental state examination are the only diagnostic tools currently available.

ICD-10 Criteria (5)

At least one of the symptoms (a)–(d) or at least two of the symptoms (e)–(i) should have been present during a period of a month or more:

a. Thought echo, thought insertion, thought withdrawal or thought broadcasting
b. Delusions of control, influence, or passivity, clearly referred to body or limb movements or specific thoughts, actions or sensations; or delusional perception
c. Hallucinatory voices, giving a running commentary on the patient's behaviour or discussing the patient among themselves or other types of hallucinatory voices coming from some part of the body
d. Persistent delusions of other kinds that are culturally inappropriate and completely impossible, such as religious or of political identity or superhuman powers and abilities
e. Persistent hallucinations in any modality, accompanied either by fleeting or half- formed delusions, without a clear affective component, or by persistent overvalued ideas occurring every day for weeks or months on end
f. Breaks or interpolations in the train of thoughts, resulting in incoherence or irrelevant speech, or neologism
g. Catatonic behaviour, such as excitement, posturing, or waxy flexibility, negativism, mutism or stupor
h. Negative symptoms such as marked apathy, paucity of speech and blunting or incongruity of emotional responses, usually resulting in social withdrawal and lowering of social performance; it must be clear that they are not due to depression or neuroleptic medication
i. A significant and consistent change in the overall quality of some aspects of personal behaviour, manifesting as loss of interest, aimlessness, idleness, a self-absorbed attitude and social withdrawal

DSM-5 Diagnostic Criteria (6)

Two (or more) of the following, each present for a significant portion of time during a 1-month period (or less if successfully treated). At least one of these must be (1), (2), or (3):

1. Delusions
2. Hallucinations
3. Disorganised speech (e.g. frequent derailment or incoherence)
4. Grossly disorganised or catatonic behaviour
5. Negative symptoms (i.e. diminished emotional expression or avolition)
    a. For a significant portion of the time since the onset of the disturbance, level of functioning in one or more major areas, such as work, interpersonal relations, or self-care, is markedly below the level achieved prior to the onset (or when the onset is in childhood or adolescence, there is a failure to achieve expected level of interpersonal, academic, or occupational functioning).
    b. Continuous signs of the disturbance persist for at least six months. This 6-month period must include at least one month of symptoms (or less

if successfully treated) that meet criterion A (i.e. active-phase symptoms) and may include periods of prodromal or residual symptoms. During these prodromal or residual periods, the signs of the disturbance may be manifested by only negative symptoms or by two or more symptoms listed in Criterion A, present in an attenuated form (e.g., odd beliefs, unusual perceptual experiences).

c. Schizoaffective disorder and depressive or bipolar disorder with psychotic features have been ruled out because either:
   i. No major depressive or manic episodes have occurred concurrently with the active-phase symptoms, or
   ii. If mood episodes have occurred during active-phase symptoms, they have been present for a minority of the total duration of the active and residual periods of the illness.
d. The disturbance is not attributable to the physiological effects of a substance (e.g., a drug of abuse, a medication) or another medical condition.
e. If there is a history of autism spectrum disorder or a communication disorder of childhood onset, the additional diagnosis of schizophrenia is made only if prominent delusions or hallucinations, in addition to the other required symptoms of schizophrenia, are also present for at least 1 month (or less if successfully treated).

Differential Diagnosis

Illicit Drugs and Psychosis

Drugs like amphetamines, MDMA (ecstasy) and cocaine can produce schizophrenia-like psychosis. However, it is short-lived and resolves within a few days after abstinence from drugs. LSD (acid), phencyclidine (angel) and acute intoxication with cannabis can also cause psychotic symptoms. There is, moreover, some evidence that cannabis abuse in early life can increase the risk of development of schizophrenia (7).

Organic Conditions

Some medical conditions can give rise to a schizophrenia-like picture. These include cerebral tumours, neurosyphilis, Wilson's disease, temporal lobe epilepsy, Huntington's disease and the adult form of metachromatic leukodystrophy. In most cases, gross brain pathology, physical signs, abnormal laboratory and other investigations suggest the correct diagnosis.

Paranoid States

These include paranoid personality disorders, delusional disorders, erotomania and morbid jealousy. In paranoid personality disorders, the person exhibits a very rigid and inflexible personality and overvalued ideas may be common. In delusional disorders, there is an elaborate delusional system, no hallucinations and an intact personality. In erotomania, a female would hold a delusional belief about a higher status male being in love with her. Morbid jealousy is usually in males who have delusions about their wives' or lovers' infidelity.

Other Psychiatric Conditions

Psychiatric illnesses which can cause symptoms suggestive of schizophrenia also include acute and transient psychotic disorders (which are short-lived) and affective disorders. The latter may be quite difficult to distinguish from schizophrenia. In fact, some patients diagnosed with schizophrenia initially have to be reclassified as having a bipolar affective disorder. In mania, which occurs as an episodic illness, affective symptoms appear first and the mood of a patient with mania is typically infectious, whereas in schizophrenia, which is a chronic illness, psychotic symptoms precede the excitation seen in mania and the mood is rather shallow and not contagious.

Epidemiology

Incidence and Prevalence

The lifetime risk of schizophrenia is about 1%, with an incidence of approximately 15 new cases per 100,000 population per annum. The prevalence is 2–4 per 1000.

Age and Sex

The disorder usually begins in late adolescence or early twenties, though it can develop at any age. It has been, for a long time, thought that males and females are equally affected. Recently some evidence has emerged that it is more common in males. The age of onset in males is earlier as well. The incidence is higher in the unmarried than the married (both sexes). Female patients generally have a better outcome. One factor for this difference could be the comparatively milder form of illness in females including fewer negative symptoms.

Fertility

Both males and females have reduced fertility rates. Even after excluding factors like fewer opportunities for relationships, and such, it has been confirmed that patients still have fewer children than normal people. The reasons are not clear.

Mortality

As compared to the general population, patients with schizophrenia have higher mortality rates. This is attributed to suicides, homicides, and physical health problems, e.g., respiratory disease, metabolic syndrome, obesity and diabetes, etc.

Developed Versus Developing Countries

Some studies have demonstrated that schizophrenia has a more acute onset and better outcome in developing countries as compared to industrialised countries (8).

Urbanicity

The incidence is greater in cities. According to the 'drift hypothesis', patients with schizophrenia drift downwards on the social scale because of their inability to function. The other explanation could be that they themselves become socially isolated in certain run-down areas of the cities. The 'social causation' theory, however, appears to be more convincing. This theory states that certain social stressors like poverty, lack of education and healthcare increases the risk for schizophrenia. Studies suggest that the incidence is higher among those born or brought up in urban areas (9). Another study highlighted an interesting finding, i.e. the period of stay and the size of the of the town proportionately increases the risk of schizophrenia (10). The importance of social support has been demonstrated by findings that the highest rates of schizophrenia were found in those areas of cities which had little social cohesion (11).

Migration and Ethnicity

Schizophrenia appears to be more common in populations that have migrated. Various studies have confirmed the observation that ethnic minority groups have higher rates of schizophrenia (12) (13).

Aetiology

Aetiology of schizophrenia still remains unclear and is one of psychiatry's greatest challenges. No single factor has been found to cause schizophrenia and the aetiology is perhaps multifactorial. The following explanations have been put forward:

Genetic Factors

The genetic predisposition to schizophrenia is well known as it has been supported by family, adoption and twin studies. However, the nature of its transmission is still unclear, and schizophrenia is not transmitted by the Mendelian pattern of autosomal dominance such as in Huntington's chorea, or recessiveness such as in cystic fibrosis (14).

Family Studies

Family members of patients suffering from schizophrenia are at a higher risk of developing the disorder as compared to the general population. The risk increases according to the proximity of the relationship. The approximate lifetime risk of developing schizophrenia in the relatives of patients suffering from schizophrenia is given below (15):

Parent	5.6%
Sibling and one affected parent	16.7%
Children (one affected parent)	12.8%
Children (both affected parents)	
Uncles/aunts/nephews /nieces	
Grandchildren	46.3%

A large family study carried out in Ireland found that the lifetime risk of schizophrenia in the first degree relatives of those with schizophrenia was 6.5% compared to 0.5% in the relatives of the control (16). This was confirmed by another study in London. This study also showed that relatives of probands who had early-onset had a higher risk than those with late-onset. In addition, relatives of female probands had an increased risk than the relatives of the male probands (17). Family studies on their own are not conclusive of genetic contribution as shared environment could play a part in familiality.

Twin Studies

Monozygotic twins are genetically identical whereas dizygotic twins share about 50% of their genes. Studies have shown a higher concordance rate (i.e. both twins suffering from schizophrenia) for MZ than DZ twins (18). As monozygotic twin studies demonstrate that the concordance rate is less than 100%, it is evident that schizophrenia is not totally genetic and environmental factors are also involved.

Adoption Studies

Since an adopted individual has genes from one family and lives with another family, adoption studies can help discriminate genetic and environmental effects. These studies have found that the rate of schizophrenia in adopted children of patients with schizophrenia is higher than the adopted children of normal parents.

A study done in Denmark confirmed the genetic basis to familial aggregation of schizophrenia (19). Similar findings have been reported from Finland.

Developmental and Environmental Factors

It seems that a combination of genetic and environmental factors leads to defective development and maturation of the brain which, later, leads to the development of schizophrenic illness.

Obstetric Complications

Studies report more obstetric complications in patients with schizophrenia than normal controls. These can be grouped into complications of pregnancy (bleeding, pre-eclampsia), fetal complications (low birth weight, congenital malformations) and delivery complications (asphyxia, uterine atony) (20).

Prenatal Factors

Another epidemiological observation of schizophrenia is excess winter-spring births found in the northern hemisphere but not in Southern Hemisphere (21). One explanation put forward for this is the teratogenic effect of infection on the fetal brain development. There have been reports that mothers of patients with schizophrenia have prenatal exposure to influenza and other findings are increased antibodies for rubella, herpes simplex and toxoplasmosis. An increased rate has also been reported in women who had food deprivation in the first trimester of pregnancy (22).

Early Developmental Delays

Longitudinal follow-up studies have demonstrated slight delays in motor, speech and intellectual milestones in some patients with schizophrenia. Developmental receptive language disorders also occur.

Heavy Cannabis Intake

Studies have shown that the use of cannabis can double the risk of developing schizophrenia.

Some Other Risk Factors

Risk increases in people with Epilepsy and also in those with low IQ. Paternal age and head injury are two other factors associated with this disorder but the evidence for head injury is quite weak.

Abnormal Family Interactions

Double-bind communication: This idea was put forward by Bateson and his colleagues in 1956. They asserted that schizophrenia develops due to distorted communications in a family. The child is exposed to excessive double-bind communication in which opposite meanings are implied, the child starts making ambiguous responses and develops schizophrenia.

Marital skew and marital schism: This concept was given by Lidz and his colleagues in 1965. In marital skew one parent yields to the other eccentricities, which dominates the family. In marital schism, parents maintain contrary views as a result of which the child develops divided loyalties.

These two theories do not have hard evidence.

High Expressed Emotion (High EE)

This finding was initially put forward by Brown and his colleagues in 1972. Subsequent studies of high expressed emotions have proved that this is a strong predictor of relapse following discharge from hospital (23). Contact with family members with high EE (features of hostility, critical comments and emotional over- involvement) for more than 35 hour a week further increases the risk of relapse (24).

Life Events

There is some evidence that life events may be important (25) and a general consensus is that major life events can precipitate schizophrenia in the predisposed people. Life events are not only relevant for the first episodes of schizophrenia but also to subsequent relapses.

Neuropsychological Factors

In schizophrenia, there is a consistent pattern and broad range of neurocognitive impairments. These include attention/information processing, processing speed, reasoning and problem-solving, verbal learning and memory, visual learning and memory, working memory and social cognition (26). One model proposes that positive symptoms arise from a failure to integrate stored memories with current stimuli (27). According to another model, in schizophrenia there is a breakdown in the internal representation of mental events (28). Patients fail to identify their own intentions and erroneously think that their thoughts and actions have an external cause.

Neurochemistry

The following neurochemical dysfunctions and neurotransmitters abnormalities are considered to be the link between underlying causal factors and the psychopathology of schizophrenia.

a. *Dopamine hypothesis*: This hypothesis sug- gests positive symptoms of schizophrenia are due to the excess of dopaminergic ac- tivity in the mesolimbic system. This could be due to excess of dopamine, deficiency of dopamine antagonists or increased sensitivity of dopamine receptors (29). The dopamine hypothesis is well-established and is supported by the observation that most antipsychotic drugs act by blocking dopamine receptors, thus lowering dopaminergic activity. Moreover, amphetamine and LSD lead to an increase in dopaminergic activity and produce a clinical picture which is similar to schizophrenia. The third evidence put forward was that chlorpromazine's side effects were like Parkinsonism disease (which results because of dysfunction of dopamine transmission).

b. *Serotonergic transmission:* This hypothesis states that serotonergic transmission may be increased in the brains of schizophrenic patients.

c. *Glutamate hypothesis*: It proposes that glutamate and glutamate receptor genes are involved in neuro-development and that abnormalities in these systems lead to schizophrenia. The evidence for this is increasing.

d. *Noradrenaline hypothesis*: There is evidence for over and underactivity of this neurotransmitter.

e. *Other neurotransmitters*: Acetylcholine is implicated in the regulation of attention, memory as well as other cognitive functions. As these are impaired in schizophrenia,there might be a possible role for this neurotransmitter. GABA interneurons may be decreased in schizophrenia.

Neurological Abnormalities

Patients with schizophrenia have grey matter reductions in the prefrontal, superior temporal and inferior parietal areas. MRI studies have also confirmed findings of enlarged ventricles, increased sulcal widening, and decreased cortical volume with greater decrease in the hippocampus, amygdala, and thalamus (30). Hippocampus, amygdala and parahippocampus are involved in emotions and memory. Male patients have been found to have greater volume reductions in the temporal lobes. Some patients have decreased blood flow in the frontal lobe (hypofrontality)(31). Although these findings are present at the onset of illness, there is some evidence that these abnormalities may appear after the onset of schizophrenia. Histological findings in the cerebral cortex in schizophrenia include reduced glial-cell density, increased neuronal density, aberrant migration of neurons, smaller neurons, loss of synapses and loss of dendritic complexity (32).

Neurophysiological Findings

In schizophrenia, there are EEG changes like increased theta activity, fast activity and paroxysmal activity. Abnormalities of evoked potentials (P300 and P50) and defective performance in tests of eye-tracking have also been reported (33).

Course and Outcome

People with schizophrenia vary in their course of illness and prognosis. It is important to consider the outcome of schizophrenia with regards to symptomatic recovery as well as the social functioning. The outcome of schizophrenia is comparatively better in developing countries than industrialised countries, although this finding has now been challenged.

There has been a lot of research regarding prognosis of schizophrenia. (34). One study found that the relapse rates were very high, with 81.9% of patients experiencing at least one further episode within five years (35). The risk of relapse is increased five times in those who discontinue antipsychotic medication. The effects of antipsychotic medication on the long-term prognosis of schizophrenia are less impressive than the short-term effects.

Suicide is the leading cause of death among people with schizophrenia. It has been estimated that 25% to 50% of schizophrenia patients attempt suicide and 4% to 13% successfully commit suicide. Risk factors associated with suicide in this population include more severe accompanying depressive symptoms, being male, earlier onset, and recent traumatic events (36). There are also premature deaths from other causes like accidents, CVS disease, obesity, and metabolic syndromes.

Poor prognostic factors include being male, gradual onset, early age of onset, poor premorbid functioning, and family history of schizophrenia . In addition, some environmental factors have been found to contribute to a worse outcome. For example, schizophrenia patients who live in homes where family members express greater negative emotions are more likely than those from warm, supportive families to have relapses. Also, exposure to stress has been found to exacerbate schizophrenia symptoms. Researchers have found an increase in the number of stressful events in the months immediately preceding a schizophrenia relapse.

The prognosis for many schizophrenia patients is poor. Only 20% to 30% are able to live independently and maintain a relationship and a job. The majority experience a more debilitating course, with 20% to 30% manifesting continued moderate symptoms and over half experiencing significant impairment for the rest of their lives. Furthermore, patients with schizophrenia often suffer from other comorbid conditions. For example, the rate of substance abuse among schizophrenia patients is very high.

Management of Schizophrenia

Although there is no cure for schizophrenia, there have been lots of advances in pharmacological and psychosocial interventions which have contributed significantly to successfully improve the treatment of schizophrenia. There have also been lots of efforts and movements in manageing patients in the community but when patients have florid psychotic symptoms as well as risks, hospital admission is indicated. Treatments are more effective when the psychopharmacology and psychosocial interventions are combined.

Pharmacological Treatment

Antipsychotic medications are the backbone and mainstays of treatment of schizophrenia (37). This is the case for both acute and maintenance treatment for minimising relapse (38). The two major classes of antipsychotic medications are: conventional, neuroleptics, first generation (FGAS) or typical antipsychotics; and novel, second generation (SGAS) or atypical antipsychotics. See the chapter 'Drugs and Other Physical Treatments' for details.

Typical Antipsychotics (FGAS)

There are both oral and injectable, long-acting depot forms of antipsychotics. The majority of typical antipsychotics are all potent dopamine D2 receptor antagonists. They do not vary much in their efficacy but differ in their side effect profile. The higher the potency of these drugs, the greater the risk of extrapyramidal symptoms; the lower the potency, the higher the incidence of sedation, hypotension, anticholinergic effects and seizures. Haloperidol, chlorpromazine, trifluoperazine, flupenthixol, pimozide, sulpiride and thioridazine are typical antipsychotics. Haloperidol and fluphenazine are high-potency drugs whereas chlorpromazine and thioridazine are low potency antipsychotics.

Extrapyramidal Side Effects (EPSE) include Parkinsonism, dystonia, akathisia and tardive dyskinesia. In dystonia, the muscles of the neck, face and tongue are usually affected. Torticollis and oculogyric crisis occurs. Anticholinergic medications resolve this, although they themselves can cause side effects like blurred vision, dry mouth and constipation. Akathisia is characterised by restlessness and mental agitation. Some patients do not respond well to anticholinergics and adding benzodiazepines can be helpful.

Tardive dyskinesia is an important long-term side effect that is characterised by slow irregular movements in the region of mouth: grimacing, smacking of the lips and protrusion of the tongue. Management of tardive dyskinesia includes reducing or stopping the anticholinergic medication, reducing the dose of antipsychotic medication and considering switching to atypical medication. There is some evidence that clozapine may actually treat tardive dyskinesia.

Neuroleptic Malignant Syndrome (NMS) is a rare but very serious side effect. It is characterised by muscle rigidity, autonomic instability (elevated pulse rate and blood pressure), and fever. NMS has to be managed in a medical unit.

Atypical Antipsychotics (SGAS)

The essential difference between atypical and typical antipsychotic drugs is that atypical have less propensity to cause EPS. They are effective at doses that do not cause EPS. They, however, can cause weight gain, metabolic syndromes dyslipidemia, and increased blood glucose levels associated with higher risk for developing diabetes.

Atypical antipsychotics are clozapine, risperidone, olanzapine, quetiapine, aripiprazole, ziprasidone, zotepine, and sertindole. All of these are not available in all countries. Clozapine is the prototype atypical antipsychotic and in contrast to typical antipsychotics, it binds to many neurotransmitter receptors (39).

Depot and Long-Acting Intramuscular Antipsychotics

Improved bioavailability and increased compliance are the main benefits of the intramuscular medications. There is, however, no established evidence regarding their superiority in efficacy. Typical antipsychotic injections are, fluphenazine decanoate, clopenthixol decanoate, flupenthixol decanoate and haldol decanoate. Atypical antipsychotics injections are risperidone, olanzapine, paliperidone and aripiprazole.

Acute Treatment

The goals of acute management include establishing a therapeutic relationship with the patients and their families, to control behavioural disturbances like agitation and aggression, to do a comprehensive risk assessment (as there is potential of harm to self and others), treatment of psychotic symptoms and any associated symptoms or disorders (e.g., drug abuse) and to draw a long-term management plan.

It is imperative to commence pharmacological treatment as soon as the diagnosis is made. There is evidence that if treatment is delayed, psychotic symptoms not only take longer to improve but this has implications for achieving remission (40). Moreover, the Duration of Untreated Psychosis (DUP) significantly determines future relapses (41).

There is evidence that SGAS may have comparative advantage over typical antipsychotic medication (42). Another meta-analysis also found that most atypical drugs are modestly superior in the treatment of positive and negative symptoms (43). Currently most guidelines recommend SGAS as the first choice of medication.

Most patients show some improvement in 2–6 weeks. The dose should be increased after 4–6 weeks and if there is still no satisfactory improvement, another atypical antipsychotic should be tried. Failing 6 weeks trial of second atypical (with an adequate dose and provided that the patient has complied), clozapine should be considered. Benzodiazepines and short-acting injectable antipsychotic formulations are used for behavioural disturbances.

Treatment-Resistant Patients

About one-third of patients are poor responders and treatment-resistant (44). Clozapine is the most effective medication for treatment-resistant schizophrenia and is the only medication currently licensed for this treatment. Meta-analytic findings have confirmed its superiority (45).

For patients who do show adequate response to clozapine, various adjunctive strategies are recommended. Adding risperidone or sulpiride to clozapine may be beneficial.

Maintenance Treatment

About 80% of patients experience further episodes of schizophrenia after the first episode. When medication is stopped there is a five times higher risk of relapsing. As it is currently not possible to know which patients would relapse after they stop their antipsychotic medication, most clinicians and researchers advocate maintenance treatment for all patients.

Treatment of Negative and Cognitive Symptoms

Negative symptoms are a major cause of the poor quality of life of patients. Moreover, relatives and carers are more burdened by negative symptoms as compared to positive symptoms. Both typical and atypical antipsychotics have some effect on the secondary negative symptoms and have limited efficacy on the primary avolitional syndrome. There is some evidence for using agents that increase the level of activity of the N-Methyl-D-Aspartate (NMDA) receptor. There is modest benefit of atypical antipsychotics on cognitive impairments. It remains unclear whether this is because they directly enhance cognitive functions or this is due to their less adverse effects.

Cariprazine, a partial agonist with strong binding to D3 receptors, has shown very encourageing and positive results regarding negative symptoms.

Electroconvulsive Therapy (ECT)

In schizophrenia, ECT is given in cases of catatonic illness or comorbid severe depression which is severe, recurrent or unresponsive to antidepressants. It can also be considered when suicidal ideation is not responding to antidepressant therapy. It should be noted that ECT should be considered as a treatment of the last resort for patients with refractory illness, as its role in the treatment of patients with schizophrenia is very limited (46).

Psychosocial Interventions

Many patients make a symptomatic recovery but remain functionally disabled. They are socially isolated as well because of stigma and lack of motivation, etc. Although antipsychotic medication is the crucial first step in the treatment of schizophrenia, there is substantial evidence that psychosocial interventions can also be beneficial for both the patient and the family. It is generally agreed that the optimal treatment approach is one that integrates pharmacologic and psychosocial interventions.

Social skills training seeks to improve the overall functioning of patients by teaching the skills necessary to improve the performance of activities of daily living, employment-related skills, and interaction with others. Some social skills programs emphasise learning new skills through modelling. Others focus more on teaching patients better strategies for solving interpersonal problems or training them to read non-verbal cues of emotion in other people. Research indicates that all of these approaches to social skills training can improve social competence.

Family Interventions

Families play an essential role in supporting and improving the lives of these patients (47). The important role of high expressed emotions has already been discussed above. Family interventions are aimed at enhancing coping strategies by educating about the illness. Family therapy includes psychoeducational and behavioural components. Family therapy has been shown to reduce the risk of relapse, reduce family burden, and improve family members' understanding of and coping with schizophrenia.

Cognitive-Behavioural Interventions and Cognitive Remediation

There is evidence that Cognitive-Behavioural Therapy (CBT) can be effective for psychotic symptoms (48). The theory is that normal psychological processes can play an important role in specific psychotic symptoms. Cognitive behaviour therapy challenges the concept that there is a discontinuity between psychotic and normal thinking. The normal cognitive mechanisms that are already being used by the patients in areas that are not psychotic, can be used to help the patients deal with their psychotic beliefs. Delusional beliefs are not directly confronted. Studies have shown that CBT is somewhat effective in reducing hallucinations and delusions.

Cognitive remediation aims to train patients on specific neuropsychological tasks and has been demonstrated to be helpful.

Relapse Prevention and Improving Compliance

Medication continues to play a significant role in preventing relapse. Complementing this by CBT, early detection of signs of relapse, and treatment of any comorbid disorder especially substance abuse, and motivational interviewing can be very helpful. In motivational interviewing, patients are encouraged to review the advantages and disadvantages by taking or rejecting medication. Similarly, the comparison between short-term pleasure of street drugs and the serious harmful effects are discussed.

The main reasons of non-compliance are adverse side effects, lack of proper information, stigma, delusional beliefs and perceived lack of efficacy. Involving family members and other carers is very important.

Social Skills Training

The beneficial role of social skills training has been increasingly recognised (49). It is based upon behavioural and learning theory techniques.

Art and Vocational Rehabilitation

Sheltered workshops and supportive work therapies have been shown to improve the quality of life (50). Similarly, art activities not only involve patients in productive activities but also enhance self-esteem.

Schizotypal (Personality) Disorder

DSM-5 considers this disorder as part of schizophrenia spectrum of disorders, but is described in detail in personality disorder category. In ICD-10, it is not classified under personality disorders but separately as schizotypal disorder.

Schizophreniform Disorder

This is a syndrome similar to schizophrenia. It is distinguished from schizophrenia by its difference in duration: the total duration of the illness is at least one month but less than six months. The disorder is most common in adolescents and young adults and is less than half as common as schizophrenia. A lifetime prevalence rate of 0.2 percent and a 1-year prevalence rate of 0.1 percent have been reported.

Patients with schizophreniform disorder respond to antipsychotic treatment much more rapidly than do patients with schizophrenia. A trial of lithium has been recommended for treatment and prophylaxis if a patient has a recurrent episode. Electroconvulsive therapy may be helpful in patients with catatonic or depressive features. Many cases with this disorder progress to full-blown schizophrenia despite treatment.

Delusional Disorder

Delusional disorder is synonymous with paranoid psychoses and paranoid states. When delusional disorder occurs in late life, it is called paraphrenia.

It is a rare condition that differs from schizophrenia in that delusions dominate the clinical picture. The delusions are persistent and non-bizarre. The content of the delusion or delusions is specific and circumscribed (51). The hallucinations and thought disorder are usually absent (or nearly absent). Hallucinations, if present, are not prominent and are related to the delusional theme. If manic or depressive episodes occur, they are relatively brief to the duration of delusional beliefs. Personality is relatively intact and many patients continue to work or function socially. The DSM- criteria is that the duration of delusion(s) has to be at least one month whereas ICD-10 requires three months duration.

The subtypes of delusional disorder are persecutory, jealous, erotomanic, somatic, grandiose, mixed and unspecified. Management is often difficult. Among antipsychotics, there is some evidence for better efficacy with pimozide (52).

Induced Delusional Disorder

This is also called shared psychotic disorder and folie a deux. In this rare disorder, there is transfer of delusions from one person to another. Both persons live in close proximity one person chronically ill with the delusion and the other having a suggestible and passive personality. In most cases, the secondary person abandons the delusion when the pair is separated but this does not happen uniformly.

Brief Psychotic Disorder

This is a DSM-5 term. It involves the sudden onset of psychotic symptoms which lasts one day or more but less than a month. For diagnostic purposes, at least one major symptom of psychoses (delusions, hallucinations, disorganised speech) must be present. Emotional volatility, strange or bizarre behaviour, screaming or muteness, and impaired memory for recent events may be present. This is generally considered an uncommon disorder that occurs more often in young persons than older persons. It has a higher incidence in females and people with low socioeconomic status. Personality disorders are the most frequent comorbid disorders.

Antipsychotic drugs and benzodiazepines are used for treatment. There is full remission and the individual is able to resume his or her premorbid level of functioning. In ICD-10 it is classified under acute and transient psychotic disorders.

Schizoaffective Disorder

In this disorder, both affective and schizophrenic symptoms are prominent within the same episode of illness, preferably simultaneously or at least within a few days of each other.

According to ICD-10, the diagnosis should only be made when both schizophrenic and affective symptoms are equally prominent and present simultaneously, or within a few days of each other. ICD-10 further classifies schizoaffective disorder by whether the mood disturbance is depressive, manic or mixed.

It is important to differentiate schizoaffective disorder from post-schizophrenic depressive disorder. In the latter, patients with an established diagnosis of schizophrenia develop depressive symptoms after the acute psychotic symptoms have improved (but still present). The requirement is that depressive symptoms have to be present for at least two weeks.

Treatment of schizoaffective disorder usually consists of a combination of an antipsychotic and a mood stabiliser. These patients usually make a good recovery, especially those with manic rather than depressive symptoms.

REFERENCES

1. Kraeplin, E. (1919). *Dementia precox and paraphrenia* (trans. Barclay, R. M.). Edinburgh: Livingstone.
2. Bleuler, E. (1951). *Dementia or the group of schizophrenia* (trans. Zinken J.). London: Allen and Unwin.
3. Crow, T. J. (1980). Molecular pathology of schizophrenia: more than one disease process? *British Medical Journal*, 280, 66–68.
4. Liddle, P. F. (1987). The symptoms of chronic schizophrenia: a re-examination of the positive- negative dichotomy. *British Journal of Psychiatry*, 151, 145–151.
5. World Health Organisation. (1992). *ICD-10 Classifications of mental and behavioural Disorders* : Clinical descriptions and diagnostic guidelines. Geneva: World Health Organisation.
6. American Psychiatric Association.(2013). *Diagnostic and statistical manual of mental disorders* (5th Edition). Arlington, VA: American Psychiatric Publishing.
7. Susser,E.andWanderling,J.(1994). Epidemiology of nonaffective acute remitting psychosis vs schizophrenia. Sex and sociocultural setting. *Archives of General Psychiatry*,51, 294–301.
8. Dean, K. and Murray, R. (2008). *Lectures in schizophrenia.* London: Current Medicine Group.
9. Lewis, G., David, A., Andreasson, S., et al. (1992). Schizophrenia and city life. *The Lancet*, 340,137–140.
10. Pederson, C. B., Mortensen, P. B. (2001). Evidence of a dose–response relationship between urbanicity during upbringing and schizophrenia risk. *Archives of General Psychiatry*, 58, 1039–1046.
11. Kirkbridge, J. B., Morgon, C., Fearon, P., et al. (2007). Neighborhood level effects on psychosis: Re-examining the role of context. *Psychological Medicine*, 37, 1413–1425.
12. Fearfon, P., Kirkbridge, J. B., Morgan, C., et al. (2006). Incidence of schizophrenia and other psychosis in ethnic minority group: results from the MRC AESOP study. *Psychological Medicine*, 36, 1541–1550.
13. Sharpley, M., Hutchinson, G., mckenzie, K., et al. (2001). Understanding the excess of psychosis among the African-Caribbean population in England. Review of current hypothesis. *British Journal of Psychiatry*, 40, 60–68.
14. Lewis, S. W. and Buchanan, R. W. (2007). *Fast facts: Schizophrenia* (3rd Edition). Oxford: Health Press Limited.
15. Murray, R. M. and McGuffin, P. (1993). Genetic aspects of psychiatric disorders. In R. E. Kendell, A.K. Zealley (Eds.), *Companion to psychiatric studies* (5th Edition). Edinburgh: Churchill- Livingstone.
16. Kendler, K. S., McGuire, M., Gruenberg, A.M. and Walsh D. (1994). Clinical heterogeneity in schizophrenia and the pattern of psychopathology in relatives: results from an epidemiologically based family study. *Acta Psychiatrica Scandinavia*, 89, 294–300.
17. Sham, P. C., Jones, P., Russell, A., et al. (1994). Age at onset, sex, and familial psychiatric morbidity I schizophrenia. Camberwell collaborative psychosis study. *British Journal of Psychiatry*, 165, 466–473.
18. Gottesman, I. I., Shields, J. and Hanson, D. R. (1982). *Schizophrenia: The epigenetic puzzle.*Cambridge: Cambridge University Press.
19. Kety, S. S., Wendler, P. H., Jacobson, B., et al. (1994). Mental illness in the biological and adoptive relatives of schizophrenic adoptees. Replication of the Copenhagen study in the rest of Denmark. *Archives of General Psychiatry*, 51, 442–452.

20. Cannon, M., Jones, P. B., Murray, R. M. (2002). Obstetric complications and schizophrenia: historical and meta-analytic review. *American Journal of Psychiatry*, 159, 1080–1092.

21. McGrath, J. J. and Welham, L. (1999). Season of birth and schizophrenia: a systematic review and meta-analysis of data from the Southern Hemisphere. *Schizophrenia Research*, 35, 237–242.

22. Susser, E. S. and Lin, S. P. (1992). Schizophrenia after perinatal exposure to the Dutch Hunger Winter of 1944–1945. *Archives of General Psychiatry*, 49, 983–988.

23. Bebbington, P. and Kuipers, L. (1994). The predictive utility of expressed emotion in schizophrenia: an aggregate analysis. *Psychological Medicine*, 24(3), 707–718.

24. Vaughn, C. and Leff, J. (1976). The measurement of expressed emotion in the families of psychiatric patients. *British Journal of Clinical Psychology*, 2, 157–165.

25. Steinberg, H. R. and Durrell, J. (1968). A stressful social situation as a precipitant of schizophrenic symptoms: an epidemiological study. *British Journal of Psychiatry*, 114, 1097–1105.

26. Lewis, S. W. and Buchanan, R. W. (2007). *Fast facts: schizophrenia* (3rd Edition). Oxford: Health Press Limited.

27. Gray, J., Feldon, J. and Rawlins, J. (1991). The neuropsychology of schizophrenia. *Behavioural and Brain Sciences*, 14, 1–84.

28. Frith, C. (1996). Neuropsychology of schizophrenia, what are the implications of intellectual and experiential abnormalities for the neurobiology of schizophrenia? *British Medical Bulletin*, 52, 618–626.

29. Carlson, A., Waters, N. and Carlson, M. L. (1999). Neurotransmitter interactions in schizophrenia-therapeutic implications. *Biological Psychiatry*, 46, 1388–1395.

30. Wright, I. C., Rabe-Hesketh, S., Woodruff, P. W., et al. (2000). Meta-analysis of regional brain volumes in schizophrenia. *American Journal of Psychiatry*, 157, 16–25.

31. Ingvar, D. H. and Franzen, G. (1974). Abnormalities of cerebral blood flow distribution in patients with chronic schizophrenia. *Acta Psychiatrica Scandinavica*, 50, 425–462.

32. Lewis, S. W. and Buchanan, R. W. (2007). *Fast facts: schizophrenia* (3rd Edition). Oxford: Health Press Limited.

33. Gelder, M., Harrison, P. and Cowen, P. (2006). *Shorter Oxford textbook of psychiatry* (5th Edition). Oxford: Oxford University Press.

34. Wing, J. K. (1982). Course and prognosis of schizophrenia. In J. K. Wing and L. Wing (Eds.), *Handbook of psychiatry*. Cambridge: Cambridge University Press.

35. Robinson, D., Woerner, M. G., Alnir, J. M., et al. (1999). Predictors of relapse following response from a first episode of schizophrenia or schizoaffective disorder. *Archives of General Psychiatry*, 56, 241–247.

36. Wiersma, D., Isometsa, E. T., Henriksson, M. M., et al. (1997). Suicide and schizophrenia: a nationwide psychological autopsy study on age-and sex specific clinical characteristics of 92 suicide victims with schizophrenia. *American Journal of Psychiatry*, 154, 1235–1242.

37. Emsley, R. and Oosthizen, P. (2004). Evidence- based psychopharmacology of schizophrenia. *International Journal of Neuropsychopharmacology*, 7, 219–238.

38. Kane, J. M. and Marder, S. R. (1993). Psychopharmacological treatment of schizophrenia. *Schizophrenia Bulletin*, 19, 287–302.

39. Richelson, E. and Souder, T. (2000). Binding of antipsychotic drugs to human brain receptors- focus on new generation compounds. *Life Sciences*, 68, 29–39.

40. Loebel, A. D., Lieberman, J. A., Alvir, J. M., et al. (1992). Duration of psychosis and outcome in first episode schizophrenia. *American Journal of Psychiatry*, 149, 1183–1188.

41. Crow, T. J., Macmillan, J. F., Johnson, A. L. and Jonstone, E. C. (1986). A randomised controlled trial of prophylactic neuroleptic treatment. *British Journal of Psychiatry*, 148, 120–127.

42. Leucht, S., Pitschel-Walz, G., Abraham, D. and Kissling, W. (1999). Efficacy and extrapyramidal side effects of the new antipsychotics olanzapine, quetiapine, risperidone, and sertindole compared to conventional antipsychotics and placebo. A meta-analysis of randomised control trials. *Schizophrenia Research*, 35, 51–68.

43. Davis, J. M., Chen, N. and Glick, I. D. (2003). A meta-analysis of the efficacy of second- generation antipsychotics. *Archives of General Psychiatry*, 60(6), 553–564.

44. Kane, J., Honigfield, G., Singer, J. and Meltzer, H. (1988). Clozapine for the treatment-resistant schizophrenia. A double-blind comparison with chlorpromazine. *Archives of General Psychiatry*, 45, 789–796.

45. Wahlbeck, K., Cheine, M. and Essali, M. A. (2000). Clozapine versus typical neuroleptic medication for schizophrenia. *Cochrane Database of Systematic Reviews*, 2, CD000059.

46. Chanpattana, W. and Kramer, B. A. (2003). Acute and maintenance ECT with flupenthixol in refractory schizophrenia: sustained improvements in psychopathology, quality of life, and social outcomes. *Schizophrenia Research*, 63(1–2), 189–193.

47. Lauriello, J., Bustillo, J., Keith and S. J. (1999). A critical review of research on psychosocial treatment of schizophrenia. *Biological Psychiatry*, 46, 1409–1417.

48. Garety, P., Fowler, D. and Kuipers, E. (2000). Cognitive-behaviour therapy for medication resistant symptoms. *Schizophrenia Bulletin*, 26, 73–86.

49. Bustillo, J., Lauriello, J., Horan, W., et al. (2001). The psychosocial treatment of schizophrenia: an update. *American Journal of Psychiatry*, 158, 163–175.

50. Lehman, A. F., Goldberg, R., Dixon, L. B., et al. (2002). Improving employment outcomes for persons with severe mental illness. *Archives of General Psychiatry*, 59, 165–172.

51. David, A. S. (1997). Atypical Psychosis. In R. Murray, P. Hill, P. Mcguffin (Eds.), *The essentials of postgraduate psychiatry* (3rd Edition). Cambridge: Cambridge University Press.

52. Munro, A. (1999). *Delusional disorder.* Cambridge: Cambridge University Press.

Personality Disorders 07

Personality Disorders represent a major public health concern, as more than 1 in 10 adults in the community meet the diagnostic criteria for at least one PD. PD diagnoses are associated with increased risk for hospitalisation, criminal behaviour, suicidal behaviour, and dysfunction at work and in relationships. Relatively few evidence-based treatments are available for PDs, which are notoriously difficult to treat and interfere with the treatment of other kinds of disorders. The wide-ranging clinical importance of normative personality traits thought to predispose personality and other forms of psychopathology is also well-documented.

The subject of personality disorders has always remained one of the most controversial issues in psychiatry, as it is difficult to draw a dividing line between normal and disordered personality. The distinction between normal and abnormal personality is debatable as it mainly relies on an arbitrary cutoff point on the continuum between two extremes of a behaviour trait.

To demark precisely where, on a continuum, a normal personality becomes problematic and changes into a personality disorder, is not only a very difficult task but, as mentioned above, also an arbitrary distinction. However, functional impairment (in personal, social or occupational domains) is usually taken as a dividing line.

Personality is difficult to define but it usually refers to those aspects of a person's behaviour, thinking and emotional reactions, which are persistent and predictable throughout a wide range of circumstances and life situations. It comprises characteristics or qualities within an individual which includes mental, emotional, social, and physical aspects. Knowing the personality of a patient is important as it affects the prognosis, management and risk of developing many physical and mental disorders. Personality influences therapeutic alliance, compliance with treatment, and coping styles. Attributes of normal personality include correct self-perception, ability to adjust, autonomy, accurate reality testing and integration.

Personality traits are enduring features of personality that are heritable, linked to specific neurobiological structures and pathways, well-characterised in terms of content and course, valid for predicting a host of important life outcomes and amenable to reliable assessment, particularly via self-report question-naires. The Five-Factor Model (FFM) currently represents the most viable model of normative personality traits, having the advantage of decades of empirical evidence. In the FFM, five normally distributed traits represent the broadest level of variation in personality: neuroticism, extraversion, openness to experience, agreeableness, and conscientiousness. These traits provide a context for all human behaviour, and certain constellations of these traits make personality pathology in general and certain forms of PD more or less likely.

One researcher has proposed five diverse concepts of personality disorder: Personality disorder as a form of major mental illness (e.g., Schizotypal personality disorder which appears to be part of the schizophrenia spectrum); As a failure to develop certain important parts of the normal adult personality; As a particular form of personality structure (e.g., borderline personality organisation which has identity diffusion and primitive defences); As a social deviance; and as an abnormality in the statistical sense (1).

Both ICD-10 and DSM-5 utilise categorical approach, which implies qualitative differences between what is normal and abnormal and whether a disorder is present or absent. Although there is sufficient evidence that the categorical approach to measuring personality has less validity than the dimensional approach (2), the categorical model is simpler and is more amenable than the dimensional one, and is therefore more popular. However, the categorical and dimensional descriptions of personality disorder are not incompatible (3).

According to DSM-5, a personality disorder is an enduring pattern of inner experience and behaviour that deviates markedly from the expectations of the individual's culture, is pervasive and inflexible, has an onset in adolescence or early childhood, is stable over time and leads to distress or impairment. DSM- 5 further emphasises that only when personality traits (enduring patterns of perceiving, relating to, thinking about the environment and oneself that are exhibited in a wide range of social and personal contexts) are inflexible and maladaptive and cause significant functional impairment or subjective distress do they constitute personality disorders.

The diagnosis of personality disorder should not be made before 16 years of age. Some less well-defined personality disorders only become overt under conditions of stress. A personality disorder is only diagnosed when physical disorders of the brain have been excluded. There are other clinicians who consider that personality disorders are more than a social problem, that some treatment approaches are effective and that some symptoms of personality disorder improve with time. One of the most serious objections against the concept of personality disorder is that it has a derogatory implication (4). Sometimes people with personality disorders are deemed as responsible for their unwanted behaviours. There have been claims that the diagnosis of personality disorder has been used as a pejorative label for those patients whom clinicians do not like (5).

There can be no doubt that personality disorders cannot be ignored as they are a predisposing factors for many other psychiatric illnesses, including substance abuse disorders, suicide, mood disorders, impulse-control disorders, and anxiety disorders.

Personality disorders carry significant costs for healthcare services. About 80 percent of criminals, and alcohol and drug abusers have personality disorders.

A common misconception regarding personality disorders is that they are untreatable. This is not entirely true. However, as mentioned above, personality disorders are very difficult disorders to treat, because they involve well-established patterns of behaviours that are integral to a patient's self-image. Nevertheless, psychosocial and pharmacological treatments can produce clinically and socially meaningful changes. In personality disorders, even small improvements in functioning and reductions in symptomatology can be important.

ICD-10 and DSM-5 Classification of Personality Disorders

Both classificatory systems have similar general definitions of personality disorders. Both systems emphasise that the fundamental pathology lies in the interpersonal relationships, perception about self and others, and emotional dysregulation. The difficulties in these areas are consistent and pervasive and have detrimental effects on the individual's functioning in various domains of life.

ICD-10 defines personality disorder as deeply ingrained maladaptive patterns of behaviour generally recognisable by the time of adolescence or earlier and continuing throughout adult life. The personality is abnormal either in the balance of its components, their quality and expression or in its total aspect. Because of this deviance the patient suffers or others have to suffer and there is an adverse effect upon the individual or on society. The disturbance of personality and behaviour is profoundly deviant from the normal cultural patterns.

ICD-10 Diagnostic Guidelines

- Markedly disharmonious attitudes and behaviour
- Abnormal behaviour pattern is enduring/long-standing
- Abnormal behaviour pattern is pervasive and maladaptive to a broad range of personal and social situations
- Appear during childhood or adolescence and continue during adulthood
- Disorder leads to considerable personal distress
- Disorder is usually associated with significant problems in occupational and social performance

DSM-5 Diagnostic Criteria

a. An enduring pattern of inner experience and behaviour that deviates markedly from the expectations of the individual's culture. This pattern is manifested in two (or more) of the following areas:
   i. Cognition (i.e. ways of perceiving and interpreting the self, other people, and events)
   ii. Affectivity (i.e. the range, intensity, lability, and appropriateness of emotional response)
   iii. Interpersonal functioning
   iv. Impulse control

b. The enduring pattern is inflexible and pervasive across a broad range of personal and social situations.

c. The enduring pattern leads to clinically significant distress or impairment in social, occupational, or other important areas of functioning.

d. The pattern is stable and of long duration, and its onset can be traced back at least to adolescence or early adulthood.

e. The enduring pattern is not better explained as a manifestation or consequence of another mental disorder.

f. The enduring pattern is not attributable to the physiological effects of a substance (e.g., a drug of abuse, a medication) or another medical condition (e.g., head trauma).

It is important to attempt to classify the personality disorder into a specific subtype, after a general diagnosis of personality disorder has been made. It should also be borne in mind that the subtypes of personality disorders are not mutually exclusive and have some overlapping characteristics. Both ICD-10 and DSM-5 classifications have the same personality disorders subtypes except for some differences. ICD-10 does not have schizotypal and narcissistic personality disorders. However, it has a category of other specific personality disorders under which narcissistic, immature and passive-aggressive personality disorders are included.

DSM-5 has a category of borderline personality disorder whereas, the equivalent personality disorder in ICD-10 is an emotionally unstable personality disorder which is further subdivided into the impulsive type and the borderline type. ICD-10 has a category of mixed personality disorder which DSM-5 does not have. DSM-5 has the categories of other specified personality disorders and unspecified personality disorders. This category is provided for two situations:

1. The individual's personality pattern meets the general criteria for a personality disorder, and traits of several different personality disorders are present, but the criteria for any specific personality disorder are not met; or
2. The individual's personality pattern meets the general criteria for a personality disorder, but the individual is considered to have a personality disorder that is not included in the DSM-5 classification (e.g., passive-aggressive personality disorder).

Finally ICD-10 includes a category of 'enduring personality changes' in which the personality changes are regarded as being permanent following psychiatric illnesses or extremely stressful experiences (e.g., experiencing disaster, torture, or any life-threatening circumstances). This diagnosis should only be made if the personality changes have persisted for more than two years. This disorder may be difficult to differentiate from a chronic post-traumatic stress disorder and the latter may precede it. There is no such equivalent category in DSM-5, but it does include personality change due to a medical condition.

- Anankastic PD
- Obsessive-Compulsive PD
- Dependent PD
- Dependent PD

Preoccupation with unsubstantiated conspiratorial explanations of events.

- Anxious/avoidant PD
- Avoidant PD
- Schizoid personality disorder

a. The general criteria for personality disorder must be met.

b. DSM-5 further places personality disorders into three groups each sharing some clinical features.
   - Cluster A (having odd, aloof and eccentric features)

     Paranoid PD, Schizoid PD, and Schi-zotypal PD
   - Cluster B (having dramatic, impulsive and erratic features)

     Antisocial PD, Borderline PD, His-trionic PD, and Narcissistic PD
   - Cluster C (having anxiety features)

     Avoidant PD, Dependent PD, and Obsessive-Compulsive PD

For diagnosis of specific personality disorders clear evidence of at least three of the traits or behaviours mentioned in the ICD-10 diagnostic guidelines is required.

Paranoid Personality Disorder

a. The general criteria for personality disorder must be met.

b. At least four of the following must be present:
   - Tenacious sense of personal rights
   - Recurrent suspicions about sexual fidelity
   - Excessive self-importance
   - Few activities provide pleasure
   - Emotional coldness
   - Limited capacity to express feelings
   - Apparent indifference to praise or criticism
   - Little interest in sexual experiences
   - Preference for solitary activities
   - Excessive preoccupation with fantasy
   - Lack of close friends
   - Insensitivity to prevailing norms

Histrionic Personality Disorder

a. The general criteria for personality disorder must be met.

b. At least four of the following must be present:
   - Self-dramatisation
   - Suggestibility
   - Shallow and labile affect
   - Excitement seeking behaviour
   - Inappropriate seductiveness
   - Over-concern with physical attractiveness

Anankastic Personality Disorder

a. The general criteria for personality disorder must be met.

b. At least four of the following must be present:
   - Excessive doubt and caution
   - Preoccupation with details and rules
   - Perfectionism
   - Excessive conscientiousness
   - Excessive pedantry
   - Rigidity and stubbornness
   - Unreasonable insistence that others do things exactly
   - Intrusion of insistent thoughts

Anxious Personality Disorder

a. The general criteria for personality disorder must be met.

b. At least four of the following must be present:
   - Persistent and pervasive feelings of tension
   - Belief that one is inferior
   - Excessive preoccupation with criticism
   - Unwillingness to become involved with people
   - Restriction in lifestyle
   - Avoidance of social or occupational activities

Dependent Personality Disorder

a. The general criteria for personality disorder must be met.

b. At least four of the following must be present:
   - Allowing others to make important decisions
   - Subordination of one's own needs to those of others
   - Unwillingness to make reasonable demands
   - Feeling helpless when alone
   - Fears of being abandoned
   - Limited capacity to make everyday decisions

Dissocial Personality Disorder

a. The general criteria for personality disorder must be met.
b. At least three of the following must be present:
   - Callous unconcern for the feelings of others
   - Disregard for social norms
   - Incapacity to form enduring relationships
   - Very low tolerance to frustrations
   - Incapacity to experience guilt or profit from experience
   - Marked proneness to blame others

Emotionally Unstable Personality Disorder

There are two sub types:

Impulsive Type

a. The general criteria for personality disorder must be met
b. At least three of the following must be present, one of which must be the first one:
   - Marked tendency for quarrelsome behaviour and conflicts with others
   - Marked tendency to act unexpectedly and without consideration of the consequences
   - Liability to outbursts of anger and violence
   - Difficulty in maintaining any course of action that offers no immediate reward
   - Unstable mood

Borderline Type

a. The general criteria for personality disorder must be met.
b. At least three of the symptoms mentioned in criterion B for impulsive type must be present. In addition at least two of the following are required:
   - Uncertainty about self-image, aims and internal preferences
   - Excessive efforts to avoid abandonment
   - Chronic feelings of emptiness
   - Intense and unstable relationships
   - Series of suicidal threats /acts of selfharm

Schizotypal Personality Disorder

a. There is a pervasive pattern of social and interpersonal deficits marked by acute discomfort with, and reduced capacity for, close relationship as well as by cognitive or perceptual distortions and eccentricities of behaviour beginning by early adulthood. These are manifested in at least five of the following contexts:
b. At least four of the following:
   - Ideas of reference
   - Odd or magical beliefs
   - Unusual perceptual experiences
   - Odd thinking
   - Suspiciousness
   - Restricted and inappropriate affect
   - Eccentric behaviour or appearance
   - No confidants
   - High levels of social anxiety with paranoid fear

Narcissistic Personality Disorder

The hallmarks of narcissistic personality disorder are a pervasive sense of grandiosity (in fantasy or behaviour), need for admiration, lack of empathy, and chronic intense envy. At least five of the following features are required:

- Grandiose sense of self-importance
- Fantasies of success, power, and beauty
- Belief that one is special and unique
- Need for excessive admiration
- Sense of entitlement i.e. unreasonable expectations of especially favourable treatment or automatic compliance with expectations
- Interpersonally exploitative
- Lack of empathy
- Envious of others
- Arrogant behaviour

Mixed Personality Disorder

In this category, the personality disorders and abnormalities are quite troublesome but do not clearly demonstrate the specific patterns of symptoms that characterise any specific personality disorder. Because of lack of predominant set of symptoms, this personality disorder cannot be categorised as one of the other personality disorders.

Psychopathy, Severe Personality Disorder, and Dangerously Severe Personality Disorder

Although the term psychopathy is quite popular, neither the ICD-10 or DSM-5 have this term or psychopathic personality disorder. Similarly, severe personality disorder or dangerously severe personality disorder are not clinical categories in these classification systems.

Psychopathy generally implies a very cold, detached, remorseless, manipulative and controlling interpersonal style. According to one operational definition (6) psychopathy is a set of core traits that are narrower than DSM-5 antisocial personality disorder or ICD-10 dissocial personality disorder.

A four factor model of psychopathy has been proposed (7): interpersonal, affective, lifestyle and antisocial behaviour facets. Although most psychopathic traits mirror the dissocial dimension, there are many psychopathic individuals who also meet the criteria for narcissistic, histrionic, paranoid and borderline personality disorder.

There is no agreed definition of severe personality disorder, and severity is generally defined by the extent of the pathology of personality disorder. This and the dangerously severe personality disorder pose a risk to the public, and are usually managed by the criminal justice system.

Epidemiology

Due to the problems and controversies with the concept and classification of personality disorders, epidemiological studies have been limited.

Personality disorders are more likely to be present in the lower social class, unstable and disadvantaged communities, urban and prison population. One study has reported the prevalence of personality disorder among prisoners as 78% (8). In primary care, prevalence rates of a personality disorder range from 13% to 30%, depending partially on the methods employed (9). Some studies have suggested prevalence of 10% in the community (10). A more recent study claims prevalence up to 11% (11). Another study (after adjusting for gender, age, social class and marital status) reported association between cluster B personality disorders and functional psychosis, affective disorders, anxiety disorders and alcohol dependence. Association was also demonstrated between cluster C personality disorders and affective and anxiety disorders. There was no association between cluster A personality disorders and psychiatric illnesses (12).

One classical study demonstrates that antisocial behaviour as a child is associated with similar behaviour in adulthood (13). There is an association of childhood abuse and Borderline Personality Disorder (BPD). 70% of BPD have been sexually abused and long-term studies have found that about 10% of BPD patients commit suicide (14). BPD patients also seem to have a higher rate of deaths from natural causes as compared to the general population. Antisocial personality disorder is diagnosed more frequently in males, whereas borderline, histrionic and dependent personality disorders are diagnosed more frequently in females.

Aetiology

Genetics, neurobiological and psychological factors have been implicated in the aetiology of personality disorders. There is now no doubt about the genetic contribution in the development of a normal personality. According to two studies, the heritability rates for normal personality traits range from 30% to 60% (15), (16). The heritable role has been found in all personality disorders in Clusters A, B, and C.

Studies have found neurobiological factors in antisocial personality disorder, borderline personality disorder and schizotypal personality disorder. Low levels of serotonin have been found in individuals with impulsive aggression. Low levels of cortisol and high testosterone are found in psychopathic individuals (17). Another study has demonstrated structural and functional abnormalities in the amygdala and orbitofrontal regions (18). In borderline personality disorder, abnormalities in the serotonin system and opiate pathways have been demonstrated (19).

Most clinicians agree that an individual's experience is significant in the development of a personality disorder. There is also agreement that there are causal links between childhood experiences, personality, and personality disorders. Risk factors for personality disorders include childhood abuse, neglect, problematic attachment to parents (especially mother), and adverse school experiences (20).

Assessment

Assessment of personality disorder should be based on as many sources of information as possible. More than one interview is very desirable, if not essential, for diagnosing a personality disorder. Emphasis should be given on details regarding relationships development and interpersonal difficulties. The diagnosis requires an evaluation of the individual's long-term patterns of functioning, and the particular personality features must be evident by early adulthood. It is essential to assess the stability of personality traits over time and across different situations. According to DSM-5, for a personality disorder to be diagnosed in an individual younger than 18 years, the features must have been present for at least 1 year. However, antisocial personality disorder cannot be diagnosed in those under 18 years.

Unstructured clinical assessments may be unreliable as many clinicians tend to under or over diagnose personality disorders. Structured or semi-structured interviews are, therefore, recommended. Millon Clinical Multiaxial Inventory (MCMI-III) is the most widely used personality disorders inventory. The inventory is intended exclusively for subjects believed to possess a personality disorder and should not be used with normals. Some other scales are: International Personality Disorders Examination, Personality Assessment Schedule (PAS), Revised Diagnostic Interview for Borderlines (DIB-R), Diagnostic Interview for Narcissism, Psychopathy Check List Revised (PCL-R) and Dimensional Assessment of Personality Pathology (21).

Treatment of Personality Disorders

Management of personality disorders is particularly challenging. Containment of disruptive behaviours, enhancing the safety of the patient as well as others, and treatment of additional psychiatric illnesses forms a major part of management strategies. Other aims of treatment include reducing subjective distress of patients and improving their relationships and social skills.

It has been observed that the subjective distress and social disability of some people with personality problems tend to improve with age. Many people with personality disorders (especially those with paranoid, schizoid and antisocial personality disorders) do not regard their lifestyles as abnormal and hence do not perceive the need for treatment. Their problems bother other people rather than themselves. Help is, however, subsequently sought when their maladaptive behaviours result in serious occupational, personal or social problems or when there are secondary anxiety, depression, substance abuse, or eating disorders.

Most patients with borderline and anxious personality disorder actively seek treatment. Although some psychiatrists believe that personality disorders are not treatable, various treatments, including pharmacological, psychoanalytic, cognitive, cognitive-analytic, dialectical behaviour therapy, emotional regulation therapy (e.g., anger management), and therapeutic communities have been advocated.

Although the evidence is not substantial, some psychotherapeutic techniques have been shown to be effective (22). As long-standing maladaptive traits are difficult to change, so it is realistic to expect some changes rather than a complete change of character.

General Issues and Measures

Much of the research regarding the management of personality disorders has been done with borderline personality disorder and antisocial personality disorders, but many of the findings may be applied to other personality disorders.

A trusting and confiding relationship (but not of dependency), is the basis of treatment, although this will not be possible with all patients and at all times. Not infrequently, patients (especially with borderline personality disorder) would sabotage the therapeutic relationship. A very conspicuous and common feature of all personality disorders is the self-defeating nature of the maladaptive traits.

It helps to do a functional analysis by looking into the abnormal personality features regarding the thoughts, feelings, behaviour, and interference in occupational, social and family relations. Patients should be involved in planning their care, and reasons for particular rules and professional boundaries should be clearly explained. They should be discouraged to have less contact with situations that provoke problems, and opportunities be provided to enhance their strengths and assets.

Personality disorder patients have to be dealt with consistently as they are notorious to cause splitting among various mental health professionals. It is important to identify clearly the roles and responsibilities of all health and social care professionals. The need for very clear and prompt communication between all the professionals involved, and a shared formulation of the case, cannot be overstated.

Short-term treatment aims as well as long- term realistic goals (such as employment) should be specified. A comprehensive crises plan that identifies potential triggers of the disruptive behaviour needs to be formulated. Self-help management strategies are very helpful.

In order to manage a crisis, maintaining a calm and non-threatening attitude and effort to understand the crisis from the patient's point of view would be helpful. Exploring the patient's reasons for acute distress and using empathic statements (including validating statements) are also helpful. As already mentioned, treating comorbid disorders is essential, and giving practical support for issues like housing, finance and childcare is beneficial. Teaching skills to deal with specific areas like anger control, self-harm ideas and, social relations is also very helpful. It needs to be emphasised that in- patient admission, although structured, goal determined and short, is sometimes needed, and it is not desirable that some patients with personality disorder are permanently banned from hospital admission. Indication for brief admission include, imminent risks to self or others, and transient psychotic episodes. Severe suicidality, non-adherence to community programmes, and treatment of comorbid disorder (e.g., major depressive episode) would be some of the reasons for longer admissions.

Psychological Treatment of Personality Disorders

Due to the inherent difficulty in research in psychotherapy and especially in personality disorders, there is an understandable paucity of randomised controlled trials regarding psychotherapeutic techniques in personality disorders. Most randomised trials have, however, been done in borderline personality disorder or mixed personality disorders (23). Both dynamic psychotherapy and schema-focused cognitive therapy have demonstrated improvement in the underlying personality disturbance (24). Cognitive Behavioural Therapy (CBT) has shown more improvement as compared to psychodynamic therapy (25). CBT has also shown to be beneficial in reducing aggression in antisocial personality disorder (26). Dialectical behavioural therapy has been successfully tried with borderline personality disorders (27). Transference–focused therapy in combination with medication has been tried with success to reduce suicidal behaviour and anxiety in borderline personality disorders (28).

Pharmacological Treatment of Personality Disorders

Just like psychotherapy, there are not many randomised controlled trials for drug treatment in personality disorder population. Some authors, in fact, argue that improvement in some cases could be attributed to the response of other coexisting mental illnesses. Although it is true that psychotropic drugs may change the mental state, they rarely induce changes in the internalized self-concepts of people with personality disorders (which are more responsive to psychological interventions). There is, however, increasing evidence that pharmacotherapy is an appropriate treatment, and will be at least as important as psychotherapy in the treatment of personality disorders (29). Pharmacotherapy is either casual, aimed at correcting neurobiological dispositions which underly deviant behaviour, or it is symptomatic, and treats target behaviours and symptoms. Drug therapy is not categorised for specific personality disorders. The main reason is that the efficacy of the drugs have been evaluated on a symptom level rather than at the syndrome level. Moreover, the target symptoms that respond to a particular drug are not unique to any specific personality disorder.

Antipsychotics reduce impulsiveness and aggression. SSRIs (in high doses) may also improve impulsivity and hostility. Lithium has a proven role in suicidality reduction, and it does this by possibly reducing the impulsivity. It may also, like some anticonvulsants, help with impulsive aggression. Lamotrigine (30) and valproic acid (31), are effective in reducing aggression, anger, hostility and interpersonal sensitivity in borderline personality disorders.

Small doses of neuroleptic medication have an important role in the management of borderline and schizotypal personality disorders. One study reported improvement with small doses of Olanzapine (2.5 mg) in affect, impulsivity and interpersonal relationships in patients with borderline personality patients (32). According to another study, small doses of risperidone (1 mg–2 mg) are effective in schizotypal personality disorder.

REFERENCES

1. Livesley, J. (2001). *Handbook of personality disorders: theory, research and treatment.* New York: Guildford Press.
2. Livesley, W. J., Schroeder, M. L., Jackson, D. Et al. (1994). Categorical distinction in the study of personality disorders: implications for classification. *Journal of Abnormal Psychology*, 103, 6–17.
3. Widiger, T. A. and Frances, A. J. (1994). Toward a dimensional model for the personality disorders. In P. T. Costa and T. A. Widiger (Eds), *Personality disorders and the five factor model of personality.* Washington DC: American Psychological Association.
4. Gunn, J and Robertson, G. (1976). Psychopathic personality: A conceptual problem. *Psychological Medicine*, 6, 631–634.
5. Lewis, G. and Appleby, L. (1988). Personality disorder: The patients' psychiatrists dislike. *British Journal of Psychiatry*, 153, 44–49.
6. Hare, R. D. (1991). *The Hare Psychopathy Checklist-Revised manual.* Toronto: Multi-Health Systems.
7. Hare, R. D. (2004). *The Hare Psychopathy Checklist-Revised manual* (2nd Edition). Toronto: Multi-Health Systems.
8. Singleton, N., Meltzer, H., Gatwood, R., et al. (1998). *Psychiatric morbidity among prisoners in England and Wales.* London: Office for National Statistics.
9. Moran, P., Jenkins, R., Tylee, A., et al. (2000). The prevalence of personality disorder among UK primary care attenders. *Acta Psychiatria. Scandanvia*, 102, 52–57.
10. Reich, J. H., Yates, W. and Nduaguba, M. (1989). Prevalence of DSM III personality disorders in the community. *Social Psychiatry*, 24, 12–16.
11. Lenzenweger, M. F. (2008). Epidemiology of personality disorders. *Psychiatric Clinics of North America*, 31, 395–403.
12. Coid, J., Tyrer, P. and Roberts, A. (2006). Prevalence and correlates of personality disorder in Great Britain. *British Journal of Psychiatry*, 188, 423–431.
13. Robins, L. N. (1966). Deviant children grown up: *A sociological and psychiatric study of sociopathic personality.* Baltimore: Williams and Wilkins.
14. Paris, J. and Zweig-Frank, H. (2001). The 27 year follow-up of patients with borderline personality disorder. *Comprehensive Psychiatry*, 42, 482–487.
15. Plomin, R., Owen, M. J. and mcguffin, P. (1994). The genetic basis of complex human behaviours. *Science*, 264, 1733–1739.
16. Bouchard Jr, T. J. and Loehlin, J. C. (2001). Genes, evolution, and personality. *Behavioural Genetics,* 31, 243–273.
17. Glenn, A. L. and Raine, A. (2008). The neurobiology of psychopathy. *Psychiatric Clinics of North America*, 31, 463–476.
18. Kiehl, K. A. (2006). A cognitive neuroscience perspective on psychopathy. Evidence for paralimbicsystem dysfunction. *Psychiatry Research*, 1442, 107–128.
19. New, A. S., Goodwin, M., Triebwasser, J., et al. (2008). Recent advances in the biological study of personality disorder. *Psychiatric Clinics of North America*, 31, 441–461.
20. Cohen, P., Crawford, T. N., Johnson, J. G., et al. (2005). The children in the community study of developmental course of personality disorder. *Journal of Personality Disorders*, 19, 466–486.
21. Livesley, W. J. (2007). A Framework for Integrating Dimensional and Categorical Classifications of Personality Disorder. *Journal of Personality Disorders*, 21, 199–224.
22. Bateman, A. W. and Tyrer, P. (2004). Psychological treatments for personality disorders. *Advances in Psychiatric Treatment*. 10, 378–388.
23. Duggan, C, Huband, N., Smailagic, N., et al. (2007). The use of psychological treatments for people with personality disorder: A systematic review of randomised control trials. *Personality and Mental Health*, 1, 95–125.
24. Beck, A. T. and Freeman, A. (1990). *Cognitive therapy and personality disorders.* New York: Guildford Press.
25. Giesson-Bloo, J., van Dyck, R., Spinhoven, P., et al. (2006). Outpatient psychotherapy for borderline personality disorder: Randomised trial of schema-focused therapy vs transference- focused therapy. *Archives of General Psychiatry*, 63, 649–658.
26. Davidson, K., Tyrer, P. and Tata, D. (2009).Cognitive Behaviour Therapy for violent men with antisocial personality disorder in the community. An exploratory randomised controlled trial. *Psychological Medicine*, 39, 569–578.
27. Linehan, M. M., Comtois, K. A., Murray, A. M., Brown, M. Z., Gallop, R. J., Heard, H. L., et al. (2006). Two-year randomised control trial and follow-up of dialectic behaviour therapy vs therapy by experts for suicidal behaviours and borderline personality disorder. *Archives of General Psychiatry*, 63(7), 757–766.
28. Levy, K. N., Clarkin, J. F., Yeomans, F. E., et al. (2006). The mechanisms of change in the treatment of borderline personality disorder with transference-focused psychotherapy. *Journal of Clinical Psychology*, 62, 481–501.
29. Sadock, B. J. and Sadock, V. A. (2007). *Kaplan and Sadock's Synopsis of psychiatry*: Behavioural sciences/ clinical psychiatry (10th Edition). Philadelphia: Lippincott Williams and Wilkins.
30. Pinto, O. C. and Akiskal, H. S. (1998). Lamotrigine as a promising approach to borderline personality disorder: An open case series without concurrent DSM-IV major mood disorder. *Journal of Affective Disorders*, 51, 333–343.
31. Frankenberg, F. R. and Zanarini, M. C. (2002).Divalproex sodium treatment of women with borderline personality disorder: a double blind placebo controlled study. *Journal of Clinical Psychiatry*, 63, 442–446.
32. Zanarini, M. C. and Frankenberg, F. R. (2001). Olanzapine treatment of female borderline personality disorder patients. A double blind placebo controlled pilot study. *Journal of Clinical Psychiatry*, 62, 849–854.

CHAPTER

08 Alcohol and Drug Dependence

People take drugs for many reasons. They can produce a so-called rush of pleasurable sensations, which is a dramatic and memorable experience. Sometimes drugs are taken because of peer pressure or stress. Related to the latter, drugs are sometimes used to self-medicate unpleasant feelings such as pain, anxiety, or depression. When addicted, users may take drugs to avoid the negative symptoms of withdrawal.

The terms addict and addiction should preferably be avoided as these have negative connotations. In addition, these terms also tend to minimise or ignore the concept of substance abuse as a medical disorder.

According to a number of clinical and epidemiological studies, substance abuse especially alcoholism, is among the most prevalent psychiatric disorders in most Western countries (1). It is extremely important to manage alcohol and drug dependence problems effectively, as a high prevalence of psychiatric disorders is found among people having drug dependence. Such comorbidity makes the management difficult and the prognosis poorer. Some studies have shown that up to 50 percent of patients having drug dependence also have a comorbid psychiatric disorder (2).

Substance abuse is a maladaptive pattern of substance use leading to significant adverse consequences manifested by psychosocial, medical, or legal problems or use in situations in which it is physically hazardous that must recur during a 12-month period (3). A drug of abuse is any substance, taken through any route of administration, that alters the mood, the level of perception, or brain functioning (4). This can be prescribed or non-prescribed medication. Misuse is similar to abuse, but usually applies to drugs prescribed by physicians that are not used properly.

Dependence is a more reliable and apparently valid diagnosis than abuse. Dependence indicates a central role that the substance plays in an individual's life. It indicates the problems relating to controlling the intake of the drug, and development of difficulties, despite which the individual continues to take the substance. It connotes a psychological and /or physical need for the drug (5). When the individual is psychologically dependent, he or she feels as if the drug is required in order to reach a maximum level of functioning or well-being. When the drug has adapted physiologically to the chronic use of the drug, it is called physical dependence.

Tolerance is a phenomenon in which, after repeated administration, a given dose of drug produces a decreased effect, or increasingly larger dose are needed to obtain the effect observed with the original dose.

Reverse tolerance, also known as sensitisation, occurs when an effect of a drug increases with repeated administration. Reverse tolerance occurs less frequently than tolerance and happens only with particular effects of certain drugs. The phenomenon of reverse tolerance is not fully understood.

Cross-tolerance refers to the ability of one drug to be substituted for another, each usually producing the same physiological and psychological effect (e.g., diazepam and barbiturates). Withdrawal is a syndrome that occurs after stopping or reducing the amount of the specific drug or substance that has been used regularly over a prolonged period of time. The syndrome is characterised by physiological signs and symptoms in addition to psychological changes, such as disturbances in thinking, feeling, and behaviour. It is also called abstinence syndrome or discontinuation syndrome.

The term intoxication is used for a reversible non-dependent experience with a substance that affects one or more of the following mental functions: memory, orientation, mood, judgment, behavioural, social, or occupational functioning.

The essential feature of a substance use disorder is a cluster of cognitive, behavioural, and physiological symptoms indicating that the individual continues using the substance despite significant substance-related problems. Overall the diagnosis of a substance use disorder includes impaired control, social impairment, risky use and pharmacological implications.

The individual may take the substance in larger amounts or over a longer period, may express a persistent desire to cut down and may report multiple unsuccessful efforts to decrease or discontinue use. The individual may spend a great deal of time obtaining the substance and all of the individual's daily activities revolve around the substance. Craving is manifested by an intense desire or urge for the drug. Social impairment is the second grouping of criteria. The individual may continue substance use despite having persistent or recurrent social or interpersonal problems caused or exacerbated by the effects of the substance.

Risky use of the substance is the third grouping of criteria. The individual may continue substance use despite knowledge of having a persistent or recurrent physical or psychological problem that is likely to have been caused or exacerbated by the substance.

Pharmacological criteria are the final grouping. This includes tolerance and withdrawal. Tolerance is signalled by requiring a markedly increased dose of the substance to achieve the desired effect or a markedly reduced effect when the usual dose is consumed. The degree to which tolerance develops varies greatly across different individuals as well as across substances (6).

The following conditions are classified as substance-induced: intoxication, withdrawal, and other substance/medication-induced mental disorders (psychotic disorders, bipolar and related disorders, depressive disorders, anxiety disorders, obsessive-compulsive and related disorders, sleep disorders, sexual dysfunctions, delirium, and neurocognitive disorders) (7).

Aetiology of Drug Dependence

Although the cause of substance dependence is multi-factorial and depends on a variety of genetic, psychological and social factors, all drugs that are taken in excess have in common direct activation of the brain reward system. Debate continues on whether substance dependence is a brain disorder. Those who consider substance dependence as a brain disorder put forward the argument that there are changes in the structure and neurochemistry of the brain of the drug user. Others insist that these brain changes are not necessary, and they are also insufficient to explain drug dependence behaviour (8). The major neurotransmitters possibly involved in developing substance abuse and substance dependence are the opioid, dopamine, and GABA.

Although there is some role of genetic factors (especially in alcohol abuse), the learning and conditioning theory is widely accepted. There is little doubt that drug use is maintained and reinforced by its (rewarding) consequences e.g. alleviation of pain, anxiety, or depression. Each episode of use of the substance results in rapid positive reinforcement. Drug availability, social acceptability, peer pressures and antisocial personality disorder are significant contributory factors. As compared to the general population, patients with substance dependence come from disturbed family backgrounds and have deviant personalities.

Alcohol-Related Disabilities and Disorders

Even though alcohol is used in many different situations, it is important to remember that alcohol is a drug — one that can prove addictive and that alters the way the brain functions.

Alcohol is defined as a colourless liquid obtained either synthetically or naturally, through the fermentation of certain carbohydrates (that is, the transformation of carbohydrates to alcohol by means of enzyme activity). The colourless liquid the one that is used in beer, wine, and other alcoholic beverages — is known as ethyl alcohol or ethanol. It is created when yeast spores cause sugars to ferment. Alcohol is most often created when fruits, grains, or vegetables are fermented. Yeast or bacteria affect the sugars in the grain, fruit, or vegetable, causing them to change chemically into alcohol.

The amount of alcohol a drink contains depends on many factors: the type of yeast used, the amount and type of sugar used, and the temperature during the process of fermentation. Different combinations produce different beverages, which contain different concentrations of alcohol. Of the three basic types of alcoholic drinks—beer, wine, and liquor—each has a different alcohol content.

Even though alcoholic beverages contain different amounts of alcohol, this does not mean that one is more dangerous or addictive than another. Distilled spirits are not somehow "worse" than beer or wine. One can become addicted to alcohol no matter how it is packaged.

Many people drink because alcohol makes them feel relaxed or happy. But alcohol is not a stimulant. It is a depressant, and it has a depressant effect on the brain's functioning. Consumption of alcohol can injure brain tissue and interfere with the parts of the brain that control memories, emotions, and thinking

There is significant variability in drinking patterns among individuals, and unfortunately, there is no universally accepted distinction between 'social drinking' and 'harmful drinking'. Guidelines regarding alcohol consumption vary in different countries. It is clear, however, that as average alcohol consumption and frequency of intoxication increase, so does the incidence of medical and psychosocial problems. Other factors like age, gender, culture, and genetics also contribute to the adverse and harmful effects of alcohol.

As alcohol causes dopamine release in the nucleus accumbens, when it is stopped, dopamine falls below normal, apparently resulting in subsequent depressed mood which is associated with early withdrawal. Alcohol also acts through GABA and excitatory amino acid receptors.

Alcohol precipitates numerous psychological symptoms as a result of intoxication, withdrawal and dependence. Moreover, there are many medical complications and cognitive impairments. The most conspicuous group of people affected by alcohol problems are those who have developed a syndrome of alcohol dependence. Other alcohol-related disorders include alcohol intoxication, alcohol withdrawal, alcohol-induced persistent amnestic disorder, alcohol-induced persistent dementia, alcohol-induced mood disorder, alcohol-induced anxiety disorder, alcohol-induced psychotic disorder, alcohol-induced sexual dysfunction disorder and alcohol-induced sleep disorder. There are other people who experience problems with their drinking. These individuals are termed as alcohol abusers, problem drinkers or harmful drinkers. If the individual has ever met the criteria for alcohol dependence, a diagnosis of abuse is not made. Many persons use alcohol for its efficacy in alleviating anxiety. About 25 to 50 percent of all persons with alcohol-related disorders also meet the diagnostic criteria for an anxiety disorder.

Alcohol use is associated with a decrease in rapid eye movement sleep (REM or dream sleep) and deep sleep (stage 4) and more sleep fragmentation, with more and longer episodes of awakening. Therefore, the idea that drinking alcohol helps persons fall asleep is a myth (9). The Mean Corpuscular Volume (MCV) is high in about 60 percent, more so in women than in men. Other laboratory test values that may be high in association with alcohol abuse are those of uric acid, triglycerides, aspartate aminotransferase (AST), and alanine aminotransferase (ALT). The interaction between alcohol and other substances can be dangerous, even fatal. Certain substances, such as alcohol and phenobarbital, are metabolised by the liver, and their prolonged use can lead to acceleration of their metabolism.

The effects of alcohol and other Central Nervous System (CNS) depressants are usually synergistic. Sedatives, hypnotics, and drugs that relieve pain, motion sickness, head colds, and allergy symptoms must be used with caution by persons with alcohol-related disorders. Because sedatives and other psychotropic drugs can potentiate the effects of alcohol, patients should be instructed about the dangers of combining CNS depressants and alcohol, particularly when they are driving or operating machinery.

As already mentioned there can be numerous neurological and medical complications as a result of alcohol use. These are listed below:

- Cerebellar degeneration
- Peripheral neuropathy
- Optic neuropathy
- Pellagra
- Central pontine myelinolysis
- Marchiafava-Bignami disease
- Fetal alcohol syndrome
- Myopathy
- Alcoholic cerebral atrophy
- Liver disease
- Hepatic encephalopathy
- Acquired (non-Wilsonian) chronic hepatocerebral degeneration
- Malabsorption
- Pancreatic encephalopathy
- Cardiomyopathy
- Arrhythmias
- Hypertension leading to cerebrovascular disease
- Anaemia
- Leukopaenia
- Thrombocytopaenia
- Hypothermia and hyperthermia
- Hypotension and hypertension
- Respiratory depression and associated hypoxia

Alcohol Dependence Syndrome

The alcohol dependence syndrome has the following main features (10):

1. Narrowing of the repertoire of drinking behaviour
2. Salience of drinking over other activities
3. Increased tolerance to alcohol
4. Repeated withdrawal symptoms
5. Repeated relief or avoidance of withdrawal symptoms by further drinking
6. Subjective awareness of a compulsion to drink
7. Reinstatement of the syndrome after abstinence

The rate of alcohol dependence varies in different countries. In UK it is 2% in women and 6% in men (11). Severity of Alcohol Dependence Questionnaire, is a short and self-rated instrument with reasonable validity which can be used to measure the severity of dependence (12). The psychiatric diagnoses most commonly associated with alcohol dependence are other substance-related disorders, antisocial personality disorder, mood disorders, and anxiety disorders.

About 30 to 40 percent of persons with an alcohol dependence suffer from major depressive disorder. Depression is more common in women than in men with these disorders. The association between alcohol and suicide is well-established. Persons with alcohol dependence and major depressive disorder are at a great risk for attempting suicide and are likely to have other substance-related disorder diagnoses.

Alcohol intoxication is characterised by behavioural, cognitive, and physiological symptoms. Symptoms of alcohol intoxication develop soon after consumption and include slurred speech, impaired coordination and balance, memory and attention problems, poor judgment, and, in severe cases, stupor or coma. Blackouts are sometimes experienced during intoxication and are characterised by amnesia for the period of intoxication. Blackouts are thought to occur when intoxication occurs rapidly, and amnesia resolves as intoxication abates.

Pathological Jealousy

People who misuse alcohol, sometimes develop delusions of jealousy. This carries a very high risk of physical violence towards the partner and in some cases separation may be indicated on urgent basis. Factors like ongoing conflicts and the partner's neglectful behaviour as a consequence of the alcohol abuse, and patients own feelings of inadequacy may further fuel the volatile situation. Sometimes pathological jealousy is a part of schizophrenic illness.

Alcohol Withdrawal Syndrome

The DSM-5 criteria for alcohol withdrawal require the cessation or reduction of alcohol use that was heavy and prolonged as well as the presence of specific physical or neuropsychiatric symptoms (autonomic hyperactivity, increased hand tremor, insomnia, nausea or vomiting, transient hallucinations, psychomotor agitation, anxiety, and generalised tonic-clonic seizures). Two or more of these symptoms are required. In addition, the criteria state that these symptoms cause significant distress or impairment in social or occupational functioning. Finally, these symptoms should not be due to another medical condition or explained by another mental disorder, including intoxication or withdrawal from another substance.

Alcohol withdrawal can be of three types: mild or simple withdrawal, alcoholic hallucinosis, or a much more severe withdrawal state called Delirium Tremens (DTs). The severity of the withdrawal symptoms reflect the quantity and duration of alcohol use, as well as the pattern of recent use.

Alcohol withdrawal, even without delirium, can be serious; it can include seizures and autonomic hyperactivity. Conditions that may predispose to, or aggravate, withdrawal symptoms include fatigue, malnutrition, medical disorders, and depressive disorder.

The hallmark of alcohol withdrawal is tremulousness, commonly called the shakes or jitters, and typically occurs in the upper limbs. The range of withdrawal symptoms is, however, quite wide and can include psychotic symptoms like delusions, hallucinations, and seizures. The withdrawal can progress to symptoms of delirium tremens. Tremors occur 6 to 8 hours after the cessation of drinking, the psychotic and perceptual symptoms begin in 8 to 12 hours, seizures in 12 to 24 hours, and DTS during 72 hours. It is imperative to remember that the syndrome of withdrawal can at times skip the usual progression and can go directly to DTs.

The tremor of alcohol withdrawal can be similar to either physiological tremor, with a continuous tremor of great amplitude and of more than 8 Hz, or familial tremor, with bursts of tremor activity slower than 8 Hz. Other symptoms of withdrawal include general irritability, gastrointestinal symptoms (e.g., nausea and vomiting), and sympathetic autonomic hyperactivity, including anxiety, arousal, sweating, facial flushing, mydriasis, tachycardia, and mild hypertension. Patients experiencing alcohol withdrawal are generally alert but may startle easily.

Seizures associated with alcohol withdrawal are stereotyped, generalised, and tonic- clonic in character. They are thought to be more common in patients with a history of epilepsy. Patients often have more than one seizure 3 to 6 hours after the first seizure. Status epilepticus is relatively rare and occurs in less than 3 percent of patients. Although anticonvulsant medications are not required in the management of alcohol withdrawal seizures, sometimes the cause of the seizures can be difficult to establish when a patient is first assessed in the accident and emergency department with limited information about the patient. Even if there is history of alcohol misuse, other causative factors for seizures such as head injuries, CNS infections, CNS neoplasms, and cerebrovascular diseases should not be overlooked.

Long-term severe alcohol abuse can result in hypoglycaemia, hyponatraemia, and hypomagnesaemia all of which can also be associated with seizures. A comprehensive medical history and careful physical examination is essential. Severity of dependence and risk of delirium tremens should be assessed.

The main medications to control alcohol withdrawal symptoms are the benzodiazepines. Benzodiazepines help control seizure activity, anxiety, tachycardia, hypertension, diaphoresis, and tremor associated with alcohol withdrawal. Benzodiazepines can be given either orally or parenterally; neither diazepam nor chlordiazepoxide, however, should be given Intramuscularly (IM) because of their erratic absorption by this route. The dosage of the benzodiazepine has to be titrated, starting with a high dosage and lowering the dosage as the patient recovers.

Carbamazepine is also effective for alcohol withdrawal and can be used instead of benzodiazepines. However, using carbamazepine and benzodiazepines together do not have any added benefit (13). Rest, adequate nutrition, and multiple vitamins, especially those containing thiamine, are parts of the management plan. Some clinicians have also recommended propranolol and clonidine, although these medications do not appear to be superior to the benzodiazepines.

Counselling or therapy can be carried out in an individual or group setting.

Relapse Prevention Strategies

Acamprosate

Many studies have shown the efficacy of acamprosate regarding reduction in relapse rates (14) as well as relapse prevention (15). Acamprosate has a half-life of 3.2 hours, and it has no active metabolite. There is no evidence of a withdrawal syndrome or abuse potential. Common side effects are diarrhoea and nausea.

Disulfiram (Antabuse)

Disulfiram is a deterrent drug, and it can be regarded as a form of exposure/response prevention therapy (16). It acts by inhibiting Aldehyde Dehydrogenase (ALDH). The symptoms of reaction include flushing, nausea, vomiting, dyspnoea, palpitations, dizziness, headache, hypertension and anxiety. The recommended dose is 200 mg daily. Except for somnolence the side effects at this dose are uncommon. It is advisable that patients carry cards with the name of this medication and they should be vigilant regarding any food or other medication that contains alcohol. Disulfiram should not be commenced within 24 hours of alcohol consumption (17).

Motivational Interviewing

Part of the relapse prevention strategy is to remind the patient about the relapses and consequent complications, to identify high-risk situations and to help develop more appropriate coping techniques.

Motivational interviewing strives to increase the individual determination or resolution to change. It has an important but limited role. Motivational interviewing is based on strategies like empathy, avoidance of argument, detection of client resistance, and highlighting the client's own dissatisfaction and discomfort with the addictive behaviour (18). The main idea is to make the clients more aware of their own concerns regarding the addiction. Although the use of this technique is widespread, the evidence for its effectiveness is not very robust (19).

Delirium Tremens

Delirium Tremens (DTs), also called alcohol withdrawal delirium, is a medical emergency, that can result in significant morbidity and mortality. It is a florid form of alcohol withdrawal. Patients who have already exhibited withdrawal symptoms should be carefully monitored to prevent progression to this serious condition, as it is generally agreed that the best treatment for DTs is prevention. Prompt administration of benzodiazepines when a patient is undergoing alcohol withdrawal, may prevent seizures and DTs. Alcohol-induced delirium can also occur during intoxication, but in alcohol withdrawal it is more common and risky. The essential feature of the syndrome is delirium occurring within 1 week after a person stops drinking or reduces the intake of alcohol.

Delirium is defined as a fluctuating change in consciousness and cognition. Symptoms include marked restlessness and agitation, autonomic symptoms like tachycardia and sweating, tremors in limbs and tongue, disorientation and hallucinations which are commonly visual but tactile or auditory hallucinations may also occur. Persecutory delusions may also occur. Because of the unpredictability of their behaviour, patients with delirium are a danger to themselves and to others. They may act on hallucinations or delusions, and be violent or suicidal. Untreated, DTs have a mortality rate of 20 percent, usually as a result of an intercurrent medical illness such as pneumonia, renal disease, hepatic insufficiency, or heart failure. As mentioned before, withdrawal seizures commonly precede the development of alcohol withdrawal delirium, but delirium tremens can appear unheralded.

Since the syndrome usually develops on the third hospital day, a patient admitted for some other medical or psychiatric condition may suddenly and unexpectedly have an episode of delirium, which may be the first sign of a previously undiagnosed alcohol-related disorder. Episodes of DTs are more common between 30 and 40 years, after 5 to 15 years of heavy drinking. The drinking pattern is typically of the binge type. Physical illness (e.g., hepatitis or pancreatitis) predisposes to the syndrome. A person in good physical health has less chance of developing DTs during alcohol withdrawal.

Patients withdrawing from alcohol who exhibit withdrawal phenomena should receive a benzodiazepine, such as 25 to 50 mg of chlordiazepoxide every 2 to 4 hours until they seem to be out of danger. Once the delirium appears, however, 50 to 100 mg of chlordiazepoxide should be given every four hours orally, or lorazepam should be given intravenously (IV) if oral medication is not possible.

Antipsychotic medications that may reduce the seizure threshold in patients should be avoided. A high-calorie, high-carbohydrate diet supplemented by multivitamins is very important.

Physically restraining patients with the DTs is risky; they may fight against the restraints to a dangerous level of exhaustion. When patients are disorderly and uncontrollable, a seclusion room can be used. Dehydration, often exacerbated by diaphoresis and fever, can be corrected with fluids given by mouth or IV. Anorexia, vomiting, and diarrhoea often occur during withdrawal. The emergence of focal neurological symptoms, lateralising seizures, increased intracranial pressure, or evidence of skull fractures or other indications of CNS pathology should prompt clinicians to examine a patient for additional neurological disease.

Alcohol Hallucinosis

The chronic ingestion of alcohol can cause hallucinations, usually voices accusing the patient of being a bad person, although at times the hallucinations can be visual or tactile. This picture can develop in the midst of a drinking bout, occur in an otherwise clear sensorium, begin during alcohol withdrawal, or have an onset within several days to several weeks if no further drinking occurs. After an episode is treated, the hallucinations may return if drinking is renewed.

In about 10 to 15% of patients, the voices do not remit. In those cases, alcohol hallucinosis needs to be differentiated from schizophrenia, as third person auditory hallucinations can occur in alcohol hallucinosis.

Premorbid adjustment, a lack of family history of schizophrenia, and absence of gross cognitive impairment are some of the features which may help clarify the diagnosis. Moreover, in majority of cases the hallucinations in alcohol hallucinosis, have prominent sensory qualities, indicating that, unlike the voices heard by patients with schizophrenia, these voices are false perceptions of environmental stimuli.

Management in a hospital may be required to minimise the risks.

As hallucinosis is a variant of withdrawal, metabolic and nutritional support is essential. Although the psychoses is likely to clear spontaneously within a few days or weeks, an antipsychotic may be indicated for a couple of weeks.

Wernicke-Korsakoff Syndrome

The most common cognitive impairments induced by alcohol are subsyndromal. The full- fledged syndrome called Wernicke-Korsakoff occurs in 3% to 5% all alcohol-related cognitive impairment disorders (20).

Wernicke's encephalopathy, also called alcoholic encephalopathy, comprises a set of acute symptoms whereas Korsakoff's syndrome is a chronic condition. Wernicke's encephalopathy is completely reversible with treatment, but with Korsakoff's syndrome only about 20 percent of patients recover. Wernicke's encephalopathy may clear spontaneously in a few days or weeks or may progress into Korsakoff's syndrome.

The pathophysiological connection between the two syndromes is thiamine deficiency, caused either by poor nutritional habits or by malabsorption problems. The neuropathological lesions are symmetrical and involve the mammillary bodies, the thalamus, the hypothalamus, the midbrain, the pons, the medulla, the fornix, and the cerebellum.

Wernicke's encephalopathy is characterised by ataxia (primarily affecting the gait), vestibular dysfunction, confusion, and a variety of opthalmic features, (horizontal nystagmus, lateral orbital palsy, and gaze palsy). These eye signs are usually bilateral but not necessarily symmetrical. Other eye signs may include a sluggish reaction to light and anisocoria. Cognitive impairment dominates this syndrome, and many patients are significantly disorientated. Although there are atypical presentations, delirium marked by confusion is the initial presenting feature in the majority of cases (21).

In the early stages, Wernicke's encephalopathy responds rapidly to large doses of parenteral thiamine, which may be effective in preventing the progression into Korsakoff's syndrome. The dosage of thiamine is usually initiated at 100 mg by mouth two to three times daily and is continued for 1 to 2 weeks.

Korsakoff's syndrome is the chronic amnestic syndrome that can follow Wernicke's encephalopathy. Most people who exhibit Korsakoff's syndrome have had previous episodes of Weneckie's syndrome. Unlike dementia and delirium in which there is global and diffuse impairment, patients with Karsakoff 's syndrome have marked deficits in anterograde and retrograde memory, but the preservation of other intellectual abilities. The patient may or may not have the symptom of confabulation, which is the production of fictitious responses to compensate for memory deficits. Confabulation is not required for diagnosis.

Treatment of Korsakoff's syndrome is also thiamine, given 100 mg by mouth two to three times daily; the treatment regimen should continue for 3 to 12 months. Although there is improvement in functioning, complete recovery is rare.

Stimulants

Stimulants encompass a variety of drugs that share the ability to stimulate the Central Nervous System (CNS), and are greatly misused. They include all forms of amphetamine (such as dextroamphetamine, methamphetamine, and a mixed dextroamphetamine-amphetamine salt), related substances such as phenmetrazine and methylphenidate, and cocaine. Amphetamines are the most commonly used stimulants, but cocaine use is increasing rapidly. Methylenedioxy-Methamphetamine (MDMA), also called ecstasy, is used mostly as a stimulating hallucinogen.

The street names of amphetamine are ice, crystal, crystal meth, speed and whizz. The crystalised form of cocaine (on the streets) is known as crack or rock. Amphetamines are used to increase performance and to induce a euphoric feeling, for example by students, long-distance truck drivers, people struggling to work with deadlines, athletes and by soldiers.

Amphetamines and cocaine work by causing release or blocking the reuptake of dopamine and norepinephrine from nerve cells. They also have effects on serotonin, acetylcholine and GABA. The combination of these changes result in feelings of marked stimulation and euphoria (22). Cocaine produces effects that are almost indistinguishable from those of amphetamines. However, cocaine has a relatively brief effect, as its half-life is 50 minutes. Traces of cocaine can be found in the urine samples for three days or longer.

Amphetamine has a half-life of 10 hours, and methamphetamine's half-life is 5 hours. Effects of amphetamines are therefore comparatively longer (23). The effects of stimulant drugs are quite similar regardless of the mode of administration. The onset of action is slow when they are orally administered as compared to IV use or when smoked. The resultant effects are increased heart rate and blood pressure, feelings of well-being and enhanced concentration. Concomitantly, there is a reduction in appetite, and an elevation of blood glucose and blood coagulation, and also an increase in muscle tension (24). There is less need for sleep, increased energy and decreased fatigue. There can be tremor of hands and restlessness.

These effects are increased with higher doses of stimulants. Many people who are dependent on amphetamines and cocaine also abuse alcohol. This results in attenuation of the cognitive impairment caused by alcohol. Combination of cocaine and alcohol produces a third active substance, called cocaethylene which increases the risk of sudden cardiac deaths in people with preexisting coronary heart disease (25).

Tolerance to stimulants develops within hours to days, cocaine being particularly notorious regarding rapid development of tolerance. The reason for this is that both the euphoric and the cardiovascular effects of cocaine decrease much more rapidly than the plasma levels (26). On the other hand sensitisation or reverse tolerance with cocaine can also occur. This is because drug actions can vary with individual's history and clinical circumstances.

Although there is cross-tolerance with most stimulants, clinicians are not sure whether this is true for cocaine. Unlike the previous school of thought, most researchers now agree that there are symptoms of physical withdrawal with stimulants (27).

Stimulants dependence can result in a rapid deterioration of a person's abilities to cope with occupational, family and social obligations. After intoxication, a crash occurs with symptoms of anxiety, tremulousness, dysphoric mood, lethargy, fatigue, nightmares, headache, profuse sweating, muscle cramps, stomach cramps, and insatiable hunger. The withdrawal symptoms generally peak in 2 to 4 days and are resolved in 1 week. The most serious withdrawal symptom is depression, which can be particularly severe after the sustained use of high doses of stimulants, and which can be associated with suicidal ideation or behaviour.

Stimulant-Induced Psychotic Disorder

This occurs gradually, in clear sensorium, usually after chronic use but can also be seen acutely with a large dose of amphetamine. The hallmark of this disorder is the presence of paranoid delusions, although auditory and tactile hallucinations (the individual feels things crawling on the skin) are usually present as well. Visual hallucinations, labile mood and compulsive behaviour can be additional symptoms. Paranoia can result in violence.

This disorder can be distinguished from paranoid schizophrenia by its several differentiating characteristics. Generally sudden onset, appropriate effect, hyperactivity, hypersexuality, confusion and incoherence, and little evidence of formal thought disorder (e.g., looseness of associations) are some features which help to differentiate. Stimulant psychosis might also have physical symptoms like weight loss, excoriations (from scratching at non-existent bugs), needle marks, and elevated blood pressure and temperature. After cessation of stimulant intake, the psychotic symptoms usually disappear within days to a week, the hallucinations disappearing first, followed by delusion (28). The treatment of stimulant intoxication is symptomatic. Antipsychotics may be prescribed for the first few days, although the psychosis is likely to clear even if no antipsychotics are given (29). Diazepam is useful to treat patients' agitation and hyperactivity. Bupropion may be of use after patients have withdrawn from amphetamine. If there is underlying depression and personality disorder, treating them is important.

Opioids

The words opiate and opioid come from the word opium, the juice of the opium poppy, Papaver somniferum, which contains approximately 20 opium alkaloids, including morphine. Opioids include naturally occuring substances (morphine), semisynthetics (heroin) and synthetics (codeine, pethidine, hydromorphone, methadone, oxycodone, meperidine, levo-alpha-acetylmethadol, dipipanone). Pentazocine and buprenorphine have opiate agonists and antagonists effect, and are also classified as opioids (30). Opioid antagonists have been synthesised (naloxone, naltrexone, nalorphine, levallorphan, and apomorphine) to treat opioid overdose and opioid dependence.

The primary effects of the opioids are mediated through the opioid receptors (mu, kappa, delta, lambda). In addition to the morbidity and mortality associated directly with the opioid- related disorders, the association between the transmission of the Human Immunodeficiency Virus (HIV) and intravenous opioid and opiate use is now a worldwide concern. It has also been demonstrated that women who are dependent on opioids during pregnancy, have more risk of having premature and low-weight babies.

Heroin, the most commonly abused opioid, is more potent and lipid soluble than morphine. Due to these properties, heroin crosses the blood brain barrier faster and has a more rapid onset than morphine. Although some people use heroin without becoming dependent, dependence and tolerance can develop rapidly with heroin, as well as with most other opioids. Apart from IV use, opioids are also administered subcutaneously and sniffed (snorted). Heroin is also heated on a metal foil and inhaled (chasing the dragon).

It should be remembered that opiate overdose is an acute, life-threatening event, although it is usually accidental rather than a suicidal attempt (31). However, about 15 percent of persons with opioid dependence attempt to commit suicide at least once. About 90 percent of persons with opioid dependence have an additional psychiatric disorder, the most common being major depressive disorder, alcohol use disorders, antisocial personality disorder, and anxiety disorders. The opioids produce analgesia, drowsiness, changes in mood, and if taken in high doses, results in a clouding of mental functioning through the depression of CNS and cardiac activity (32). The acute intake of opioids, especially when taken intravenously (IV), is highly reinforcing. There is rush of feelings in the lower abdomen, warm flushing of skin, euphoria, decrease in respiratory rate, constipation and decrease in pupillary size (with the exception of meperidine) (33).

Although there is initial euphoria after opioids intoxication, subsequently there is apathy, dysphoria, low libido, psychomotor agitation or retardation, drowsiness, slurred speech, impaired judgement, and impairment in occupational and social functioning. In some cases, coma and even death (due to a combination of respiratory depression and pulmonary and/or cerebral oedema) may occur. Intoxication may last for several hours after the last opioid intake (34).

The treatment of acute opioid toxicity is supportive monitoring, ensuring adequate ventilation and IV administration of opioid antagonist, naloxone. Doses of naloxone of less than 0.5 mg may be adequate to reverse respiratory depression.

Withdrawal symptoms of opioids include strong craving, restlessness, insomnia, pain in muscles and joints, running nose and eyes, abdominal cramps, vomiting, diarrhoea, piloerection, sweating dilated pupils, increased pulse rate, and disturbance of temperature control (35). In addition, there can be irritablity, loss of appetite, yawning, chills, ejaculation, gooseflesh (hence the term cold turkey), and tremor. The onset of withdrawal usually begins at the time of the next habitual drug dose, ranging from 4 to 6 hours for heroin to a day or more for methadone. The clinical picture (especially its intensity) varies directly with the dose, the duration of use, the time the dose is postponed, and inversely with the general health of the individual. In the acute phase of withdrawal, the symptoms alleviate in intensity, and are significantly alleviated by the fifth day. There is considerable improvement in 7 to 10 days (36).

Symptomatic treatment is indicated when the daily amount of opioids used is low. In these cases, opioids can be withdrawn rapidly. Loperamide or metoclopramide can be use for gastrointestinal symptoms, and analgesics for aches and pain. Some clinicians suggest that lofexidine (which has a similar action as clonidine, but causes less hypotension) is equally effective in withdrawal syndrome as methadone (37).

In cases where the daily dose of heroin is high, it is preferable to prescribe an opioid such as methadone. Methadone is the current gold standard in the treatment of opioid dependence. Because it has a long half-life (1–2 days), symptoms of withdrawal begin only after 36 hours, and reach a peak after 3–5 days. For this reason, methadone is frequently used for heroin dependent patients (38). The initial dose of methadone (given in liquid form) is between 10 and 40 mg daily, depending on the patient's daily intake of heroin. If there are still withdrawal symptoms after four hours, an extra dose of methadone can be given. A rapid withdrawal regime can be completed in about ten days to three weeks, but in some cases, very gradual regime (several months) may be needed (39). Potential side effects of methadone include sedation, sweating, sleep disorder, impaired libido, depression, constipation, impaired concentration and loss of appetite.

Buprenorphine is a potent opioid analgesic, which can be dispensed on an outpatient basis. It can be given IV, IM or sublingually. Buprenorphine 0.5 mg is equal to morphine 10 mg. Clinicians need special training in its use, as because of its agonist action, acute withdrawal may be precipitated especially in patients with higher doses of methadone or heroin (40). The daily dose of 8 to 10 mg is used. After repeated administration, buprenorphine attenuates or blocks the subjective effects of parenterally administered heroin or morphine.

For the maintenance treatment of opioid dependence, methadone is the drug of choice, and there is lot of evidence to support this (41). Methadone reduces the chance of spreading HIV through contaminated needles. Secondly, methadone produces minimal euphoria and rarely causes drowsiness or depression when taken for a long time, and thirdly, methadone maintenance has been associated with decreased criminal activity (42). It has been shown that pregnant women who are on methadone maintenance programme, have better pregnancy outcomes than those who are not (43). Daily dosage of 20 to 80 mg is usually used, although it is advisable to start at lower daily doses (10–40 mg), and to increase gradually over a number of weeks. In some cases daily doses up to 120 mg have been used. Methadone maintenance is continued until the patient can be withdrawn from methadone, which itself causes dependence. An abstinence syndrome occurs with methadone withdrawal, but patients are detoxified from methadone more easily than from heroin. Clonidine (0.1 to 0. 3 mg three to four times a day) is usually given during the detoxification period (44). After patients have been detoxified from opioids, naltrexone, a long-acting opioid antagonist (also used for the treatment of alcoholism) may be used to help prevent relapse. Naltrexone 50 mg can block the opioid receptor for at least 24 hours. It can be given orally daily (50 mg) or three times a week (100–150 mg) (45). However, it has not been widely used in the community, and therefore the evidence is limited. Some individuals may benefit from individual psychotherapy, behavioural therapy, cognitive-behavioural therapy, family therapy, support groups, and social skills training.

Cannabinoids

Cannabis is derived from the plant Cannabis Sativa, the principal and most active ingredient of cannabis being delta-9-tetrahydrocannabinol (THC). Marijuana is the term applied to the cut and dried upper leaves, tops and stems of the plants (other names for marijuana are grass, pot, weed, joint, reefer and dube). Hashish and charas are names for the dried resinous exudate of the cannabis leaves. Bhang is the less potent form, from the dried leaves and flowering shoots. Ganja is derived from resin and dried flowers.

Tolerance to cannabis develops, and psychological dependence has been found, although the evidence for physical dependence is weak. Neither tolerance nor physical dependence is a major problem with cannabis. It is, however, important to bear in mind that the mild level of cross-tolerance with alcohol is clinically important issue. Withdrawal symptoms including irritability, restlessness, insomnia, anorexia mild nausea appear when a person abruptly stops taking high doses of cannabis.

When cannabis is smoked, the euphoric effects appear within minutes, peak in about 30 minutes, and last 2 to 4 hours. Cannabis seems to exaggerate the preexisting mood, whether elation or low mood (46). Some motor and cognitive effects last 5 to 12 hours. Cannabis can also be taken orally when it is prepared in food. About two to three times as much cannabis must be taken orally to be as potent as cannabis taken by inhaling its smoke (47). The two most common physical effects of cannabis are, dilation of the conjunctival blood vessels (red eye) and mild tachycardia. Dry mouth, fine shakes or tremors, a slight decrease in body temperature, a decrease in muscle strength and balance, headache, nausea, and a decreased level of motor coordination have also been reported. At high doses, orthostatic hypotension may appear. THC may also precipitate seizures in epileptics (48).

The most serious potential adverse effects of cannabis use are those caused by inhaling the same carcinogenic hydrocarbons present in conventional tobacco, and data indicate that heavy cannabis users are at risk for chronic respiratory disease and lung cancer.

Cannabis intoxication usually heightens sensitivities to external stimuli (e.g., makes colours seem brighter and richer) and subjectively slows the appreciation of time. In high doses, there may be depersonalisation and derealisation. Impaired motor skills can interfere with driving and the operation of machinery. If alcohol is concomitantly used, these effects are additive.

The delirium associated with cannabis intoxication is characterised by marked impairment of cognition and performance tasks. Even modest doses of cannabis impair memory, reaction time, perception, motor coordination, and attention. The longer the period of heavy cannabis use, the more pronounced the cognitive impairment.

Most researchers agree that cannabis can modify the course of schizophrenia in an adverse way (e.g., it can cause more psychotic episodes and relapses) (49). There is, however, ongoing debate whether cannabis can predispose to the later development of schizophrenia. Some authors believe that heavy use of cannabis can increase the risk of development of schizophrenia about six times (50) while another study showed the risk to increase two-fold (51).

According to another study, female teenagers who use cannabis, are at increased risk of developing depressive disorder (52). Cannabis- induced psychotic disorder is rare, although transient paranoid ideation is more common. Cannabis use rarely causes a bad-trip experience. Panic attacks may, however, be induced, and the anxiety symptoms are correlated with the dose. Sleeping difficulties or sexual dysfunction usually resolve within days or a week, after cessation of cannabis intake. The flashbacks with cannabis only occur, when there is concomitant use of hallucinogens, or when cannabis has been tainted with Phencyclidine (PCP).

Amotivational syndrome has been associated with long-term heavy use of cannabis. The person lacks motivation to persist in a task that needs sustained attention. A person becomes apathetic, gains weight, and complains of lack of energy.

Abstinence can be achieved through hospitalisation, or by careful monitoring on an outpatient basis. Cannabis can be detected in urine for up to four weeks after use.

Psychoeducation can be helpful. Support can be achieved through the use of individual, family, and group psychotherapies. For some patients, an antianxiety drug may be useful for short-term relief of withdrawal symptoms. Antidepressant treatment is indicated for underlying depressive disorder.

Hallucinogens

Hundreds of species of plants contain the chemical substances we call hallucinogens and have been altering the thoughts, moods, and perceptions of animals and people all over the world for thousands of years. A hallucinogen user may "see" a song, "hear" purple, or hold seemingly coherent conversations with family pets or house plants. A minute can feel like hours, and hours can feel like seconds. A user might become intrigued by a piece of furniture that appears to walk about the dining room, a wall that seems to breathe, or a rainbow of colours that appears streaming from his or her outstretched hand.

The ability to see visions, become more creative, discover deep insights, or witness "shadow" selves — the part of our inner selves that holds our darkest secrets — are often motivations to use hallucinogens. Some users report strong feelings of love and "connectedness" with all people, nature, and the planet, while others report feelings of depression, despair, and anxiety. Whether specifically used for healing and self-revelation, in religious ceremonies, or for pure pleasure and entertainment, hallucinogens create a mind-altering experience that advocates seek out while others swear "never again."

Besides inducing hallucinations, these substances also affect the mood, result in loss of contact with reality and also cause an experience of expanded and heightened sensory perception. Colours appear more vivid, there is sharpened sense of hearing, altered body images, and a decreased ability to distinguish between oneself and the surroundings.

Although some of the effects are common, the chemical structures of various hallucinogens are quite different. Hallucinogens include psilocybin (from some mushrooms) and mescaline (from peyote cactus), harmine, harmaline, ibogaine, 2, 5-Dimethoxy-4-Methylamphetamine (STP), Phencyclidine (PCP), and Dimethyltryptamine (DMT). The classic synthetic hallucinogen is Lysergic Acid Diethylamide (LSD). LSD is the most famous and potent hallucinogen that produces frank hallucinations at very low dose (53). Some researchers classify 3, 4-Methylenedioxymethamphetamine (MDMA), which is structurally related to amphetamine, as a hallucinogen. The street names of hallucinogens are: LSD (acid, fry), psilocybin (magic mushrooms, shrooms), morning glory seeds (heavenly blue), mescaline (mesc, big chief, peyote), STP (serenity, tranquility, peace), and PCP (angel dust, hog).

Most hallucinogens are well-absorbed after oral ingestion, although some are ingested by inhalation, smoking, or intravenous injection. Tolerance for LSD and other hallucinogens develops rapidly and is virtually complete after 3 or 4 days of continuous use. Tolerance also reverses quickly, usually in 4 to 7 days.

Neither physical dependence nor withdrawal symptoms occur with hallucinogens, but psychological dependence occurs. Long-term hallucinogen use is not common and hallucinogen intoxication usually lacks a withdrawal syndrome. Patients present with hallucinogenic intoxication, when there is maladaptive behavioural and perceptual changes, and certain physiological signs. The treatment for hallucinogen intoxication is talking down, reassuring the patients that the symptoms are drug-induced, and preventing the patients from physically harming themselves or others. An antipsychotic or diazepam can be used for a limited time.

Long after ingesting a hallucinogen, a person can experience a flashback. Flashbacks are spontaneous, transitory recurrences of the substance-induced experience. They are episodes of visual distortion, geometric hallucinations, hallucinations of sounds or voices, false perceptions of movement in peripheral fields, flashes of colour, trails of images from moving objects, positive after images and halos, macropsia, micropsia, and time expansion. The episodes usually last a few seconds to a few minutes, but sometimes last longer. Most often, even in the presence of distinct perceptual disturbances, the person has insight into the pathological nature of the disturbance. The intensity, frequency and duration of flashbacks diminish over time (54).

The most common adverse effect of LSD and related substances is a bad trip (in contrast to the usual good trip), in which the perceptual and hallucinatory experiences become frightening. Although the LSD user will usually have insight and will not lose contact with reality, sometimes there is a risk of suicide (55). The bad trip generally ends, when the immediate effects of the hallucinogen wear off.

Phencyclidine (PCP) intake results in a sense of detachment from the body, as well as sensations of numbness and of floating and sometimes of a dreamlike. PCP is readily absorbed by mouth, IV route or when smoked or snorted, and has a long half-life. Compared with the other hallucinogens, PCP is more likely to cause 'bad trips' and also has a higher risk of violence. The street name of PCP is angel dust.

The chemical structure of MDMA (Ecstasy) has properties that are similar to both amphetamines and hallucinogens. These chemical similarities are directly responsible for the psycho active, mind-altering effects of the drug. The use of Ecstasy is very common among teenagers, because of the combined hallucinogenic and stimulant properties. Apart from these problems, MDMA also carries the additional potential danger of possible longer-term effects (56). Repeated Ecstasy use leads directly to a long-lasting depression in many people. Another striking characteristic of chronic Ecstasy use is an impairment of memory. The most significant long-term biological effect of Ecstasy use in the brain is the prominent and extreme damage caused to serotonin neurons.

As mentioned above, amphetamines are psychostimulants, which means they cause a "rush" or "high," increased energy, and wakefulness. In structure (and in name), MDMA is actually most similar to methamphetamine, or "speed". MDMA also has similarities with psychedelic or hallucinogenic drugs such as LSD and mescaline. While it does not usually cause overt hallucinations like LSD, the psychedelic properties of Ecstasy do cause altered perceptions and feelings of peacefulness, empathy, and acceptance.

When taken in tablet form, as it usually is, MDMA is readily absorbed into the bloodstream, enters the brain quite easily, and begins to have its effect within 20–60 minutes after ingestion. As could be inferred from its name, users of Ecstasy describe the feeling as intense and emotional. They feel energetic and confident, yet calm because of a lack of worries or problems. One has heightened sensations of touch, smell, vision, taste, and hearing. While some people have strong negative reactions to MDMA, such as confusion, paranoia, and anxiety, most people report experiencing strong positive emotional feelings. Users of Ecstasy (especially at raves) often spend entire weekends without sleep—80 hours at a time—binging on the drug. They may take an Ecstasy tablet every few hours, in order to maintain their high, and may not be able to sleep because of the stimulant qualities of the drug. What follows is a very well-characterised "crash," including extreme tiredness, listlessness, and depression in most people. After coming down off of an Ecstasy high, it is very common for people to have problems concentrating. In essence, Ecstasy feeds its own use; it brings on a depression that makes people feel like they need more Ecstasy in order to free themselves from that very depression. People also describe serious body pain during the "crash".

Solvents

The solvents or inhalants are volatile hydrocarbons such as toluene, n-hexane, methyl butyl ketone, trichloroethylene, trichloroethane, dichloromethane, gasoline, and butane. These are present in glues, aerosols, cleaning solutions, nail polish removers, lighter fluids, paints, paint thinners, hair spray and petroleum products. Inhalants are rapidly absorbed through the lungs and rapidly delivered to the brain. The effects appear within 5 minutes and can last for 30 minutes. Their misuse is mainly in young men of lower socioeconomic class (57).

Solvents can cause serious damage to various body organs and they are extremely dangerous, as their acute intoxication can cause coma and death. For this reason, harm reduction is not considered an option, and the advice is to abstain (58). There is evidence that people who use these substances do so only on a short-term basis and then, fortunately, give up (59).

In small initial doses, inhalants can produce feelings of euphoria and excitement. High doses cause intoxication and can result in blurring of vision, slurring of speech, incoordination, staggering gait, anxiety, and psychotic symptoms, especially hallucinations in various modalities. There is potential for serious physical injuries because of confusion.

There is limited evidence of dependence syndrome and specific withdrawal. When withdrawal syndrome does occur, there can be sleep disturbance, irritability, jitteriness, sweating, nausea, vomiting, tachycardia, and (sometimes) delusions and hallucinations (60). Treatment is symptomatic.

Caffeine and Nicotine

Caffeine is the most widely consumed psychoactive substance in the world. It is contained in drinks, foods, prescription medicines, and over-the-counter medicines. A cup of coffee generally contains 100 to 150 mg of caffeine; tea contains about one-third as much. Cocoa, chocolate, and soft drinks contain significant amounts of caffeine.

The half-life of caffeine is 3 to 10 hours, and the time of peak concentration is 30 to 60 minutes. Caffeine acts primarily as an antagonist of the adenosine receptors. Single low to moderate doses of caffeine (i.e. 20 to 200 mg) can produce feelings of well-being, energy, increased concentration, and more motivation to work.

In high doses, caffeine can produce marked anxiety features. An overdose of caffeine tends to be relatively mild, and death is exceptionally rare (61).

Both physical and psychological dependence occurs. The withdrawal syndrome starts about 12–24 hours, peaks at one to two days and usually lasts up to a week. Withdrawal symptoms include craving, headache, fatigue, anxiety and impaired psychomotor performance (62).

Nicotine is one of the most highly addictive and heavily used drugs around the world. It causes lung cancer, emphysema, and cardiovascular disease. Nicotine affects the Central Nervous System (CNS) by acting as an agonist at the nicotinic receptors.

Withdrawal symptoms can develop within two hours of smoking the last cigarette; they generally peak in the first 24 to 48 hours and can last for weeks or months. The common symptoms include an intense craving for nicotine, tension, irritability, difficulty concentrating, drowsiness and paradoxical trouble sleeping, decreased heart rate and blood pressure, increased appetite and weight gain, decreased motor performance, and increased muscle tension (63).

Some management strategies are restriction on smoking in public areas, development of less harmful cigarettes, behavioural approaches (like cue aversion), and provision of chewing gum, skin patch or nasal spray (64).

Sedatives and Hypnotics

Benzodiazepines

Benzodiazepines include lorazepam, alprazolam, diazepam, chlordiazepoxide, temazepam, triazolam clonazepam, and triazolam.

Benzodiazepines have a hypnotic, sedative and anxiolytic effect, and therefore have a potential for abuse and dependence. However, craving and drug-seeking behaviour are not florid and conspicuous manifestations (65).

Benzodiazepines are most predominantly prescribed for anxiety, and to treat insomnia. They are also prescribed as muscle-relaxants, as anticonvulsants for seizures, and for the management of alcohol withdrawal and delirium tremens. They can be divided into three groups: short-acting, intermediate-acting and long-acting, according to their half-lives. Regardless of the length of the half-life, all produce a similar effect within a range of intensity and have the potential for tolerance.

Common side effects are usually mild, and include drowsiness, dizziness, weakness, confusion, slurred speech, ataxia, and impairment of psychomotor skills.

The intensity of the withdrawal symptoms is dependent on the length of use, dosage, and which benzodiazepine the individual has been taking. Short-acting benzodiazepines produce withdrawal symptoms sooner than long-acting benzodiazepines. Withdrawal results in anxiety symptoms like irritability, sweating, tremor, insomnia. Other symptoms are depersonalisation, derealisation, twitches, vomiting, yawning, hypertension and dizziness.

In cases of long-term dependence and high- dosage, there is more likelihood of experiencing severe withdrawal symptoms like muscle pain, mood disturbance and psychosis. There is, moreover, also a higher risk that abrupt cessation of use can result in convulsions and delirium tremens.

Treatment of dependence is gradual withdrawal over at least 8 weeks. It is advisable to reduce the dose of benzodiazepine by one-eighth every fortnight (66). Uncomfortable symptoms of withdrawal can be diminished or completely eliminated with dosage tapering or switching to long-acting benzodiazepines before tapering. In cases of dependence on short-acting benzodiazepines, a long-acting benzodiazepine, like diazepam is used.

For benzodiazepine acute intoxication, flumazenil (a benzodiazepine antagonist)is used to reverse the respiratory depression (67). Death resulting from an overdose of benzodiazepines alone is very rare, but the risk is greatly increased when benzodiazepines are combined with other CNS depressants (e.g., alcohol, barbiturates). In spite of this, benzodiazepines are generally considered safe if used with caution and with consistent monitoring. There are many authors who believe that the dependence potential and the dangers of benzodiazepines have been exaggerated. There is likelihood of dependence when benzodiazepines have been taken at a therapeutic dose for more than six months (68).

Barbiturates

Barbiturates' potential for abuse, together with the more recent development of safer medicines to treat anxiety and insomnia, have made the drugs rare in medical practice today. Their illicit use is becoming rare (69).

Barbiturates are a class of drugs that, even more than benzodiazepines, bear strong resemblances to alcohol. They mainly act on GABA neurotransmitters, and lower inhibitions, anxiety, and feelings of restlessness. However, the visible effects of barbiturates are not always calming, as they tend to exaggerate the preexisting mood of users rather than simply sedating them.

REFERENCES

1. Fitcher, M. M., Narrow, N. E., Roper, M. T., et al. (1996). Prevalence of mental illness in Germany and the United States. Comparison of the Upper Bavarian study and the epidemiological catchment area program. *Journal of Nervous and Mental Disease*, 184, 598–606.
2. Sadock, B. J. and Sadock, V. A. (2007). *Kaplan and Sadock's Synopsis of psychiatry*: Behavioural sciences/ clinical psychiatry (10th Edition). Philadelphia: Lippincott Williams and Wilkins.
3. Jerald, K. and Allan, T. (2006). *Essentials of psychiatry*. Chichester: John Wiley and Sons Ltd.
4. Mello, N. K. and Griffiths, R. R. (1987). *Alcoholism and drug abuse*: An overview. In H. Y. Meltzer (Ed.), *Psychopharmacology: the third generation of progress* (pp. 1511–1514). New York: Raven Press.
5. Schuckit, M. A. (1995). *Drug and alcohol abuse. A clinical guide to diagnosis and treatment* (4th Edition). New York: Plenum Medical Book Company.
6. American Psychiatric Association.(2013). *Diagnostic and statistical manual of mental disorders* (5th Edition). Arlington, VA: American Psychiatric Publishing.
7. American Psychiatric Association.(2013). *Diagnostic and statistical manual of mental disorders* (5th Edition). Arlington, VA: American Psychiatric Publishing.
8. Sadock, B. J. and Sadock, V. A. (2007). *Kaplan and Sadock's Synopsis of psychiatry*: Behavioural sciences/ clinical psychiatry (10th Edition). Philadelphia: Lippincott Williams and Wilkins.
9. Sadock, B. J. and Sadock, V. A. (2007). *Kaplan and Sadock's Synopsis of psychiatry*: Behavioural sciences/ clinical psychiatry (10th Edition). Philadelphia: Lippincott Williams and Wilkins.
10. Edwards, G. and Gross, M. M. (1976). Alcohol dependence: provisional description of a clinical syndrome. *British Medical Journal*, 1, 1058–1061.
11. Mason, P. and Wilkinson, G. (1996). The prevalence of psychiatric morbidity. *British Journal of Psychiatry*, 168, 1–3.
12. McKenna, R. G. (1997). Alcoholism in clinical neuropsychiatry. In T. H. Jobe, M. Gaviria and A. Kovilparambil (Eds), *Clinical neuropsychiatry* (pp. 1511–1514). Massachusetts: Blackwell.
13. Stockwell, T., Murphuy, D. and Hodgson, R. (1979). The severity of alcohol dependence questionnaire: its use, reliability, and validity. *British Journal of Addiction*, 78, 145–155.
14. Whitworth, A. B., Fisher. F., Lesch, O. M., et al. (1996). Comparison of acamprosate and placebo in long-term treatment of alcohol dependence. *The Lancet*, 347, 1438–1842.
15. Pelc, I., lebon, O. and Verbanck, P. (1994). Acamprosate in the treatment of alcohol dependence: a six month post-detoxification study. *Alcoholism: Clinical and Experimental Research*, 133–142.
16. Brewer, C. (1990). Combining pharmacological antagonists and behavioural psychotherapy in treating addictions: why it is effective but unpopular. *British Journal of Psychiatry*, 157, 34– 40.
17. Cantwell, R and Chick, J. (1994). Alcohol misuse: clinical features and treatment. In H. Chick and R. Cantwell (Eds.), *Alcohol and drug misuse* (pp 126–155). London: Royal College of Psychiatrists.
18. Miller, W. and Rollnick, S. (1991). *Motivational interviewing*; Preparing people to change addictive behaviour. New York: Guildford Press.
19. Cantwell, R and Chick, J. (1994). Alcohol misuse: clinical features and treatment. In H. Chick and R. Cantwell (Eds.), *Alcohol and drug misuse* (pp 126–155). London: Royal College of Psychiatrists.
20. Lingford-Hughes, A. R. and Welch, S. (2004). Evidence based guidelines for the treatment of substance misuse, addiction and cormobidity: recommendations from the British Association for Psychopharmacology. *Journal of Psychopharmacology*, 18(3), 293–335.
21. Strub, R. L., Black, F. W. (1981). *Organic brain syndromes*: An introduction to neurobehavioural disorders. Philadelphia: Davis.
22. Angrist, B., Corwin, J., Bartlick, B. and Cooper,T. (1987). Early pharmacokinetics and clinical effects of oral D-amphetamine in normal subjects. *Biological Psychiatry*, 22, 1357–1368.
23. Jaffe, J. H. (1990). Drug addiction and drug abuse. In A. G. Gilman, T. W. Rall and P. Taylor (Eds.), *Goodman and Gilman's The pharmacological basis of therapeutics* (8th Edition, pp. 523–573). New York: Macmillan.
24. Winger, G., Hofmann, F. G. and Woods, J. H. (1992). *A handbook on drug and alcohol abuse* (3rd Edition). New York: Oxford University Press.
25. Randall, T. (1992). Cocaine, alcohol mix in body to form even longer lasting, more lethal drug. *Journal of the American Medical Association*, 267, 1043–1044.
26. Jaffe, J. H. (1990). Drug addiction and drug abuse. In A. G. Gilman, T. W. Rall and P. Taylor (Eds.), *Goodman and Gilman's The pharmacological basis of therapeutics* (8th Edition, pp. 523–573). New York: Macmillan.
27. Schuckit, M. A. (1995). *Drug and alcohol abuse. A clinical guide to diagnosis and treatment* (4th Edition). New York: Plenum Medical Book Company.
28. Segal, D. S. and Schuckit, M. A. (1982). Animal models of stimulant induced psychosis. I.Creese (Ed.), *Stimulants: Neurochemical, behavioural, and clinical perspectives* (pp. 131-168). New York: Raven Press.
29. Roberts, D. C., Dalton, J. C. and Vickers, G. J. (1987). Increased self-administration of cocaine following haloperidol: Effects of ovarectomy, oestrogen replacement, and estrous cycle. *Pharmacology, Biochemistry and Behaviour*, 26, 37–43.
30. American Psychiatric Association.(2000). *Diagnostic and statistical manual of mental disorders* (4th Edition, Text Rev.). Washington DC: American Psychiatric Association.
31. Jaffe, J. H. (1990). Drug addiction and drug abuse. In A. G. Gilman, T. W. Rall and P. Taylor (Eds.), *Goodman and Gilman's The pharmacological basis of therapeutics* (8th Edition, pp. 523–573). New York: Macmillan.
32. Schuckit, M. A. (1995). *Drug and alcohol abuse. A clinical guide to diagnosis and treatment* (4th Edition). New York: Plenum Medical Book Company.
33. Jaffe, J. H. (1990). Drug addiction and drug abuse. In A. G. Gilman, T. W. Rall and P. Taylor (Eds.), *Goodman and Gilman's The pharmacological basis of therapeutics* (8th Edition, pp. 523–573). New York: Macmillan.
34. American Psychiatric Association.(2013). *Diagnostic and statistical manual of mental disorders* (5th Edition). Arlington, VA: American Psychiatric Publishing.
35. Gelder, M., Harrison, P. and Cowen P. (2006). The misuse of alcohol and drugs. In P. Cowen,P. Harrison and T. Burns

(Eds.), *Shorter Oxford textbook of psychiatry* (pp. 429–469). Oxford: Oxford University Press.

36. Schuckit, M. A. (1995). *Drug and alcohol abuse. A clinical guide to diagnosis and treatment* (4th Edition). New York: Plenum Medical Book Company.
37. Gowing, L., Ali, R. and White, J. (2004). Buprenorphine for the management of opioid withdrawal. *Cochraine Database of Systematic Reviews*, 4, CD002025.
38. Gelder, M., Harrison, P. and Cowen P. (2006).The misuse of alcohol and drugs. In P. Cowen, P. Harrison and T. Burns (Eds.), *Shorter Oxford textbook of psychiatry* (pp. 429–469). Oxford: Oxford University Press.
39. Gelder, M., Harrison, P. and Cowen P. (2006). The misuse of alcohol and drugs. In P. Cowen,P. Harrison and T. Burns (Eds.), *Shorter Oxford textbook of psychiatry* (pp. 429–469). Oxford: Oxford University Press.
40. Gowing, L., Ali, R. and White, J. (2004). Buprenorphine for the management of opioid withdrawal. *Cochraine Database of Systematic Reviews*, 4, CD002025.
41. Mattick, R. P., Kimber, J., Breen, C., et al. (2003). Buprenorphine maintenance versus placebo or methadone maintenance foropioid dependence. *Cochraine Database of Systematic Reviews*, 2, CD002207.
42. Sadock, B. J. and Sadock, V. A. (2007). *Kaplan and Sadock's Synopsis of psychiatry*: Behavioural sciences/ clinical psychiatry (10th Edition). Philadelphia: Lippincott Williams and Wilkins.
43. Ward, J., Hall, W. and Mattick, R. P. (1999). Role of maintenance treatment in opioid dependence. *The Lancet*, 353, 221–226.
44. Sadock, B. J. and Sadock, V. A. (2007). *Kaplan and Sadock's Synopsis of psychiatry*: Behavioural sciences/ clinical psychiatry (10th Edition). Philadelphia: Lippincott Williams and Wilkins.
45. Michael, S. (1999). The pharmacological treatment of substance abuse. In M. Lader and D. Naber (Eds.), *Difficult clinical problems in psychiatry* (pp. 155–179). London: Martin Dunitz.
46. Gelder, M., Harrison, P. and Cowen P. (2006). The misuse of alcohol and drugs. In P. Cowen, P. Harrison and T. Burns (Eds.), *Shorter Oxford textbook of psychiatry* (pp. 429–469). Oxford: Oxford University Press.
47. Sadock, B. J. and Sadock, V. A. (2007). *Kaplan and Sadock's Synopsis of psychiatry*: Behavioural sciences/ clinical psychiatry (10th Edition). Philadelphia: Lippincott Williams and Wilkins.
48. Feeney, D. M. (1997). Marijuana and epilepsy. *Science*, 197, 1301–1302.
49. Hall, W. and Solowji, N. (1998). Adverse effects of cannabis. *The Lancet*, 352, 1611–1616.
50. Andreasson, S., Allebeck, P., Engstrom, A., et al. (1987). Cannabis and schizophrenia. A longitudinal study of Swedish conscripts. *The Lancet*, 2, 1483–1486.
51. Arseneault, L., Cannon, M., Witton, J., et al. (2004). Causal association between cannabis and psychosis: Examination of the evidence. *British Journal of Psychiatry*, 184, 110–117.
52. Patton, G. C., Coffey, C., Carlin, J. B., et al. (2002). Cannabis use and mental health in young people: A cohort study. *British Medical Journal*, 2325, 1195–1198.
53. Jaffe, J. H. (1990). Drug addiction and drug abuse. In A. G. Gilman, T. W. Rall and P. Taylor (Eds.), *Goodman and Gilman's The pharmacological basis of therapeutics* (8th Edition, pp. 523–573). New York: Macmillan.
54. Frankel, F. H. (1994). The concept of flashbacks in historical perspective. *International Journal of Clinical and Experimental Hypnosis*, 42, 321–336.
55. Jaffe, J. H. (1990). Drug addiction and drug abuse. In A. G. Gilman, T. W. Rall and P. Taylor (Eds.), *Goodman and Gilman's The pharmacological basis of therapeutics* (8th Edition, pp. 523–573). New York: Macmillan.
56. Peroutka, S. J. (1990). *Ecstasy: The clinical pharmacological, and neurotoxicological effects of the drug MDMA*. Boston: Kluwer Academic Publishers.
57. Gelder, M., Harrison, P. and Cowen P. (2006). The misuse of alcohol and drugs. In P. Cowen, P. Harrison and T. Burns (Eds.), *Shorter Oxford textbook of psychiatry* (pp. 429–469). Oxford: Oxford University Press.
58. Bruce, M. and Chick, J. (2004). Misuse of, and dependence on alcohol and other drugs. In E. Johnstone, D. C. Owens, S. Lawrie, M. Sharpe and A. C. P. Freeman (Eds.), *Companion to psychiatric studies* (pp. 353–389). Edinburgh: Churchill Livingstone.
59. Ives, R. (2000). *Disorders relating to the use of volatile substances*. Oxford: Oxford University Press.
60. Sadock, B. J. and Sadock, V. A. (2007). *Kaplan and Sadock's Synopsis of psychiatry*: Behavioural sciences/ clinical psychiatry (10th Edition). Philadelphia: Lippincott Williams and Wilkins.
61. Schuckit, M. A. (1995). *Drug and alcohol abuse. A clinical guide to diagnosis and treatment* (4th Edition). New York: Plenum Medical Book Company.
62. Marks, J. (1994). Dependence on prescribed and socially tolerated substances. In H. Chick and R. Cantwell (Eds.), *Alcohol and drug misuse* (pp 53–74). London: Royal College of Psychiatrists.
63. Sadock, B. J. and Sadock, V. A. (2007). *Kaplan and Sadock's Synopsis of psychiatry*: Behavioural sciences/ clinical psychiatry (10th Edition). Philadelphia: Lippincott Williams and Wilkins.
64. Marks, J. (1994). Dependence on prescribed and socially tolerated substances. In H. Chick and R. Cantwell (Eds.), *Alcohol and drug misuse* (pp. 53–74). London: Royal College of Psychiatrists.
65. Marks, J. (1994). Dependence on prescribed and socially tolerated substances. In H. Chick andR. Cantwell (Eds.), *Alcohol and drug misuse* (pp. 53–74). London: Royal College of Psychiatrists.
66. Gelder, M., Harrison, P. and Cowen P. (2006). The misuse of alcohol and drugs. In P. Cowen,P. Harrison and T. Burns (Eds.), *Shorter Oxford textbook of psychiatry* (pp. 429–469). Oxford: Oxford University Press.
67. Bruce, M. and Chick, J. (2004). Misuse of, and dependence on alcohol and other drugs. In E. Johnstone, D. C. Owens, S. Lawrie, M. Sharpe and A. C. P. Freeman (Eds.), *Companion to psychiatric studies* (pp. 353–389). Edinburgh: Churchill Livingstone.
68. Lingford-Hughes, A. R., Welch, S. and Nutt, D. J. (2004). Evidence based guidelines for the treatment of substance misuse, addiction and cormobidity: Recommendations from the British Association for Psychopharmacology. *Journal of Psychopharmacology*, 18(3), 293–335.
69. Gelder, M., Harrison, P. and Cowen P. (2006). The misuse of alcohol and drugs. In P. Cowen, P. Harrison and T. Burns (Eds.), *Shorter Oxford textbook of psychiatry* (pp. 429–469). Oxford: Oxford University Press.

Psychiatry and Medicine 09

There is a traditional separation of psychiatric services from the rest of medicine, although psychiatry is an integral part of medicine.Psychiatric disorders are very common in all areas of medical practice. Moreover, outside psychiatric services, somatic symptoms are often the presenting feature of psychiatric disorder. Finally, psychiatric disorders frequently coexist with medical illnesses. A significant number of patients in the surgical and medical outpatients department as well as in the wards have psychiatric issues. Some psychiatric disorders like depression and anxiety have physical symptoms as well.

There is a lot of evidence of association between psychiatric and physical illness, and there is a significantly increased rate of psychiatric disorders in the medically ill. Psychosomatic medicine is concerned with the relationship between psychological factors and physiological phenomenon in general and disease pathogenesis in particular. Liaison psychiatric services were developed from psychosomatic medicine.

The rate of psychiatric morbidity among general hospital patients, is higher than in the general population (1). It has also been well-established that psychological factors play an important role in causing, or at least contributing significantly to the causation of certain medical problems. Psychological factors result in physiological changes, and these changes, in turn, lead to physical pathology. The role of these psychological factors can, however, vary for various medical problems. They can play a direct role in causing medical problems, can precipitate an underlying vulnerability for a certain medical condition, may aggravate an existing medical problem, or play an adverse role in the prognosis of a physical illness. Personality characteristics have been traditionally thought to be important in the development of three psychosomatic illnesses: peptic ulcer, ulcerative colitis and irritable bowel syndrome.

Research indicates that psychological factors may affect the clinical expression of asthma in several ways: altered awareness of airway resistance, suggestibility to airway constriction, and comorbidity with panic disorder and depression (2). It has also been observed that the psychological response to a physical illness is rarely static: different problems emerge at different stages of the illness (3).

Some of the factors explaining the conspicuous association between psychiatric and medical disorders include stressful life events and ongoing stress, certain personality traits, the effects of mental illness and behaviour on physical health, physical illness causing organic mental reactions, the emotional impact of physical illness, adjustment disorders, anxiety disorders, depressive disorders, acute transient psychosis, elaboration of physical symptoms, and drug-induced disease population (4).

The concept of stress has been central in the development of psychosomatic medicine. The way in which a person copes with stress is critical in determining the subsequent physiological and pathological changes. The capacity to adapt to a threatening event influences the nature and severity of the response. It is a common observation that people perceive the same event or stress differently. Events are deemed stressful only when the person perceives the stress as threatening.

The basic hypothesis is that stressful events are risk factors for the development of physical illness. Many studies have demonstrated a probable relationship between stressful life events and chances of having a physical illness.

One study found an excess of life events during three weeks period in men who had an acute myocardial infarction, as compared to the control group (5). On the other hand the incidence of myocardial infarction is increased in those patients who suffer from phobic anxiety (6), or depressive disorder (7). Another study (8) confirmed that depression can increase the risk of cardiovascular disease, especially for men. Type A behaviour, characterised by personality traits such as ambition, hostility, and a chronic state of time urgency (9) has been associated with ischaemic heart disease.

Medically unexplained symptoms are common in the general population and also in people seen in the primary care. They are more frequent in women than in men (10). There are number of patients with psychiatric problems who present with various somatic symptoms which are medically unexplained. These include pain, fatigue, neurological symptoms, cardio-respiratory symptoms, gastrointestinal symptoms, dermatological symptoms, body image disturbance, and genito-urinary symptoms (11). Pain in the head, chest and abdomen is a common presenting symptom in people suffering from mood disorders, anxiety disorders and personality disorders. Psychogenic pain is usually indefinite in nature, has vague onset, its boundaries are not specific, and it may respond to alcohol or psychotropic medication (monoamine oxidase inhibitors and tricyclic antidepressants).

Some patients suffer from significant fatigue which is not explainable or confirmed by any physical reason. Patients suffering from depressive or anxiety disorders may consult neurologists for headaches, dizziness, sensory loss, motor weakness or movement disturbances. Similarly, no adequate neurological cause is established for symptoms which arise in response to emotional conflicts, e.g., dissociative psychiatric disorders. There is, however, a clinical need to differentiate these symptoms which result because of unconscious motives from intentional production (malingering).

Psychogenic fits have to be distinguished from epilepsy but it is also important to remember that psychogenic fits can coexist with epilepsy (12). Dissociative amnesia starts suddenly after an emotionally traumatic event, in which the patient usually does not remember the personal details.

The common cardio-vascular symptoms due to psychological reasons are mainly due to autonomic arousal associated with anxiety. These include palpitations, central chest or left mammary pain, breathlessness, tiredness, decreased exercise tolerance, and irritability (13). Loss of appetite, non-ulcer dyspepsia, and persistent vomiting are common gastro- intestinal problems. It has been found in one study that about 40–50% of patients attending hospital clinics with irritable bowel syndrome have a psychiatric disorder (14). Another study (15) showed patients with depressive disorder, presenting dermatological symptoms like itching, burning, excessive redness, hair loss and hirsutism. Genito-urinary symptoms without an adequate medical cause include menstrual irregularities, dysuria, and frequency and urgency of urine.

The most common psychiatric disorders in general practice are somatoform disorders, depressive disorders, anxiety and stress-related disorders, and substance misuse. Patients with psychoses are uncommon (16). Psychiatric disorders that are common in the medically ill include adjustment disorders, major depressive disorder, generalised anxiety disorder, panic disorder, phobic disorder, acute stress disorder, post-traumatic stress disorder, somatoform disorder, substance abuse, eating disorder, sleep disorder, factitious disorder, and sexual disorder (17).

A comorbid psychiatric disorder in the medically ill person, can influence the impact and outcome of medical conditions like ischaemic heart disease (18) and diabetes (19). Apart from chance association, the two reasons for psychiatric comorbidity in the medically ill are: the psychiatric disorder may have cause the medical condition (e.g., alcohol dependency causing cirrhosis of the liver) and the medical condition causing the psychiatric disorder (chronic infections causing depressive disorder). Medical conditions that may cause psychiatric disorder include chronic obstructive disease, infections, hyperventilation, hypoglycaemia, hypothyroidism, hyperthyroidism, drug withdrawal, systemic lupus erythematosus and carcinoma.

Chronic obstructive disease can cause anxiety. Hyperthyroidism can present with symptoms that resemble panic disorder, generalised anxiety disorder, social and specific phobias. In some cases, hyperthyroidism may produce severe agitation resembling a manic state (20). Hypogylycaemia, diabetes, dehydration and pheochromocytoma can also produce symptoms of autonomic hyperarousal. Hypothyroidism can cause depression, poor concentration, and impaired memory. Females with high pathological hyperprolactinemia can have higher levels of depression and anxiety.

Other endocrine abnormalities like Cushing's disease cause depression, emotional lability, irritability, decreased libido, and anxiety.

Rheumatoid arthritis, systemic lupus erythematosus and fibromyalgia are the three common musculoskeletal disorders seen in psychiatric practice.

There are also certain drugs for medical problems, which can give rise to psychological side effects (21). Anticholinergic drugs (e.g., Benzhexol, benztropine, and procyclidine) can cause disorientation, agitation, confusion, and visual hallucinations. L-Dopa can cause acute organic syndrome and psychotic symptoms. Antihypertensive drugs (e.g., methyldopa, calcium-channel blockers and clonidine) can produce tiredness, and low mood. Impotence and low mood can be caused by sympathetic blockers. Digitalis can cause disorientation, confusion and mood disturbance, while the use of diuretics can result in weakness, apathy, and depression. Analgesic, like salicylamide can produce confusion, agitation and amnesia, whereas dementia can result because of chronic use of phenacetin. Antituberculous drugs, e.g., isoniazid, can cause acute organic syndrome and mania whereas cycloserine can produce confusion and schizophrenia-like syndrome.

REFERENCES

1. Lloyd, G. C. (1997). Liaison Psychiatry. In R. Murray, P. Hill and P. Mcguffin (Eds.), *The essentials of postgraduate psychiatry*. Cambridge: Cambridge University Press.
2. Morgan, M. G. (2000). Respiratory disorders. Psychological factors affecting medical conditions. In B. Saddock and V. Saddock (Eds.), *Kaplan and Saddock's comprehensive textbook of psychiatry*. Philadelphia: Lippincott Williams and Wilkins.
3. Agkagi, H. and House, A. (2007). Psychiatry in the general hospital. In G. Stein and G. Wilkinson (Eds.), *Seminars in general adult psychiatry*. London: Royal College of Psychiatrists.
4. Lloyd, G. C. (1997). Liaison Psychiatry. In R. Murray, P. Hill and P. Mcguffin (Eds.), *The essentials of postgraduate psychiatry*. Cambridge: Cambridge University Press.
5. Connolly, J. (1976). Life events before myocardial infarction. *Journal of Human Stress*, 2, 3–17.
6. Haines, A. P., Imeson, J. D. and Meade, T. W. (1987). Phobic anxiety and ischaemic heart disease. *British Medical Journal*, 295, 297–299.
7. Appels, A. (1990). Mental precursors of myocardial infarction. *British Journal of Psychiatry*, 156, 465–471.
8. Wulsin, L. R., Vaillant, G. E. and Wells, V. E. (1999). Systematic review of the mortality of depression. *Psychosomatic Medicine*, 61, 6–17.
9. Friedman, M. and Roseman, R. H. (1959). Association of specific overt behaviour pattern with blood and cardiovascular findings. *Journal of American Medical Association*, 169, 1085–1096.
10. Gureje, O., Ustun, T. B, Simon, G. E., et al. (1997). The syndrome of hypochondriasis: a cross-national study in primary care. *Psychological Medicine*, 27, 1001–1010.
11. Lloyd, G. C. (1997). Liaison Psychiatry. In R. Murray, P. Hill and P. Mcguffin (Eds.), *The essentials of postgraduate psychiatry*. Cambridge: Cambridge University Press.
12. Fenton, G. W. (1986) Epilepsy and hysteria. *British Journal of Psychiatry*, 149, 28–37.
13. Lloyd, G. C. (1997). Liaison Psychiatry. In R. Murray, P. Hill and P. Mcguffin (Eds.), *The essentials of postgraduate psychiatry*. Cambridge: Cambridge University Press.
14. Creed, F. and Guthrie, E. (1987). Psychological factors in the irritable bowel syndrome. *Gut*, 28, 1307–1318.
15. Cotterill, J. A. (1981). Dermatological non disease: A common and potentially fatal disturbance of acutaneous body image. *British Journal of Dermatology*, 104, 611–619.
16. Ansseau, M., Dierick, M., Buntinkx, F., et al. (2004). High prevalence of mental disorders in primary care. *Journal of Affective Disorders*, 78, 49–55.
17. Gelder, M., Harrison, P. and Cowen, P. (2006). Psychiatry and medicine. In M. Gelder, P. Harrison, and P. Cowen (Eds.), *Shorter Oxford textbook of psychiatry*. Oxford: University Press.
18. Lesperance, F., Frasur-Smith, N., Talagic, M., et al. (1996). Major depression before and after myocardial infarction: its nature and consequences. *Psychosomatic Medicine*, 58, 99–110.
19. Ludman, E. J., Katon, W., Russo, J., et al. (2004). Depression and diabetes symptom burden. *General Hospital Psychiatry*, 26, 430–436.
20. Hendrick, V. C and Garrick, T. R. (2000).Endocrine and Metabolic disorders. Psychological factors affecting medical conditions. In B. Saddock and V. Saddock (Eds.), *Kaplan and Saddock's comprehensive textbook of psychiatry*. Philadelphia: Lippincott Williams and Wilkins.
21. Gelder, M., Harrison, P. and Cowen, P. (2006). Psychiatry and medicine. In M. Gelder, P. Harrison, and P. Cowen (Eds.), *Shorter Oxford textbook of psychiatry*. Oxford: University Press.

CHAPTER

10 Dissociative (Conversion) and Somatoform Disorders

Somatoform disorders present as physical symptoms that do not have a medical basis. The individuals are very distressed by their symptoms as there is significant functional impairment. They visit doctors very frequently, and repeatedly insist on investigations despite having no medical basis for their symptoms. ICD-10 lists five categories: somatisation disorder, undifferentiated somatoform disorder, hypochondriacal disorder, somatoform autonomic dysfunction and persistent somatoform pain disorder.

According to DSM-5, dissociative disorders are characterised by a disruption of and/or discontinuity in the normal integration of consciousness, memory, identity, emotion, perception, body representation, motor control, and behaviour.

Somatoform and dissociative disorders are classified in different ways in DSM-5 and ICD-10. Both conversion and dissociative disorders are placed under one umbrella in ICD-10. In DSM-5, dissociative disorders are classified separately, while conversion disorder is mentioned under a new category: Somatic Symptoms and Related Disorders. Other disorders under this category include anxiety disorder, psychological factors affecting other medical conditions, factitious disorder, other specified somatic symptoms and related disorders, and unspecified somatic symptoms and related disorders. As the majority of individuals with these problems present in primary care rather than mental health settings, it was reported that the non-psychiatric physicians were finding somatoform diagnoses difficult to understand.

It was agreed by the writers of DSM-5, that the DSM-IV term somatoform disorders were confusing, as there was a great deal of overlap across somatoform disorders and a lack of clarity about the boundaries of diagnoses.

Conversion refers to a loss or alteration in bodily function the cause of which is assumed to be of psychological origin. It implies that an unpleasant effect, engendered by the problems and conflicts that the patient cannot solve, is somehow transformed into the symptoms. Dissociation implies disturbance or disruption in the integrative functions of the mind e.g., consciousness, memory, identity and perception. The term, conversion disorder is used in place of the older term hysteria in both classifications. Because of its negative connotation, the term hysteria is also not acceptable to patients.

Conversion disorder occurs in a setting of stress, and produces bodily dysfunction which does not conform with the physiology of the central or the peripheral nervous system. The presenting physical symptoms do not have a detectable physical cause and the aetiology is attributed to psychological reasons.

Dissociative (Conversion) Disorders

The essential characteristic of dissociative disorders is a loss of a normal mental or physical function. According to ICD-10, the common theme shared by dissociative (or conversion) disorders is a partial or complete loss of the normal integration between memories of the past, awareness of identity and immediate sensations, and control of bodily movements. The ability to have a conscious degree of control over the memories is impaired. The extent of this impairment is variable and it becomes difficult to accurately assess the amount of loss of functions that might be under voluntary control. The presentation of dissociative disorders is often dramatic, perplexing, and highly variable, both within and across individuals. The hallmarks of dissociation are profound and often unpredictable shifts in consciousness, the sense of self, and perceptions of the environment. According to DSM-5, the dissociative disorders share a common feature: they are frequently manifested in the wake of trauma and are influenced by their proximity to trauma.

The ICD-10 diagnostic guidelines for these disorders (apart from clinical features of individual disorders) include a lack of evidence for any physical cause, and presence of evidence of psychological causation, in the form of clear temporal association with stressful events, problems or disturbed relationships. For the purpose of diagnosis, it is not essential for patients to admit this association.

According to one study, the annual incidence is 22 cases per 100,000 (1). The same study suggests that conversion disorders are more common in rural areas, among uneducated people and in the lower social class. Conversion disorders appear to be more common in women than in men and one study suggests that conversion symptoms are more common in young women (2). There is no agreement regarding its increased prevalence in certain cultures as altered mental and physical states may not be regarded as medical conditions but as manifestations of religious phenomenon (3). Although it is generally believed that conversion symptoms are more common on the left side of the body, this view is not substantiated by evidence (4).

Management of Conversion Disorders

It is imperative that a therapeutic alliance is established and recovery is facilitated with dignity and it is crucial that these patients are not labelled as manipulative, dependent or as exaggerating their symptoms. Some conversion reactions are transient, whereas others are very persistent (5). Following encouragement and explanation, conversion symptoms may resolve spontaneously especially when they are acute. Some patients with chronic and entrenched symptoms may require admission. They usually have underlying depression and occasionally psychosis. In these patients, medication is combined with cognitive-behavioural approaches as well as physiotherapy.

Psychotherapy, family therapy, hypnosis and abreaction has been tried successfully in many cases.

Dissociative Amnesia

Dissociative amnesia is marked by an inability to recall important autobiographical information, usually of a traumatic or stressful nature inconsistent with ordinary forgetting. This condition most often consists of localised or selective amnesia for a specific event or events, or generalised amnesia for identity and life history. The key feature of this disorder, as already stated, is loss of memory which cannot be explained by ordinary forgetfulness or fatigue and there is no evidence of any organic mental disorder. There is typically sudden onset of memory loss for important personal information such as name and address. Usually, the important recent events are forgotten as well. The amnesia for them is partial and selective. Although it is important to bear in mind the possibility of acute neurological symptoms especially stroke, the perseveration of other mental symptoms would strongly support dissociative amnesia. Complete and generalised amnesia is rare.

DSM-5 further classifies dissociative amnesia into five types:

1. Localised amnesia, in which the individual fails to recall events that occurred during a specified period of time, usually the first few hours following the traumatic event. This is the most common form of disassociative amnesia.
2. Selective amnesia, in which, the person can recall some, but not all, of the events during a specified period in time.
3. Generalised amnesia, in which the person cannot remember anything about his life. This has an acute onset, and the individual can wander about in a perplexed and disorientated state of mind. This is rare.
4. Continuous amnesia, in which the patient forgets each new event as it occurs.
5. Systematised amnesia, in which there is loss of memory for certain categories of information, such as all memories relating to one's family or a particular person, or childhood sexual abuse.

The peak incidence is in the third and fourth decade and the sex incidence is relatively equal. Intensity, duration and age of exposure to the traumatic event are critical factors in the development of dissociative amnesia; generally the stronger, longer, and earlier the exposure, the worse the amnesia. Childhood abuse, rape, incest, war experience and threats of violence are commonly reported events.

In differential diagnosis, amnestic disorder caused by organic conditions, amnesia in depression, and amnesia in substance abuse, should be considered.

Recovery is usually complete if the amnesia is localised or selective but it is slow and gradual in generalised amnesia.

Group therapy and hypnosis are helpful. Usually there is little role of medication.

Dissociative Fugue

Dissociative fugue, previously known as psychogenic fugue, is quite a rare type of dissociative disorder. The person has amnesia for the period of fugue. Dissociative fugue is characterised by amnesia for one's identity and there is sudden, unexpected travelling. The person disclaims knowledge of his or her previous identity.

The journey from home or place of work is apparently purposeful, and self-care is adequately maintained during it. Both of these two features are required for its diagnosis. Moreover, the disturbance should not be due to the effects of substance misuse or general medical conditions. The place where the person travels to is usually known or has an emotional significance. In most fugues, the individual does not appear to be confused and in fact, the person's behaviour appears to be normal to other people.

It is important to consider postictal fugue particularly after temporal lobe epilepsy, in the differential diagnosis. Other conditions to bear in mind include brain tumour, head trauma, migraine, cerebrovascular accidents, hypertensive neuropathy, limbic system dysfunction, hypoglycaemia, uraemia, dementia and malaria. It is also advisable to keep the possibility of conscious simulation or malingering, although it is fairly difficult to differentiate as this is associated with the same stressors as dissociative fugue. Hypnosis or amobarbital (amylobarbitone) interviews may be useful in making the differential diagnosis.

Organic fugue states may be caused by a wide variety of medications including hallucinogenic drugs, steroids, barbiturates, phenothiazines and triazolam. Sometimes alcohol blackouts can be easily confused with dissociative fugue. Fugues occur during and after traumatic or stressful events like wars, natural disasters, bankruptcy, impending divorce, or other legal battles. Most fugues occur in the second through fourth decades of life. Unlike what is generally said, fugues do not appear to occur more in men. Most fugues last from few days to few weeks. Although many cases have spontaneous recovery, dissociative fugues may be recurrent.

The main treatment is psychodynamic psychotherapy, but abreaction is indicated in cases where acute traumatic events have precipitated the fugue. After the amnesia has been uplifted, continued psychotherapy is indicated to support the individual to cope with the underlying psychological conflicts that were initially responsible for precipitating the fugue.

Dissociative Stupor

Stupor is diagnosed on the basis of a profound diminution or absence of voluntary movement and normal responsiveness to external stimuli such as light, noise and touch. In dissociative stupor the investigations find no physical cause for the stupor. There is, in fact, evidence for psychogenic causation in the form of recent stressful events or significant interpersonal or social problems. The person remains motionless for long periods of time, but maintains normal muscle tone, posture and eye movements. Although there is some degree of disturbed consciousness, the individual is neither asleep nor unconscious.

Before a definite diagnosis of dissociative stupor is made, the absence of a medical or psychiatric disorder has to be established. Moreover, there has to be clear evidence of recent stressful events or current problems. Differential diagnosis includes catatonic stupor, depressive stupor, manic stupor and organic stupor.

Trance and Possession Disorders

In these disorders, there is a temporary loss of both the sense of personal identity and full awareness of the surroundings. The person may act if she or he has been taken over by another personality, spirit or force. There is often a limited but repeated set of movements, postures and utterances. Only trance disorders that are involuntary or wanted, and intrude into ordinary activities by occurring outside religious or other culturally accepted situations should be included here.

Dissociative Disorders of Movement and Sensation

In these disorders, there is a loss of or interference with movements or loss of sensations (usually cutaneous). There is no evidence found for the physical disorder. The patient's concept of physical disorder may be at variance with physiological or anatomical principles.

Dissociative Motor Disorders

Some authors have emphasised that in order to diagnose hysteria, there should not only be absence of relevant organic cause but also the presence of positive signs of hysteria (6). Positive signs include, a history of hypochondriasis, secondary gain, la belle indifference (an inappropriate lack of emotion or concern regarding the disability), non-anatomical sensory loss with a split of the midline by pain or vibration stimulation, diminished sensitivity to pain, and give-away weakness.

Loss of speech or hysterical aphonia is one of the commonest motor presentations. Patients are unable to whisper but are still able to cough loudly. The explanation for this disparity is that from a psychological perspective, the resonant sound of the cough is not related to the intentional and articulated speech. In one study, mixed and depressive disorder was the most common, comorbid psychiatric disorder (7).

Another common dissociative motor presentation is loss of ability to move the whole or part of a limb or limbs. This is called flaccid paralysis. Paralysis may be partial, with movements being weak or slow, or complete.

Various forms and variable degrees of unsteadiness or incoordination (ataxia) may be evident, particularly in the legs. Patients may present with striking difficulties in walking or standing, even though all leg movements can function normally in the lying or sitting position. This results in bizarre gait or inability to stand unaided, and is called astasia-abasia. There may also be exaggerated trembling or shaking of one or more extremities or the whole body. Patients may also, at times, exhibit movements that most normal individuals would not be able to do so.

In a hysterical spasm on the same side of the body both the arm and leg are contracted. The patient may actually resist the movement of the limb in the direction in which the contraction is supposed to be occurring. In hysterical tremor there is repeated movement of the voluntary type but it varies in intensity and rapidity. Interestingly, when the patient's attention is drawn elsewhere and he or she is engaged in another activity, the tremor ceases. However, the possibility of tremors being caused by anxiety or any medical condition should be kept in mind.

Dissociative Convulsions

These may mimic epileptic seizures very closely in terms of movements, but tongue biting and incontinence of urine are absent. However, injury can very occasionally occur due to falling. The corneal reflex is preserved and the plantar response is flexor. Unlike epileptic seizures, in dissociative seizures, the person does not fall rapidly towards the ground, but gradually, and there may be opisthotonos. Moreover, loss of consciousness is absent or replaced by a state of stupor or trance.

Non-epileptic (hysterical) seizures occur only in the presence of other people or at least when they are close by. Non-epileptic seizures, however, also occur in patients with epilepsy and sometimes more commonly if there are ongoing emotional problems or if they have toxic levels of anticonvulsant medication. There is an absence of post-ictal type of confusional state in hysterical fits. After an epileptic fit, the raised level of prolactin is a useful discriminatory measure (8).

Dissociative Anaesthesia and Sensory Loss

In this presentation, the anaesthetic areas of the skin do not follow the anatomical or medical boundaries, but are associated with the patient's own ideas about bodily functions. The loss of sensation can involve half the body from head to toe, or from right to left. Sometimes the whole of the limb is involved and characteristically has a glove or stocking distribution on the arms or legs respectively. Patients may not feel touch, firm pressure or pinpricks sensation. There may be differential loss between the sensory modalities which cannot be due to a neurological reason. Sensory loss may be accompanied by complaints of paraesthesia.

Deafness as a dissociative symptom may be incomplete and can be detected during sleep, as the noise usually awakens the patient. Help in diagnosis can also be obtained from inconsistent responses on audiological testing.

Dissociative blindness is more common than deafness and is often partial rather than complete. The usual presentation is that of blurred vision or difficulty in reading.

Mixed Dissociative Disorders

Mixtures of disorders explained above are classified under this heading.

Other Dissociative Disorders

Ganser's Syndrome

This disorder is characterised by patients giving 'approximate answers', to straightforward and simple questions, usually accompanied by several other dissociative motor and sensory symptoms. Ganser syndrome patients have clouding of consciousness with impairment of attention and concentration, hallucinations, perplexity, and anxiety. Approximate answers or talking past the point, however, is the cardinal feature. It is considered that this dissociative disorder results because of patient's efforts to avoid a difficult and stressful situation (9). The syndrome is quite rare and it has been suggested that it might be helpful to distinguish between the Ganser symptom (approximate answers) and Ganser syndrome (multiple symptoms, including approximate answers) (10).

Differential diagnosis includes dementia, pseudodementia, and malingering. Sometimes patients with schizophrenia can also give Ganser-like answers. Ganser syndrome can occur in patients with organic brain disease e.g.head injury and strokes. Ganser syndrome is much more common in men than in women. Hospitalisation may be indicated in some cases but the outcome is generally favourable. Apart from treating the comorbid conditions, a structured, protective and supportive environment; and exploration of the precipitating stressors is recommended, as it usually leads to resolution of the syndrome.

Multiple Personality Disorder (Dissociative Identity Disorder)

This disorder is marked by a disruption of identity characterised by two or more distinct personality states and recurrent gaps in the recall of everyday events, personal information, and/or traumatic events that are inconsistent with ordinary forgetting.

There has been a lot of controversy regarding the existence and validity of this rare condition but is now considered a legitimate psychiatric disorder (11). The key feature, as mentioned above, is the existence of two or more distinct personalities that exchange executive control over the individual's behaviour. In addition, in most patients, there is dissociative amnesia, a loss of memory for personal history, which is unexplainable by ordinary forgetfulness or organic reasons. Only one personality becomes evident at one time. Each personality is complete, with its own memories, behaviour, and preferences; these may be in marked contrast to the single premorbid personality. In the common form with two personalities, one personality is usually dominant. But neither has access to the memories of the other and the two are almost always unaware of each other's existence. Change from one personality to another in the first instance is usually sudden and closely associated with traumatic events. Subsequent changes are often limited to dramatic or stressful events, or occur during sessions with the therapist that involve relaxation, hypnosis, or abreaction.

This disorder is strongly linked to severe experience of early childhood traumas. Physical and sexual abuse, usually in combination, are the most frequently described trauma (12).

Although there is very little information available about the course and prognosis of this disorder, some undiagnosed or untreated persons are thought to be involved in abusive relationships. This may result in the traumatisation of their children, with the potential for additional family transmission of this condition. Similarly, some of these may die by suicide or as a consequence of their risky behaviours.

Even though there is no pathognomonic presentation of multiple personality disorder in the forensic setting, the assessment of those who are involved in criminal proceedings should be very in-depth, and structured. Conducting a longitudinal life-history interview is essential.

Current treatment involves a phase of symptom stabilisation, a phase of focussed attention to the trauma, and an integration phase (13). Psychoanalytic psychotherapy, cognitive-behaviour therapy and hypnotherapy are useful treatments.

Somatoform Disorders

These are a group of disorders that include physical symptoms (for example pain, nausea and dizziness) for which a sufficient medical explanation cannot be found. The presence of physical symptoms is unexplained by physical disease, but the patient continues to complain of variable degrees of discomfort and loss of function.

The physical symptoms result in making the patient emotionally distressed and cause disruption in his social and occupational life. The patient presents repeatedly with physical symptoms and requests for medical investigations in spite of repeated negative findings and reassurances. Even if any physical disorders are present and detected, they do not sufficiently explain the nature and severity of presenting symptoms or the distress and preoccupation exhibited by the patient.

Although psychological factors merely contribute to the symptoms onset, severity and duration, they are not the result of conscious malingering or factitious disorders. The term 'medically unexplained symptoms' is now often applied to these problems.

ICD-10 Classification of Somatoform Disorders

- Somatisation disorder

- Undifferentiated somatoform disorder
- Hypochondriacal disorder
- Somatoform autonomic dysfunction
- Persistent somatoform pain disorder
- Other somatoform disorders
- Somatoform disorder, unspecified

Somatisation Disorder

In this disorder, patients complain of persistent and recurrent multiple physical symptoms which start in early adult life, with a considerable history of numerous medical and/or surgical investigations without having any beneficial outcome. There is usually a high rate of disability.

The presence of multiple somatic symptoms cannot be adequately explained on the basis of physical examination and laboratory investigations. The patient complains of multiple, recurrent and frequently changing physical symptoms. Gastrointestinal symptoms include abdominal pain, belching, regurgitation, nausea, vomiting, etc. Abnormal skin sensations such as burning, tingling, numbness, soreness and blotchiness are very common. Sexual and menstrual symptoms are also reported.

According to ICD-10, for a definite diagnosis, the presence of all the following is required:

a. At least two years of multiple and variable physical symptoms for which no adequate physical basis has been determined.

b. There is a persistant refusal to understand and accept the advice or reassurance of several doctors that there are no sufficient grounds for these symptoms.

c. Presence of some degree of disturbance of social and family functioning as a result of the nature of symptoms and subsequent behaviour.

When the complete or typical clinical picture of somatisation disorder is not met, the term undifferentiated somatisation disorder is used.

The term, somatisation, includes multiple psychosomatic disorder, and Briquet's syndrome has also been one of the predecessors to the current diagnosis of somatisation disorder. There have, however, been studies that have demonstrated only a modest degree of diagnostic concordance between Briquet's syndrome and somatisation disorder (14).

The differential diagnosis of somatisation disorder includes physical disorders, depressive and anxiety disorders, hypochondriacal disorder and delusional disorders. Apart from the initial exclusion, medical disorders have to be ruled out again if there is a change or stability of the physical symptoms as this may suggest the possibility of a physical disease.

Although some depressive or anxiety symptoms with varying degree of intensity are commonly present, the diagnosis of depressive or anxiety disorders can only be made if the complete criteria is fulfiled.

In hypochondriacal disorder patient's worry is focused on the possibility of underlying physical disease and the persistent demand for carrying out investigations for ascertaining the disease, whereas in somatisation, the emphasis is on the symptoms and their consequent adverse effects. These patients seek treatment for removal of these symptoms.

Delusional disorders can be differentiated by the bizarre quality of their beliefs plus the presence of fewer physical symptoms of constant nature.

Somatisation disorder is chronic in nature, is more common in women (male and female ratio is 1:30) and usually the onset is before the age of 30 years. The lifetime prevalence of somatisation disorder is 0.13 percent of the general population. People who meet the criteria of somatisation disorder are typically unmarried, less educated and are from rural backgrounds. Comorbid disorders are anxiety disorders, depressive disorders, substance abuse and personality disorders. There is no specific personality disorder with which somatisation disorder is associated, although one study demonstrated that the most frequent types in order were avoidant, paranoid, self-defeating, obsessive-compulsive, schizotypal, and histrionic personality disorders. Many patients with somatisation disorder also have conversion disorders. Although suicide is quite rare, suicidal threats are common. Patients have chaotic and disturbed family and social relations and have difficulty in maintaining jobs.

Regarding aetiology, numerous theories have been postulated. Somatisation has been thought to be a form of social communication to manipulate and control relationships. For example, a patient with unexplained bodily pain may succeed in enhancing the attention and care by the spouse or parents. Some patients may be unable to verbally express their emotions and may, therefore, use physical symptoms to communicate the emotions. As in conversion disorders, bodily symptoms may also be used symbolically for emotional communication. Similarly, medical symptoms can be used to cope with stress. According to psychoanalytical theory, hysterical symptoms are substitution for repressed instinctual impulses. Neuropsychological tests have demonstrated equal bifrontal impairment of the cerebral hemispheres and non-dominant hemispheric dysfunction in patients with somatisation disorder. Another biological explanation is the abnormality in cortical functioning. There is evidence of abnormal auditory-evoked potentials. In contrast to controls, patients with somatisation disorder, respond similarly to relevant and irrelevant stimuli. This demonstrates impairment in selective attention. There is data to suggest that patients with somatisation come from more disturbed family and social backgrounds as compared to controls. There is more sexual and physical abuse in their families.

Treatment

Somatisation is usually a chronic and relapsing disorder with no specific treatment. An episode usually lasts for 6 to 9 months. Typically, patients keep on developing a new symptom or symptoms when under stress.

A trusting doctor-patient relationship is the cornerstone for achieving success in manageing a somatisation patient. Somatisation disorder patients should be preferably treated by one physician who should see the patient at regular intervals. There is evidence that this approach plus doing only the pertinent investigations results in improvement (15). It is important to avoid confrontations at the initial interview and clear information is given about clinical findings at clinical examination. The relevant investigations should be arranged systematically and the results explained clearly to the patient. During subsequent appointments, even though the patient would like to elaborate on physical symptoms, emphasis should be emphatically shifted to discuss on psychosocial issues. Patients should be made aware of the possibility that psychological factors are involved in the symptoms. Psychotherapy, both individual and in groups, can be beneficial.

Psychotropic medication has a limited role and, if used, careful monitoring should be done, as the patients tend to use them erratically.

Undifferentiated Somatoform Disorder

As mentioned before, when physical symptoms are multiple, varying and persistent, but th complete criteria of somatisation is not met, the category of undifferentiated somatoform disorder should be considered. In other words this is a lesser version of somatisation disorder. Undifferentiated somatoform disorder is characterised by one or more unexplained physical symptoms. These symptoms cause hinderance in family, social or vocational domains and there is an association with stress.

It is thought to be more common than somatisation disorder and it typically affects women. It is associated with lower socioeconomic class and older age. About 50 percent of patients with this disorder have comorbid psychiatric disorders including depressive, anxiety, and personality disorders.

The course and prognosis of this disorder is generally chronic and relapsing and similar to somatisation disorder (although in some cases there is no recurrence after a single episode). The management approach is same as for somatisation disorder.

Hypochondriacal Disorder

In this disorder, there is a persistent preoccupation with the possibility of having one or more serious and progressive physical disorders. The preoccupation persists despite appropriate medical evaluation and reassurance. In this disorder, patients inaccurately perceive physical symptoms as sensations and become fearful and preoccupied that they have a serious illness even though no known medical cause can be found. This results in significant distress to the patients and adversely affects their personal, social and occupational lives. Patients persistently refuse to accept the advice and reassurances of several different doctors that there is no physical illness or abnormality underlying the symptoms. However, the belief does not have delusional intensity (although there can be hypochondriacal delusions as part of psychotic depression or other psychotic illnesses). There is substantial evidence that hypochondriasis is often a symptom of another psychiatric disorder especially anxiety (16).

Unlike somatisation disorder, where the emphasis is on symptoms, patients with hypochondriacal disorder worry about underlying progressive and serious disease and its consequences. Moreover, in the latter, patients insist on repeated investigations. Marked anxiety and depressive symptoms are not uncommon.

ICD-10 Criteria

For a definite diagnosis, both of the following should be present:

a. Persistent belief in the presence of at least one serious physical illness underlying the presenting symptom or symptoms, even though repeated investigations and examinations have identified no adequate physical explanation, or a persistent preoccupation with a presumed deformity or disfigurement;

b. Persistent refusal to accept the advice and reassurance of several different doctors that there is no physical illness or abnormality underlying the symptoms.

This term includes hypochondriasis, body dysmorphic disorder, and dysmorphobia (non- delusional). This disorder occurs in both men and women and rarely presents after the age of 50 years. The degree of disability varies and some individuals are able to function almost normally.

One study has reported high prevalence of personality disorders in patients with hypochondriasis as compared to controls (17). Adverse childhood environment has also been implicated as a predisposing factor for causing hypochondriasis (18). Differential diagnosis includes somatisation disorder, depressive disorders, anxiety disorders and delusional disorders.

Hypochondriacal disorder is a chronic, relapsing condition with waxing and waning symptoms. The disorder usually persists for several years but there is often some remission in between the episodes. 50 percent of patients show improvement.

Treatment

Hypochondriacal patients are usually quite difficult to treat. Physical examinations and relevant investigations have to be carried out, the worries and concerns of patients are rarely alleviated. Only those investigations should be carried out which are medically indicated and not what would satisfy the patients. The patients should be helped with constructive ways to deal with their symptoms and stress without reinforcing their illness behaviour, and their use of the sick role as a solution to the problem.

Drugs have a limited role and are usually helpful only if there is underlying anxiety or depressive disorder. When these comorbid conditions are treated, the hypochondriasis will often improve. SSRIs have some role in treating hypochondriacal disorder. Cognitive-behavioural treatment has shown beneficial effect (19). Group therapy is also helpful, as it decreases anxiety by providing social support and interaction. Higher social impairment and more severity of the disorder results in poor response (20).

Somatoform Autonomic Dysfunction

Here, the patients present the symptoms as if they were due to a physical disorder that is mainly under autonomic innervations and control, i.e. the cardiovascular, gastrointestinal or respiratory. The symptoms are usually of two types, neither of which indicates a physical disorder of the organ or system concerned. The first type is characterised by complaints based on objective signs of autonomic arousal, such as non-specific symptoms like the sensations of fleeting aches and pains, burning, heaviness and tightness, etc.

ICD-10 Diagnostic Criteria

The definite diagnosis requires all of the following:

a. Symptoms of autonomic arousals such as palpitations, sweating, tremor, flushing, that are persistent and troublesome.
b. Additional subjective symptoms referred to a specific organ or system.
c. Preoccupation with and distress about the possibility of a serious disorder of the stated organ or system.
d. No evidence of a significant disturbance of structure or function of the stated system or organ.

The disorder can be further classified according to the organ or system regarded by the patient as the origin of the symptoms.

Cardiovascular system includes Cardiac neurosis, and Neurocirculatory asthenia.

Gastrointestinal system includes Gastric neurosis, Psychogenic hiccough, Dyspepsia, Psychogenic flatulence, Diarrhoea gas syndrome.

Genitourinary system includes Psychogenic increase in frequency of micturition and dysuria. Differential diagnosis includes generalised anxiety disorder and somatisation disorder. In generalised anxiety disorder, there is marked fear and anxiety. In somatisation disorder, the autonomic symptoms are neither persistent nor prominent.

Persistent Somatoform Pain Disorder

This disorder includes psychogenic backache or headache and somatoform pain disorder. Persistent pain disorder is characterised by persistent, severe, and distressing pain, which cannot be explained fully by a physiological process or a physical disorder. Psychological factors are thought to play an important role in the onset, severity, exacerbation or maintenance of the pain. There is a significant association of pain with emotional stress.

When organic pathology is present, the severity of pain or the subsequent social or occupational disability is not proportionate to the medical cause. There is usually a significant increase in support and attention, either personal or medical.

Pain which is presumed to be of psychogenic origin occurring during the course of depressive disorder or schizophrenia should not be included here. Typical sites and types of pain are headache, atypical facial pain, low back pain, and chronic pelvic pain.

Differential diagnosis includes depressive disorder, conversion disorder, psychosis, and malingering. The management of pain disorder involves family support and individually tailored approach. Treatment of any associated psychiatric or physical disorder is essential. Cognitive-behavioural treatment has shown beneficial effects (21). Group therapy with anti-depressant medication has been shown to be more effective than individual therapy with antidepressant medication (22).

Other Somatoform Disorders

In this group, those disorders are categorised in which there are somatoform symptoms, but they do not fulfil the criteria for the specific somatoform categories.

Examples include:

1. Pseudocysis: A false belief of being pregnant that is associated with objective signs of pregnancy like abdominal enlargement (although the umbilicus does not become everted) decreased menstrual flow, amenorrhea, subjective sensation of fetal movement, nausea, breast engorgement and secretions, and labour pains at the expected date of delivery.
2. A disorder involving, non-psychotic hypochondriacal symptoms of less than 6 months duration.
3. A disorder involving unexplained physical complaints (e.g., fatigue or body weakness) of less than six months' duration that are not due to another mental disorder.

Factitious Disorder and Malingering

In DSM-5, factitious disorder is included under the umbrella of somatic symptoms and related disorders. In ICD-10, factitious disorder is a category in a residual grouping of other disorders of adult personality and behaviour. Factitious disorder includes hospital hopper syndrome and Munchausen syndrome, but excludes battered baby syndrome, malingering, and Munchausen by proxy.

In factitious disorder, in the absence of confirmed physical or mental disorder patients deliberately feign or create symptoms with the aim of being regarded as sick and given medical treatment. There is an intentional simulation, exaggeration, aggravation, or induction of physical or psychological symptoms. Patients may even inflict cuts or abrasions to produce bleeding or may inject themselves with toxic substances. Consequently repeated investigations and operations may be performed at several different places, with negative findings.

Patients consciously perpetrate their deceptive behaviours although their underlying motivations are unconscious. Patients who readily acknowledge that they have produced their own medical signs are not diagnosed with factitious disorder. These patients often have other personality problems and relationship difficulties as well.

Factitious disorder is differentiated from malingering that patients who malinger have an obvious motive for their behaviour. The common motives for malingering are financial or sickness benefits, evading criminal proceedings, and avoiding unlikeable duties, etc.

Factitious disorders and malingering are differentiated from somatoform disorders, on the basis that in somatoform disorders patients do not intentionally produce the symptoms. Factitious disorder is rare. There is no evidence for a specific genetic basis but many patients with factitious disorder have comorbid psychiatric disorders e.g., mood disorders, personality disorders or substance abuse disorders (which are genetically influenced).

There is no specific treatment for factitious disorder. Management primarily aims at preventing undue investigations and treatment, reduce patient's disease dissimulation by confronting the patient with evidence that the symptoms and signs have been fabricated. It is, however, not helpful to reject the patient as a fraud, and effort and treatment should be directed at the comorbid disorder. It should be remembered that many patients may have a personality disorder and a tendency for acting-out behaviours including self-harm attempts. Taking a multidisciplinary approach is invaluable.

Neurasthenia

In many countries (including USA), neurasthenia is not used as a diagnostic category but is present in ICD-10 under the heading of other neurotic disorders. ICD-10 diagnosis of neurasthenia includes Chronic Fatigue Syndrome (CFS), but excludes post-viral fatigue syndrome. The term myalgic encephalomyelitis has also been used vaguely in literature. Controversy continues whether CFS is a psychiatric illness or a somatic one with emotional components. Some authors are of the view that the distinction between neurasthenia and CFS is more a matter of illness attribution than symptoms—whereas neurasthenia is usually seen as a psychological disorder, CFS is felt more as having a physical cause (23). In fact many patients believe they only have a physical illness, e.g., a chronic viral infection or some sort of immune dysfunction. These patients may be understandably reluctant or ambivalent to see a psychiatrist.

Neurasthenia is more common in women. Between half and three-quarters of patients with CFS meet the criteria for identifiable psychiatric diagnosis. For the majority of the patients seen in secondary mental health services, investigations will be normal, and any physical causes will have been diagnosed. Although fatigue is one of the most common symptoms in all medical practice, patients with CFS complain that they become easily fatigued after minor exertions. They typically insist that this exhaustion is not the everyday tiredness that normal people have. Other symptoms include headache, pain, flu-like symptoms, disturbed sleep (hyper-somnia and daytime drowsiness).

ICD-10 Diagnostic Criteria

Requires the following:

a. Either persistent and distressing complaints of increased fatigue after mental effort, or persistent and distressing complaints of bodily weakness and exhaustion after minimal effort.
b. At least two of the following:
   - Feelings of muscular aches and pains
   - Dizziness
   - Tension headaches
   - Sleep disturbance
   - Inability to relax
   - Irritability
   - Dyspepsia
c. Any autonomic or depressive symptoms present are not sufficiently persistent and severe to fulfil the criteria for any of the more specific disorders in this classification.

Differential diagnosis includes depressive disorder, anxiety disorder and somatoform disorders. In CFS, patients consistently emphasise fatiguability and weakness and are concerned about their decreased mental and physical efficiency. In somatoform disorders patients focus on bodily complaints and are preoccupied with the possibility of physical disease.

The prognosis of CFS is generally poor. Fewer than 10% of CFS patients referred to specialist services make a full recovery (24). The occupational and social life of many patients is impaired

Aetiology

A variety of physical and psychological causes have been implicated in CFS and some researchers believe that there is a complex interaction of various factors including physiological, cognitive, behavioural and affective,which are responsible not only for causing CFS but also have a role in its maintenance (25). It has been suggested that patients with CFS have premorbid perfectionism traits and they consistently strive to excel in work. Stress, negative life events and infection have all been associated as predisposing factors (26). Fear and avoidance behaviour, play an important role in the maintenance of CFS.

Management

Engagement and therapeutic alliance are paramount. As patients are sensitive to being disbelieved, it is unhelpful to tell them their symptoms are 'psychological'. Patients should be encouraged to carry out their own rehabilitation with support and guidance from their therapist. A graded but consistent schedule is charted out to increase the activities (which include a mixture of social, work and leisure). Cognitive-behavioural techniques are employed. Unhelpful and negative thoughts are coped with cognitive strategies. Patients are advised to keep account of their daily activities and sleep patterns and are also asked to enlist any apprehensions or fears regarding their activities or exercises. There is a lot of evidence for the efficacy of CBT (27). Unless there is comorbid depressive disorder, there is a limited role of antidepressant therapy.

Depersonalisation-Derealisation Syndrome

Depersonalisation symptoms include experiences of unreality; feelings of detachment or being an outside observer of one's thoughts, feelings, sensations, or actions; an unreal or absent sense of self; physical and emotional numbing; and time distortion. in contrast, derealisation experiences involve feelings of unreality or detachment with respect to one's surroundings that include the experience of individuals or objects as unreal, dreamlike, foggy, visually distorted, or lifeless.

In this syndrome, patients complain of their perceptions being changed in qualitative sense which leads them to feel that they and their environment are not real. They describe the detached feelings and their inability to feel emotions. Patients feel as if they are no longer doing their own thinking, and somehow do not own their own movements and behaviour. Their surrounding seems plain and colourless to them. Some patients have reported feeling as if they are seeing themselves from a distance in a detached way. Elements of depersonalisation and derealisation can occur in healthy people when they have fatigue and sensory deprivation or when they are under the influence of hallucinogens.

Commonly the symptoms of depersonalisation and derealisation are part of anxiety disorders. They also need to be differentiated from psychotic symptoms. Depersonalisation and derealisation can also occur as part of temporal lobe epilepsy, depressive disorder, phobic disorder, obsessive-compulsive disorder, or schizophrenia. In dissociative disorders similar change in personality is present but there is lack of awareness of change. There is no specific treatment for depersonalisation and derealisation and the treatment is directed at the main disorder.

Other Specified Neurotic Disorders (Culture-Bound Syndromes)

This includes mixed disorders of behaviour, beliefs and emotions which are of uncertain aetiology and nosological status and which occur with particular frequency in certain cultures. These are not regarded as delusional beliefs as there is a strong association with cultural beliefs. Such syndromes are seen as illnesses in particular cultures, but are not recognised outside those cultures. People in those cultures are widely aware of the existence of these disorders and are usually treated by folk medicine of those cultures.

The concept of culture-bound syndromes is problematic and controversial, as it suggests that only some and not all mental illness is culturally influenced. In fact, some authors even insist that the term culture-bound is redundant because all reactions are to an extent influenced and determined by cultures (28).

Although culture-bound syndromes are mentioned in both ICD-10 and DSM-5, neither of these classification systems are very clear or specific about their classification status. The ICD-10 definition demands that the following two central features should be present:

1. They are not easily accommodated by the categories in established and internationally used psychiatric classifications.
2. They were first described in, and subsequently closely or exclusively associated with, a particular culture or geographical population.

The following syndromes are the most common one recognised.

Dhat Syndrome

This occurs mostly in the Indian subcontinent and is known as Shen-kui in China. In this there is premature ejaculation or impotence and people are worried and hypochondriacal about the detrimental effects of the passage of semen in urine and the discolouration of the urine. They attribute this to excessive masturbation or nocturnal emissions, and feel guilty. Symptoms include fatigue, exhaustion, muscular pains, low or loss of libido, low mood and anxiety symptoms.

Possession States

These states occur in the Indian subcontinent and West Indian cultures and are transient. There is a dramatic change in behaviour. Sufferers believe they are possessed by a spirit leading to overactivity and voice changes. Unusual desires are expressed. A ritual can be used to induce them. It is important to consider possession states in the differential diagnosis of psychoses, and delusions of control.

Susto

This syndrome occurs in Mexico, and Central and South America. There are appetite and sleep disturbances, low mood, agitation, confusion, demotivation state, aches and pains, feelings of uncleanliness, and diarrhoea. This is attributed to a frightening event that causes the soul to leave the body. The condition is chronic and the sufferers believe that it can be fatal.

Pibloktoq

It is also called 'Arctic hysteria'. It is an acute episode of chaotic and disruptive behaviour with complaints of irritability, confusion and low mood. The sufferer becomes increasingly agitated and indulges in bizarre behaviour like tearing off the clothes and exhibits echolalia, echopraxia, and coprophagia. He runs around frantically and plunges into snowdrifts or climbs into icebergs. After collapsing with exhaustion or being caught by others, he falls asleep for a prolonged duration. There is complete amnesia of the event.

Koro

This occurs mostly in Southeast Asia and it often occurs in epidemics. In China, this syndrome is called shook yang. It can occur in other cultures including Thailand (called rok joo), and Assam in India (called jinjina bemar).

This mostly occurs in males. Episodes of intense anxiety occur, lasting from 30 minutes a day to a day or two. Most episodes occur at night, sometimes after sexual activity. There are palpitations, sweating, pericardial discomfort and trembling. There is a fear that the penis will retract into the abdomen or disappear suddenly, and cause death. The person resorts to remedial action like tying the penis with strings and also enlisting the help of friends and family members. In females, there is fear that the breasts or the genitalia will retract.

Bouffée Délirante

This occurs in Haiti. There is a sudden outburst of agitated, aggressive behaviour, confusion, and psychomotor excitement. Hallucinosis or paranoia can also occur.

Windigo (Wihtigo)

This syndrome occurs among Indians of the Cree, Ojibwe and Saulteaux tribe of North America. There is an initial period of dislike of food and when it does not subside, an intense anxiety develops. The sufferer perceives this as evidence that he or she is transforming into a giant cannibalistic spirit.

Taijin Kyofusho

This occurs in Japan. There is an intense fear that the body is offensive to others.

Latah

This is often seen in females in Malaysia and Indonesia but also occurs in Siberia, Thailand and Japan. In this syndrome, which usually occurs after a frightening experience, there is coprolalia, echopraxia, echolalia, hypersensitivity to fright, and automatic response behaviour. Dissociative or trance-like behaviour also occurs.

This is also seen in other geographical areas like Burma (called yuan), Thailand (called bah- tsche), Philippines (called mali-mali), Siberia (myriachit), Lapland (Lapp panic) among the Ainu of Japan (called imu) and the French Canadians of Maine (called jumpers) (29).

Amok

This is seen in the Philippines and Malaysia. A male perceives a real or imagined threat, undergoes a spell of brooding for several hours, and then in an extremely aggressive and volatile mode tries to kill every living thing he encounters. He stops only when captured or killed. Sometimes suicides occur. The violent behaviour arises out of extremely heightened emotions but there is no evidence of a mental illness. There is amnesia for the behaviour. He is not held responsible and is consequently not punished.

REFERENCES

1. Stephansson, J. G., Messina, J. A. and Meyerowitz, S. (1976). Hysterical neurosis, conversion type: clinical and epidemiological considerations. *Acta Psychiatrica Scandanavica*, 53, 119–138.
2. Lazare, A. (1981). Current concepts in psychiatry: conversion symptoms. *New England Journal of Medicine*, 305, 745–748.
3. Sharpe, M., Baldwin, D. and Walker, J. (2010). Neurotic, stress–related and somatoform disorders. In E. C. Johnstone, D. C. Owens,S. M. Lawrie, A. M. Mcintosh and M. Stone, *Companion to psychiatric studies* (8th Edition). Edinburgh: Churchill Livingstone Elsevier.
4. Stone, J., Sharpe, M., Carson, A., et al. (2002).Are functional motor and sensory symptoms really more frequent on the left? A systematic review. *Journal of Neurology, Neurosurgery and Psychaitry*, 73, 578–581.
5. Ford, C. V. and Folks, D. G. (1985). Conversion disorders: An overview. *Psychosomatics*, 26, 371–383.
6. Head, H. (1922). An address on the diagnosis of hysteria. *British Medical Journal*, 1, 827–829.
7. Bhatia, M. S. and Vaid, I. (2000). Hysterical aphonia-an analysis of 25 cases. *Indian Journal of Medical Sciences*, 54, 335–338.
8. Trimble, M. R. (1978). Serum prolactin in epilepsy and hysteria. *British Medical Journal*, 2, 1682.
9. Enoch, M. D. and Trethowan, W. (1991). *Uncommon Psychiatric Syndromes*. Oxford: Butterworth-Heinemann.
10. Scott, P. D. (1965). The Ganser Syndrome. *The British Journal of Criminology*, 5, 127–131.
11. Putmnam, F. W. and Loewenstein, R. J. (2000). In B. J. Sadock and V. A. Sadock, *Kaplan and Saddock's comprehensive textbook of psychiatry* (7th Edition). Philadelphia: Lippincot Williams and Wilkins.
12. Putmnam, F. W. and Loewenstein, R. J. (2000). In B. J. Sadock and V. A. Sadock, *Kaplan and Saddock's comprehensive textbook of psychiatry* (7th Edition). Philadelphia: Lippincot Williams and Wilkins.
13. Putmnam, F. W. and Loewenstein, R. J. (2000).In B. J. Sadock and V. A. Sadock, *Kaplan and Saddock's comprehensive textbook of psychiatry* (7th Edition). Philadelphia: Lippincot Williams and Wilkins.
14. Putmnam, F. W. and Loewenstein, R. J. (2000).In B. J. Sadock and V. A. Sadock, *Kaplan and Saddock's comprehensive textbook of psychiatry* (7th Edition). Philadelphia: Lippincot Williams and Wilkins.
15. Smith Jr, G. R. (1995). Treatment of patients with multiple symptoms. In R. A. Mayou, C. Bass and M. Sharpe (Eds.), *Treatment of functional somatic symptoms*. Oxford: Oxford University Press.
16. Barsky, A., Wyshak, G. and Klerman, G. (1992). Psychiatric comorbidity in DSM III hypochondriasis. *Archives of General Psychiatry*, 49, 101–108.
17. Barsky, A. J., Cleary, P. D., Wyshak, G., et al. (1992). A structural diagnostic interview for hypochondriasis: a proposed criterion standard. *Journal of Nervous and Mental Disease*, 180, 20–27.
18. Barsky, A. J., Cleary, P. D., Wyshak, G., et al. (1992). A structural diagnostic interview for hypochondriasis: a proposed criterion standard. *Journal of Nervous and Mental Disease*, 180, 20–27.
19. Clark, D. M., Salkovskis, P. M., Hackman, A., et al. (1998). Two psychological treatments for hypochondriasis. A randomised controlled trial. *British Journal of Psychiatry*, 173, 218–225.
20. Hiller, W., Leibbrand, R., Rief, W., et al. (2002). Predictors of course and outcome in hypochondriasis after cognitive-behavioural treatment. *Psychotherapy and Psychosomatics*, 71, 318–325.
21. Morley, S., Eccleston, C. and Williams, A. (1999). Systematic review and meta-analysis of randomised control trials of cognitive therapy and behaviour therapy for chronic pain in adults, excluding headache. *Pain*, 80, 1–13.
22. Putmnam, F. W. and Loewenstein, R. J. (2000). In B. J. Sadock and V. A. Sadock, *Kaplan and Saddock's comprehensive textbook of psychiatry* (7th Edition). Philadelphia: Lippincot Williams and Wilkins.
23. Wessely, S. (1994). Neurasthenia and chronic fatigue syndrome: theory and practice in Britain and America. *Transcultural Psychiatry*, 31, 173–209.
24. Vercolulen, J., Swanink, C., Fennis, J., Galama, J., Van der Meer, J. and Bleijenberg, G. (1996). Prognosis in chronic fatigue syndrome: a prospective study on the natural course. *Journal of Neurology, Neurosurgery and Psychiatry*, 60, 489– 494.
25. Chalder, T., Alicia, D. and Wessely, S. (1999). Treatment of chronic fatigue syndrome. In L. Malcom and D. Naber (Eds.), *Difficult clinical problems in psychiatry*. London: Martin Dunitz.
26. Ware, N. and Klienman, A. (1992). Culture and somatic experience—the social course of illness in neurasthenia and chronic fatigue syndrome. *Psychosomatic Medicine*, 54, 546–560.
27. Sharpe, M., Hawton, K., Simkin, S., et al. (1996). Cognitive behaviour therapy for chronic fatigue syndrome; a randomised controlled trial. *British Medical Journal*, 312, 22–26.
28. Littlewood, R. (1990). From categories to contexts: a decade of the 'new cross-cultural psychiatry'. *British Journal of Psychiatry*, 156, 308– 327.
29. Simons, R. C. (1980). The resolution of the Latah paradox. *Journal of Nervous and Mental Disease, 168, 195–206.*

Neuro and Old Age Psychiatry

CHAPTER 11

Neurocognitive disorders involve structural or functional disturbances of brain function leading to impairments in memory, abstract thinking, or judgment. Their underlying pathology—and their aetiology—is often known. Although the terms neuropsychiatry and organic psychiatry are sometimes used synonymously, there is a difference between the two. Psychiatric disorders that result because of defects or abnormalities in the brain structure and function come under the heading of neuropsychiatry, whereas organic psychiatry is a broader term and it comprises those psychiatric disorders that are due to medical conditions outside the brain (e.g., metabolic and endocrine disorders) (1).

Amnestic Disorders

In amnestic disorders there is circumscribed deficit in memory. The amnestic disorders are a broad group of disorders that present with an amnestic syndrome which can be due to various conditions. There is a primary impairment in the ability to create new memories (anterograde amnesia), but retrograde amnesia (inability to recall past events) is also present. The patient's social and occupational life is adversely affected.

The amnestic disorder can be caused by a general medical condition (e.g., hypoglycaemia, head trauma, cerebral tumours, multiple sclerosis), or it can be substance-induced (e.g., caused by carbon monoxide poisoning, chronic alcohol consumption, neurotoxins). Commonest cause of amnestic syndrome is Korsakoff's syndrome. In some cases, the aetiology is unknown or unclear. Unlike dementia, there is no generalised intellectual dysfunction. Amnestic disorder is termed as transient when the duration is less than one month, and chronic when it persists beyond one month.

The major neuroanatomical structures involved in memory and in the development of an amnestic disorder are the dorsomedial and midline nuclei of the thalamus, hippocampus, the mamillary bodies and the amygdala.

Korsakoff's Syndrome

Korsakoff's syndrome is the commonest cause of amnestic syndrome. Recent memory is affected more than remote memory but this is not always the case. Other features include confabulation, apathy, and passivity. This syndrome is caused by thiamine deficiency, most commonly associated with chronic alcohol abuse but can also be caused by severe starvation, gastric carcinoma, hemodialysis and hyperemesis gravidarum.

Korsakoff's syndrome is often associated with Wernicke's encephalopathy (an acute syndrome), in which there is delirium, truncal ataxia, pupillary abnormalities, ophthalmoplegia, nystagmus and peripheral neuropathy. When Wernicke's encephalopathy is not treated, Korsakoff's syndrome develops in a majority of cases.

Patients with Korsakoff's syndrome display a lack of initiative and interest, and executive function deficits involving attention and planning (2).

With treatment, patients may remain amnestic for up to three months and then there is gradual improvement. Although thiamine may prevent the development of additional amnestic symptoms, the treatment is usually unsuccessful in reversing the severe amnestic symptoms. However, approximately one-third to one-fourth of all patients recover completely.

Organic Hallucinosis, Organic Catatonic Disorder and Organic Delusional Disorder

In organic hallucinosis, there are visual or auditory hallucinations in clear consciousness, which are due to a specific organic cause. There might be secondary delusions. Common causes are hallucinogens, sensory deprivation, brain damage, seizures, and alcohol withdrawal. Common causes of organic catatonic disorder are: brain tumours, encephalitis, hypercalcaemia, liver failure and diabetic ketoacidosis.

Clinical features include decreased (stupor) or increased psychomotor activity associated with catatonic activity. The central feature of stupor is the absence or reduction of action and speech. According to Bleuler (3) the patient with a catatonic stupor has lost his will to exercise his speech, motor systems, and consciousness. Organic delusional disorder is a schizophrenia-like disorder with an organic aetiology.

Frontal Lobe Syndrome

In frontal lobe lesion, there are prominent changes in personality but IQ, memory and other cognitive functions are commonly preserved (4). The frontal lobe has functions for motor activation, intellect, conceptual planning, and aspects of personality and language production. Because of the dysfunction of the prefrontal and orbital cortex, there is disinhibition, facetious humour, euphoria, over-talkativeness, inappropriate sexual behaviour, impulsivity, apathy, loss of initiative, and slowing of thought and motor activity.

Temporal Lobe Syndrome

Temporal lobes have an important role in language, memory and emotions. Various syndromes result because of dysfunction of temporal lobes, depending on which lobe is affected or whether lesions involve both the lobes. Dominant lobe lesions cause auditory agnosia, sensory dysphasias, contralateral upper quadrant, homonymous hemianopia and prosognosia. Bilateral lesions cause global amnesia. Unilateral lesions on the dominant side cause impaired verbal memory and non- dominant unilateral lesions result in impaired non-verbal (spatial) memory. Bilateral lesions of the medial and lateral temporal lobes can cause Kluver-Bucy syndrome. Its features are: hyperorality, visual agnosia, loss of fear or anger, hypermetamorphosis (irresistible impulse to touch objects), and changes in sexual activities.

Parietal Lobe Syndrome

Due to lesions in the parietal lobes, there are a number of features.

The important ones are: cortical sensory loss, stereognosis, sensory Jacksonian fits, sensory inattention, constructional apraxia, dressing apraxia, hemiasomatognosia, anosognosia and features of Gerstmann's syndrome.

Occipital Lobe Lesions

Dysfunction of occipital lobes can cause cortical blindness, contralateral homonymous hemianopia, loss of visual perception, visual object agnosia, and alexia without agraphia.

Disorders/Symptoms due to Regional Lesions

Aphasia and Dysphasia

Aphasia is an acquired disorder of language. It is not due to dysarthria. Although the dominant hemisphere is involved in speech, there is some involvement of the non-dominant hemisphere. Broca's aphasia causes motor aphasia and expressive aphasia. Broca's aphasia causes great frustration as patients find it difficult to interact socially.

In Wernicke's aphasia, there is fluent aphasia and receptive aphasia. There is marked irritability, and no insight. Lesion in the arcuate fasciculus (that connect the Broca and Wernekie's area) results in conduction aphasia. Due to global aphasias (infarction of entire hemisphere), all language abilities are lost. The term dysphasia strictly means congenital or developmental disorders that interfere with the proper functioning of language.

Agraphia

In agraphia, there is an inability to write, subsequent to possessing the ability to write. It always accompanies aphasia.

Alexia and Dyslexia

Alexia is the inability to comprehend written words. Alexia is commonly associated with aphasia. In alexia with agraphia, disturbances of reading appear as letter and numerical plus word blindness, and all aspects of writing are affected. In alexia without agraphia, only reading is affected and writing and spelling are intact (5). Dyslexia is a developmental reading disorder. It is a very commonly recognised reading disorder. Dyslexia is characterised by difficulty with reading to read fluently and with precise comprehension. The intelligence is normal or above average.

Apraxia

Apraxia is the inability to carry out small tasks and specific movements in response to stimuli that usually elicit the tasks and the movements. In ideomotor apraxia, the person is unable to do a trivial task e.g., hammering a nail. In ideational apraxia, there is inability to perform a sequence of movements e.g., put letter in an envelope, close it and place a stamp. In constructional aphasia, the person cannot draw or copy a geometric design or to arrange toy building blocks. Inability to dress is present in dressing apraxia.

Anomia

In anomia the person is unable to name objects e.g., a comb. The function of that object is, however, described.

Word Deafness

The patient cannot understand spoken words, although the ability to write, read and speak is intact.

Agnosia

This is a disorder of recognition of objects. In auditory agnosia there is inability to recognise non-verbal sounds e.g., car horns or music (Amusia). In visual agnosia, there is inability to recognise a previously recognizable object, by visual inspection alone In tactile agnosia, the person is unable to recognise objects by touching. Prosopagnosia is the inability to recognise faces and to learn the new ones. This is due to bilateral lesions.

Anosognosia

This means a lack of awareness of disease. In anosognosia, there is partial or complete awareness of the deficit. The commonest unawareness is for hemiplegia. Anosognosia occurs more often in right-sided lesions.

Aprosody

Due to non-dominant frontal lobe lesion, there is an inability to inflect speech or affect. Lesion in the posterior non-dominant region results in losing the ability to comprehend the prosody of another person's speech.

Gerstmann Syndrome

Lesions in the dominant parietal lobe results in this syndrome. The prominent features include finger agnosia, right-left disorientation, dyscalculia and dysgraphia.

Epilepsy

Epilepsy is the most common chronic neurological disease in the general population. A substantial number of patients with epilepsy have psychiatric difficulties sometime during the course of their illness. A conspicuous change in personality is quite common. Psychosis and violence in patients with epilepsy do not occur as often as is generally believed.

Epilepsy can be defined as a disturbance in the central nervous system resulting from excessive neuronal discharge. An epileptic seizure involves proximal cerebral neuronal firing. However, this does not necessarily result in disturbance of consciousness, perceptual abnormalities or motor symptoms.

The term 'convulsion' refers to any seizure in which motor manifestations predominate (6). Incidence rates of 20–70 per 100,000 per year and point prevalence rates of 4–100 per 1000 in the general population have been found. Both incidence and prevalence rates are greatest for children in early childhood, decline between 5–16 years of age and rise again in the elderly population (7).

The various causes include genetic causes, birth trauma, congenital malformations, neurological disorders, trauma or physical agents, alcohol and drug abuse, metabolic and nutritional disorders, neoplasms, degenerative disease, febrile seizures and various other neuro-chemical abnormalities.

Generalised seizures include tonic-clonic (grand mal) seizures and absence (petit mal) seizures, and they can be primary or secondary in occurrence. Primary generalised seizures are generalised from the beginning of the ictus and show no warning symptoms, whereas secondary seizures are frequently preceded by warnings or auras. Tonic-clonic (grand mal) seizures are characterised by a sudden loss of consciousness followed by a period of tonic rigidity in which the entire body usually becomes rigid in extension, the patient falls to the ground from a standing or sitting posture, sometimes with a cry, and may urinate. After the period of tonic rigidity, clonic, rhythmic jerking of the face, trunk and limbs ensue. Consciousness gradually returns and is often accompanied by a post-ictal state of confusion, headache and drowsiness. EEG shows bilaterally synchronous poly-spikes and slow-wave bursts during the seizure.

Absence (petit mal) seizures are manifested by brief attacks of unconsciousness. They usually occur in childhood between 4 and 8 years of age. Most of the seizures are simple absence attacks in which the patient does not lose body tone or fall. They last 5–10 seconds. The EEG shows bilateral, synchronous 3–4 per second spike and slow-wave discharges. The patient is rarely aware of these attacks, so history from an observer is not only helpful but mandatory as well.

Partial seizures arise from a particular focal region of the brain. A partial seizure may remain partial, spreading to neighbouring cortical regions without loss of consciousness (Jacksonian seizures) or become a generalised convulsion (8). Partial seizures can be simple or complex. Consciousness is preserved in simple partial seizures, whereas the person's consciousness is impaired in complex partial seizures. Simple partial seizures are usually motor seizures that involve clonic movement or a muscle or loss of muscle tone on the side of the body contralateral to the seizure focus, but patients may also exhibit sensory symptoms such as abdominal pain, pain localised elsewhere, proximal autonomic discharges (for example experiencing sudden cold), or hallucinations which may be visual, auditory, olfactory or gustatory.

Complex partial seizures may be temporal or extra-temporal in origin. Complex partial seizures can be divided into the following six categories:

1. Impairment of consciousness only
2. Psychomotor symptoms
3. Psychosensory symptoms
4. Cognitive symptoms
5. Emotional symptoms
6. Mixed symptoms

Psychomotor symptoms, or automatisms, often start with repetitive movements of the hands or shuffling of the feet. Automatic behaviours can include simple movements of the hands and feet to more complex tasks like dressing. There can be visual and auditory hallucinations and perceptual changes in shape and size. Changes in the intensity of sound, taste or smell also occur. The patient also has intense anxiety, sadness and feelings of happiness. Cognitive experiences such as déja-vu and jamais-vu are also experienced. Most of the time psychosensory symptoms occur as auras, but may also occur during the ictus or after or between ictus (9).

Epilepsy and Behavioural Disturbances

One author (10) described the psychiatric disturbances that occur in epilepsy patients as follows:

1. Behavioural disturbances that are related to structural defects in the brain that cause both epilepsy and behavioural disturbances, such as psychosis in intellectual disability patients who also suffer from seizures
2. Disturbances that are related to the ictus (seizure) itself, for example, automatisms
3. Behavioural problems occurring inter- ictally that may or may be related to the epileptic process

Another author (11) has proposed the following two mechanisms to explain the behavioural disturbances that occur:

1. A positive seizure effect in which an ictal discharge in a specific brain area elicits behaviour represented in that area
2. A negative seizure effect in which an ictal discharge in a specific brain area interferes with the expression of behaviours that are generated in other brain areas

Behavioural Disturbances

Peri-ictal events readily precede the seizure and take the form of a prodrome or aura. The epileptic prodrome consists of dysphoria (sadness and irritability) and occasionally hallucinations and may last several days, sometimes more than a week. Ictal events are associated with mental state changes that are sometimes mistaken for classic psychotic behaviours. The most common ictal behavioural disturbances are psychomotor symptoms (automatisms). Aggressive behaviour during an ictus is rare and usually not directed towards a person or object. In some patients, status epilepticus can resemble major psychiatric disorders. Post-ictal psychosis is the most common epileptic psychosis encountered in clinical practice.

Inter-Ictal Behavioural Changes

Epileptic psychosis can resemble schizophrenia-like psychosis or bipolar-like psychosis. Depression can occur and there can be personality changes as well. The issue of violence in epilepsy is highly controversial (12). No increase in violence has been observed for epileptics in the general population. Ictal aggression is extremely rare.

Prolactin Levels

Although there is a significant increase in the level of prolactin after a tonic clonic seizure, it is important to remember that a rise in prolactin level is not necessary for establishing a diagnosis of epileptic seizures (13).

Treatment of Seizures

Conventional anticonvulsants drugs include carbamazepine, sodium valproate (valproic acid), phenytoin, phenobarbital, clonazepam, ethosuxemide and primidone. New anticonvulsant drugs include felbamate, gabapentin and vigabatrin for the treatment of behavioural symptoms. Lithium has been used in low levels to control behavioural disturbances. Regarding the use of neuroleptic medication, it must be remembered that these drugs tend to promote epileptic seizures in patients both with and without epilepsy. However, fluphenazine and haloperidol are considered safer drugs. Phenothiazines are more at risk.

Head Injury

Head trauma can result in an array of mental symptoms and lead to a diagnosis of dementia due to head trauma or to a mental disorder not otherwise specified due to a general medical condition (e.g., post-concussional disorder). Head trauma most commonly occurs in people 15 to 25 years of age and has a male-to-female predominance of approximately 3 to 1. Gross estimates based on the severity of the head trauma suggest that virtually all patients with serious head trauma, more than half of patients with moderate head trauma, and about 10 percent of patients with mild head trauma have ongoing neuropsychiatric sequelae resulting from the head trauma.

Head trauma can be divided grossly into penetrating head trauma (e.g., trauma produced by a bullet) and blunt trauma, in which there is no physical penetration of the skull. Blunt trauma is far more common than penetrating head trauma. Motor vehicle accidents account for more than half of all the incidents of blunt Central Nervous System (CNS) trauma; falls, violence, and sports-related head trauma account for most of the remaining cases.

Head injuries may be categorised by the type of injury produced by the trauma, that is, as either a closed head injury or an open head injury. The following may be found as consequences of the trauma: skull fractures, cranial nerve injuries, concussions, contusions, haemorrhages, shearing lesions, and haematomas. Other less common lesions include penetrating lesions, compressions, lacerations, and vascular occlusions and dissections. The secondary effects of such trauma, which complicate the neuropsychiatric sequelae and rehabilitation, include hypoxemia, hypotension, hypercapnia, anaemia, hyponatremia, hypoglycaemia, infection, and seizures. Personality changes that occur in brain-injured patients may persist for years after the injury. Depression with typical vegetative signs has been noted in brain-injured patients.

Management and Treatment

The treatment of the cognitive and behavioural disorders in patients with head trauma is basically similar to the treatment approaches used in other patients with these symptoms. One difference is that patients with head trauma may be particularly susceptible to the side effects associated with psychotropic drugs; therefore, treatment with these agents should be initiated in lower dosages than usual, and they should be titrated upward more slowly than usual. Standard antidepressants can be used to treat depression, and either anticonvulsants or antipsychotics can be used to treat aggression and impulsivity. Other approaches to the symptoms include lithium, calcium channel blockers, and β-adrenergic receptor antagonists.

Tic Disorders

Tic disorders are distinguished by the type of tic symptoms, their frequency, and the pattern in which they emerge over time. Tics are abnormal movements or vocalisations that most commonly affect the muscles of the face and neck, such as eye-blinking, head-jerking, mouth-grimacing, or head-shaking. Typical vocal tics include throat-clearing, grunting, snorting, and coughing. Tics are defined as rapid and repetitive muscle contractions resulting in movements or vocalisations that are experienced as involuntary. Children and adolescents may exhibit tic behaviours that occur after a stimulus or in response to an internal urge. Tic disorders, a group of neuropsychiatric disorders, generally begin in childhood or adolescence with a stable or fluctuating course in childhood and generally wane by adolescence. Although tics are not volitional, in some individuals they may be suppressed for periods. The most widely known and most severe tic disorder is Gilles de la Tourette syndrome, also known as Tourette's disorder (for more details, please refer to this topic in the chapter 'Child and Adolescent Psychiatry').

Multiple Sclerosis (MS)

A demyelinating disorder of the central nervous system, MS causes some degree of cognitive impairment in almost half of cases and can present with unexplained subcortical dementia. The disorder can also cause and occasionally present with affective disorders. MS is characterised by multiple episodes of symptoms, pathophysiologically related to multifocal lesions in the white matter of the CNS. The cause remains unknown, but studies have focused on slow viral infections and disturbances in the immune system. The disease is much more frequent in cold and temperate climates than in the tropics and subtropics and more common in women than in men; it is predominantly a disease of young adults. In most patients, the onset occurs between the ages of 20 and 40 years.

The neuropsychiatric symptoms of MS can be divided into cognitive and behavioural types. Research reports have found that 30 to 50 percent of patients with MS have mild cognitive impairment and that 20 to 30 percent of them have serious cognitive impairments. Although evidence indicates that patients with MS experience a decline in their general intelligence, memory is the most commonly affected cognitive function. The severity of the memory impairment does not seem to be correlated with the severity of the neurological symptoms or the duration of the illness.

The behavioural symptoms associated with MS are varied and can include euphoria, depression, and personality changes. Psychosis is a rare complication. Approximately 25 percent of persons with MS exhibit a euphoric mood that is not hypomanic, but somewhat more cheerful than their situation warrants and not necessarily in character with their disposition before the onset of MS. Only 10 percent of patients with MS have a sustained and elevated mood, although it is still not truly hypomanic. Depression, however, is common; it affects 25 to 50 percent of patients with MS and results in a higher rate of suicide than is seen in the general population. Risk factors for suicide in patients with MS are male sex, the onset of MS before age 30, and a relatively recent diagnosis of the disorder. Personality changes are also common in patients with MS; they affect 20 to 40 percent of patients and are often characterised by increased irritability or apathy.

Human Immunodeficiency Virus (HIV) infection

The Human Immunodeficiency Virus (HIV) produces primary and secondary effects in the Central Nervous System (CNS), resulting in numerous neuropsychiatric syndromes. The initial presentation in approximately 10% of HIV-infected patients, consists of overt neuropsychiatric complaints and findings. An organic cognitive or mental disorder will develop in approximately 70% of HIV-infected people during their illness.

The most common neuropsychiatric syndromes associated with HIV infection include dementia, delirium, depression, and apathy. The AIDS Dementia Complex (ADC) is the most common chronic neuropsychiatric syndrome in AIDS patients.

Neurosyphilis

Neurosyphilis (also known as general paresis) appears 10 to 15 years after the primary Treponema infection. Since the advent of penicillin, neurosyphilis has become a rare disorder, although AIDS is associated with reintroducing neurosyphilis into medical practice in some urban settings. Neurosyphilis generally affects the frontal lobes and results in personality changes, development of poor judgment, irritability, and decreased care for self. Delusions of grandeur develop in

10 to 20 percent of affected patients. The disease progresses with the development of dementia and tremor, until patients are paretic. The neurological symptoms include Argyll-Robertson pupils, which are small, irregular, and unequal and have light-near reflex dissociation, tremor, dysarthria, and hyperreflexia. Cerebrospinal Fluid (CSF) examination shows lymphocytosis, increased protein, and a positive result on a Venereal Disease Research Laboratory (VDRL) test.

Chronic Meningitis

Chronic meningitis is now seen more often than in the recent past because of the immunocompromised condition of people with AIDS. The usual causative agents are Mycobacterium tuberculosis, Cryptococcus, and Coccidioides. The usual symptoms are headache, memory impairment, confusion, and fever.

Prion Disease

Prion disease is a group of related disorders caused by a transmissible infectious protein known as a prion. Included in this group are Creutzfeldt-Jakob disease (CJD), Gerstmann-Straussler-Scheinker disorder (GSS), and kuru. Collectively, these disorders are also known as subacute spongiform encephalopathy because of shared neuropathological changes that consist of (1) spongiform vacuolisation, (2) neuronal loss, and (3) astrocyte proliferation in the cerebral cortex. Amyloid plaques may or may not be present.

Prions are transmissible agents, but differ from viruses in that they lack nucleic acid. Creutzfeldt-Jakob disease is an invariably fatal, rapidly progressive disorder that occurs mainly in middle-aged or older adults. It manifests initially with fatigue, flu-like symptoms, and cognitive impairment. As the disease progresses, focal neurological findings such as aphasia and apraxia occur. Psychiatric manifestations are protean and include emotional lability, anxiety, euphoria, depression, delusions, hallucinations, or marked personality changes. The disease progresses over months, leading to dementia, akinetic mutism, coma, and death.

The rates of CJD range from 1 to 2 cases per 1 million persons a year, worldwide. The infectious agent self-replicates and can be transmitted to humans by inoculation with infected tissue and sometimes by ingestion of contaminated food. Iatrogenic transmission has been reported via transplantation of contaminated cornea or dura mater or to children via contaminated supplies of human growth hormone derived from infected persons. Neurosurgical transmission has also been reported.

Diagnosis requires pathological examination of the cortex, which reveals the classic triad of spongiform vacuolation, loss of neurons, and astrocyte cell proliferation. The cortex and basal ganglia are most affected. No known treatment exists for Creutzfeldt-Jakob disease. Death usually occurs within six months after diagnosis.

In 1995 a variant of CJD appeared in the United Kingdom. At autopsy, prion disease was found. The disease was attributed to the transmission in the United Kingdom of BSE between cattle and from cattle to humans in the 1980s. No cure exists, and death usually occurs within 2 to 3 years after diagnosis. Prevention is dependent on careful monitoring of cattle for disease and feeding them grain instead of meat by-products.

Kuru is an epidemic prion disease found in New Guinea that is caused by cannibalistic funeral rituals in which the brains of the deceased are eaten. Women are more affected by the disorder than men, presumably because they participate in the ceremony to a greater extent. Death usually occurs within two years after symptoms develop. Neuropsychiatric signs and symptoms consist of ataxia, chorea, strabismus, delirium, and dementia. Pathological changes are similar to those with other prion diseases: neuronal loss, spongiform lesions, and astrocytic proliferation. The cerebellum is most affected.

Gerstmann-Straussler-Scheinker disease is characterised by ataxia, chorea, and cognitive decline leading to dementia. The disease is inherited, and affected families have been identified over several generations. Genetic testing can confirm the presence of the abnormal genes before onset. Pathological changes characteristic of prion disease are present: spongiform lesions, neuronal loss, and astrocyte proliferation. Amyloid plaques have been found in the cerebellum. Onset of the disease occurs between 30 and 40 years of age. The disease is fatal within five years of onset.

Normal Pressure Hydrocephalus

Hydrocephalus (HC) is dilatation of the ventricles within the brain caused by elevation of the pressure of the CSF synthesised within them. It is 'communicating' when the block to CSF flow occurs outside the ventricular system and non-communicating when the block is within the ventricles.

Hydrocephalus can cause a wide range of neurological and psychiatric symptoms and signs. Manifestations include enlargement of the head (if present in infancy), headache, and sudden death due to hydrocephalic attacks with acute elevation of intracranial pressure, progressive visual failure, gait disturbances (often 'gait apraxia'), incontinence and subcortical cognitive impairment progressing to dementia. 'Normal pressure hydrocephalus' in older people is classically associated with the triad of gait apraxia, incontinence and cognitive decline.

Subdural Haematoma

Subdural haematomas are accumulations of blood and blood products in the space between the fibrous dura mater and the more delicate arachnoid membrane which encloses the brain. Acute subdural haematomas are by definition diagnosed close to the time of trauma as a result either of symptoms present at the time— headache, depressed level of consciousness, focal neurological signs—or from a CT scan. Chronic subdurals give rise to more gradually evolving symptoms and signs. While they can also cause headache, depressed consciousness and focal signs, they sometimes result in predominantly cognitive features, including confusion and dementia.

Delirium

Delirium is also known as an acute confusional state, an acute brain syndrome, a toxic confusional state, and an acute organic psychosis.

In delirium, there are three essential clinical features:

1. There is impairment of consciousness.
2. Change in cognition (e.g., memory deficit, disorientation, language disturbance) or the development of a perceptual disturbance that is not because of a pre-existing dementia.
3. The disturbance develops over a short time (usually within hours to days) and typically fluctuates during the day.

Delirium has many causes, but the resultant clinical presentation is more or less similar as all signs and symptoms are related to the patient's level of consciousness and cognitive disturbance. Patients may become hyperaroused, overactive and restless (14). In addition there are mood symptoms, perceptual abnormalities, and neurological symptoms like tremor, asterixis, nystagmus, incoordination, and urinary incontinence. Helpful initial indicators which should arouse suspicion of delirium include changes in cognitive function (e.g., worsening of concentration), visual or auditory hallucinations, reduced mobility, restlessness, agitation, appetite and sleep disturbances, social withdrawal, and changes in mood (15). If delirium is identified, then the short Confusion Assessment Method (CAM) (16) should be used to confirm the diagnosis. CAM-ICU (17) is used for those patients who are in critical care or the recovery room after surgery.

The point prevalence of delirium in the general population is 0.4 percent for people 18 years of age and older, and 1.1 percent for people 55 and older. It occurs in about 10–20% of all hospitalised patients, and in 10–42% of elderly patients upon admission to the hospital; the incidence is 11–31% after admission (18).

The causes of post-operative delirium include the stress of surgery, post-operative pain, insomnia, pain medication, electrolyte imbalances, infection, fever, and blood loss. Delirium develops in 80 percent of terminally ill patients. Advanced age and male gender are risk factors for the development of delirium. Other predisposing factors are: post-cardiotomy patients, burn victims, brain damage patients (dementias, stroke and brain injuries), and drugs withdrawal.

DSM-5 Diagnostic Criteria for Delirium Due to General Medical Conditions (19)

a. Disturbance in attention (i.e. reduced ability to direct, focus, sustain, and shift attention) and awareness (reduced orientation to the environment).

b. The disturbance develops over a short period of time (usually hours to a few days), represents a change from baseline attention and awareness, and tends to fluctuate in severity during the course of a day.

c. An additional disturbance occurs in cognition (e.g., memory deficit, disorientation, language, visuospatial ability, or perception).

d. The disturbances in Criteria A and C are not better explained by another pre-existing established, or evolving neurocognitive disorder and do not occur in the context of a severely reduced level of arousal, such as coma.

e. There is evidence from the history, physical examination, or laboratory findings that the disturbance is a direct physiological consequence of another medical condition, substance intoxication or withdrawal (i.e. due to a drug of abuse or to a medication), or exposure to a toxin, or is due to multiple aetiologies.

Mini-Mental State Examination is helpful in the assessment of delirium. The presence of a known physical illness or a history of head trauma or alcohol or other substance dependence increases the likelihood of the diagnosis. The laboratory tests should include standard blood tests and urine analysis. In delirium, the EEG characteristically shows a generalised slowing of activity and may be useful in differentiating delirium from depression or psychosis. The EEG sometimes shows focal areas of hyperactivity.

Common Causes of Delirium

Central nervous system disorder

Seizure (post-ictal, non-convulsive status)

Migraine

Head trauma, brain tumour, subarachnoid haemorrhage, subdural, epidural haematoma, abscess, intracerebral haemorrhage, cerebellar haemorrhage, non-haemorrhagic stroke, transient ischaemia

Metabolic Disorder

Electrolyte Abnormalities

Diabetes, hypoglycaemia, hyperglycaemia, or insulin resistance

Systemic Illness

Infection (e.g., sepsis, malaria, erysipelas, viral, plague, Lyme disease, syphilis, or abscess)

Trauma

Change in fluid status (dehydration or volume overload)

Nutritional deficiency

Burns

Uncontrolled pain

Heat stroke

Medications

Pain medications (e.g., post-operative morphine)

Antibiotics, antivirals, and antifungals

Steroids Anaesthesia

Cardiac medications

Antihypertensives

Antineoplastic agents

Anticholinergic agents

Cardiac

Cardiac failure, arrhythmia, myocardial infarction, cardiac assist device, cardiac surgery

Pulmonary

Chronic obstructive pulmonary disease, hypoxia, SIADH

Endocrine

Adrenal crisis or adrenal failure, thyroid abnormality, parathyroid abnormality

Haematological

Anaemia, leukaemia, blood dyscrasia, stem cell transplant

Renal

Renal failure, uraemia, SIADH

Hepatic

Hepatitis, cirrhosis, hepatic failure

Drugs of Abuse

Intoxication and withdrawal

Toxins

Heavy metals and aluminium.

In treating delirium, the main goal is to treat the underlying cause and the presenting symptoms. The other important goal of treatment is to provide physical, sensory, and environmental support. The two major symptoms of delirium that may require pharmacological treatment are psychosis and insomnia. A commonly used drug for psychosis is haloperidol. Phenothiazines should be avoided in delirious patients because these drugs are associated with significant anticholinergic activity. Use of second-generation antipsychotics, such as risperidone, clozapine, olanzapine, quetiapine, ziprasidone, and aripiprazole, may be considered for delirium management.

Insomnia is best treated with benzodiazepines with short or intermediate half-lives. Benzodiazepines with long half-lives and barbiturates should be avoided.

Course and Prognosis

Although the onset of delirium is usually sudden, prodromal symptoms (e.g., restlessness and fearfulness) can occur in the days preceding the onset of florid symptoms. Delirium generally lasts less than a week. When the causative factors are treated, the symptoms of delirium usually recede over a 3 to 7 day period, but in patients, some of the symptoms may take up to two weeks to resolve completely. The older the patient and longer the patient has been delirious, the longer the delirium takes to resolve. Because of the various associated medical conditions that lead to delirium, delirium can have a high mortality rate.

Assessment and Management of Psychiatric Disorders in Old Age

Although the principles of assessment of elderly patients do not differ significantly from those of adult patients, there is more emphasis on certain areas. As there is a high prevalence of cognitive disorders in older persons, it should be ascertained at the very onset whether a patient understands the nature and purpose of the examination. There is a more significant role of physical examination and laboratory investigations. Assessments take a longer time, there is more need for information from the informant(s), and a detailed knowledge of a patient's psychosocial situation. With elderly patients, a single mental state examination may not be reliable because of fluctuations. Finally, the needs of the carers have also to be taken into account.

It is very important to bear in mind that elderly persons have a higher risk for suicide than any other population. Various reasons for suicide include loneliness, financial problems, poor medical health, or depression (which is the main psychiatric illness in suicide cases). About 60 percent of those who commit suicide are men; 75 percent of those who attempt suicide are women. Older patients with major medical illnesses or a recent loss should be evaluated for depressive symptomatology and suicidal ideation.

Regarding the pharmacological treatment of old age people, it is imperative to remember that because of the altered pharmacokinetics and higher incidence of medical problems, care needs to be exercised when prescribing medications and low doses should be preferred.

As for adults, psychological treatments are also relevant and effective for older people.

Dementia

In dementia there is acquired global impairment of intellectual functions which is usually (but not always) progressive. This occurs in a setting of clear consciousness. The syndrome of dementia is caused by a number of diseases of which 50–60% is attributed to Alzheimer's type. ICD-10 defines dementia as a syndrome due to a disease of the brain, usually of a chronic or progressive nature, in which there is disturbance of multiple higher cortical functions; including memory, thinking, orientation, comprehension, calculation, learning capacity, language and judgment while consciousness in not clouded. The cognitive impairments are commonly accompanied and occasionally preceded, by deterioration in emotional control, social behaviour and motivation.

The clinical picture is much determined by the premorbid personality of the patient (20). The intellectual impairment or dementia develops gradually over a time period. There are characteristic changes in cognition, memory, language, and visuospatial functions. Behavioural disturbances include agitation, restlessness, wandering, angry outbursts, disinhibited behaviour, impulsiveness and sleep disturbances. Delusions and hallucinations subsequently develop in about 75 percent of patients. There are various causes of cognitive impairment e.g., brain injuries, cerebral tumours, alcohol, medications, infections, chronic pulmonary diseases, and inflammatory diseases. It should be remembered that in one patient there may be more than one cause (21).

ICD-10 Diagnostic Criteria for Dementia

- Evidence of a decline in both memory and thinking which is sufficient to impair personal activities and activity of daily living. At least six months' history is required.
- A decline in other cognitive abilities characterised by deterioration in judgement and thinking, such as planning and organising, and in the general processing of information.
- At least six months' history is required.
- Evidence of clear consciousness (it is not clouded).
- There is a decline in emotional control or motivation, or change in social behaviour. This can manifest as emotional lability, irritability, apathy or coarsening of social behaviour.

DSM-5 Diagnostic Criteria for Dementia (Major Neurocognitive Disorder)

a. Evidence of significant cognitive decline from a previous level of performance in one or more cognitive domains (complex attention, executive function, learning and memory, language, perceptual-motor, or social cognition) based on:
   i. concern of the individual, a knowledgeable informant, or the clinician that there has been a significant decline in cognitive function; and
   ii. a substantial impairment in cognitive performance, preferably documented by standardised

neuropsychological testing or, in its absence, another quantified clinical assessment.

b. The cognitive deficits interfere with independence in everyday activities (i.e. at a minimum, requiring assistance with complex instrumental activities of daily living such as paying bills or manageing medications).

c. The cognitive deficits do not occur exclusively in the context of delirium.

d. The cognitive deficits are not better explained.

Dementias can be classified as reversible and irreversible, although the number of patients having reversible dementias is small. It needs to be mentioned that some dementias are arrestable rather than reversible (22). About 10 to 15 percent have potentially treatable conditions.

The treatable causes of dementia are:

- Normal pressure hydrocephalus
- Subdural haematoma
- B1, B6, and B12 deficiency
- Endocrine disorders e.g., hypothyroidism, Cushing's syndrome, and Addison's disease
- Infections e.g., syphilis
- Alcohol-related dementias (early stage)
- Wilson's disease
- Transient global amnesia

Dementias are also classified as cortical and subcortical, depending on the site of the cerebral lesion. A subcortical dementia occurs in Huntington's disease, Parkinson's disease, normal pressure hydrocephalus, vascular dementia, and Wilson's disease. The subcortical dementias are associated with movement disorders, gait apraxia, psychomotor retardation, apathy, and akinetic mutism, which can sometimes be confused with catatonia. The cortical dementias are Alzheimer's type, Creutzfeldt-Jakob disease (CJD), and Pick's disease, which frequently manifest aphasia, agnosia, and apraxia.

Clinical Presentation

Usually there is a gradual onset, but dementia may come into attention after an acute exacerbation. There is memory impairment and personality changes occur. Speech symptoms include syntactical errors, dysphasia, confabulation and muteness in the late stages. There is disorientation in time, place, and person. Frontal lobe dysfunctions include loss of planning abilities, inappropriate behaviour, organic orderliness, shrinkage of milieu, and catastrophic reaction. Parietal lobe functions are affected, there is an impaired sense of direction and difficulty in object recognition. Regarding mood, there can be anxiety, depression and irritability, restlessness. Thinking is slow and rigid and judgement becomes impaired. Persecutory delusions and abnormal perceptual experiences like hallucinations, illusions and mirror signs occur.

Common concurrent physical illnesses include infection, metabolic disturbances, anaemia, cardiac problems, drug toxicity, hypothermia, and malnutrition. Psychiatric symptoms include anxiety and depressive symptomatology, hallucinations and delusions. Physical disabilities like poor hearing, pain, poor vision, incontinence and arthritis, may develop.

Assessment

When dementia is suspected, it needs to be ascertained, whether it is reversible or not, what type of dementia it is, and what support would be needed for the patient as well as the carer. As patients with dementia have a risk of self- neglect, wandering, and abuse, it is important that risk assessment is carried out routinely for these patients. The risk of driving also needs to be looked into.

A very comprehensive cognitive assessment and a detailed physical examination are mandatory. Brain CT scan is needed is less inconvenient than MRI, although an MRI scan can help better in differentiating between Alzheimer's and vascular dementia. Brain imageing helps exclude space-occupying lesions. X-ray chest and EEG are important investigations. In AD, EEG shows diffuse theta and delta activities with slowing of the alpha rhythm. Less than 5% of AD patients have normal EEG. SPECT scan shows decreased blood flow in temporal and parietal lobes. On PET scan there is decrease glucose and O2 consumption by 50%. Full blood count, ESR, U and E,

Cortical and Subcortical Dementias

Features	Cortical	Subcortical
Alertness	Normal	Slow down
Motor speed	Normal	Slowed
Attention	Intact in early stages	Impaired
Episodic memory	Severe amnesia	Recognition better than recall
Executive functions	Normal until late	Impaired from onset
Language	Early dysphasia	Late dysphasia
Praxis	Impaired	Normal

lfts, tfts, blood glucose, serum B12 and folate, and urine examination are the routine investigations. There are many tests for cognitive testing. Although a score of less than 24 on Mini-Mental State Examination (MMSE) helps in the diagnosis, a definitive diagnosis of dementia should only be made after a complete clinical history and mental state examination.

Other tests are Abbreviated Mental Sate Test Score (AMTS), Clock drawing test, Cambridge Examination for Mental Disorders of the Elderly (CAMDEX), and Comprehensive Assessment and Referral Evaluation (CARE) (23). Dementia Rating Scale (DRS) and Dementia Behaviour Disturbance Scale (DBDS) help in assessing behavioural disturbances, whereas Instrumental Activities of Daily Living, Clifton Assessment Procedures for Elderly (CAPE), and Quality of Life Scale (QOL) assess the functioning of patients with dementia (24).

Differential Diagnoses

Differential diagnoses of dementia include normal ageing, delirium, depression, schizophrenia, fictitious disorder, amnesia, and intellectual disability. Normal ageing is not necessarily associated with any significant cognitive decline, but minor memory problems can occur as a normal part of ageing. These normal occurrences are sometimes referred to as benign senescent forgetfulness or age-associated memory impairment. They are distinguished from dementia by their minor severity and because they do not interfere significantly with a person's social or occupational behaviour.

Sometimes it may be difficult to differentiate between delirium and dementia. But it should be noted that delirium may sometimes be superimposed on dementia.

Some patients with depression have symptoms of cognitive impairment difficult to distinguish from symptoms of dementia. The clinical picture is sometimes referred to as pseudodementia. Patients with depression-related cognitive dysfunction generally have prominent depressive symptoms, more insight into their symptoms than do demented patients, and often a history of depressive episodes.

Factitious disorder can sometimes be confused with dementia. Persons who attempt to simulate memory loss, as in factitious disorder, do so in an erratic and inconsistent manner. In true dementia, memory for time and place is lost before memory for person, and recent memory is lost before remote memory.

Although schizophrenia can be associated with some acquired intellectual impairment, its symptoms are much less severe than are the related symptoms of psychosis and thought disorder seen in dementia. Intellectual disability can occur in childhood which does not include memory impairment, occurs in childhood. Amnestic disorder is characterised by circumscribed loss of memory and no deterioration.

Epidemiology

The prevalence of dementia (and of the common subtype, Alzheimer's disease) rises exponentially with age. The overall prevalence of dementia in people aged 65 years and over is around 6% (25). The incidence of

Differential Diagnoses of Delirium and Dementia

Features	Delirium	Dementia
Onset	Abrupt	Insidious
Course	Fluctuating	Stable/progressive
Duration	Days/weeks	Months/years
Appearance	Frightened	Unkempt
Speech	Usually incoherent	Normal except word-finding difficulties and perseveration
Consciousness	Reduced/fluctuating	Clear
Orientation	Impaired	Intact initially
Attention	Globally impaired	Normal except in severe cases
Affect	Irritable/anxious	Labile
Memory	Recent memory markedly impaired	Both recent and remote memories are usually impaired
Hallucinations	Usually visual	Usually no hallucination
Delusions	Random, fleeting	Usually none, sometimes paranoid
Reversibility	Often reversible	Usually not reversible

Following Distinguishing Features are Helpful

Dementia	Pseudodementia
No diurnal variation	Worse in the morning
Normal sleep	Early insomnia
Wrong answer	'I do not know' answer
History of depression is not necessary	History of depression is suggestive
Psychomotor agitation	Psychomotor retardation
No guilt feelings	Guilt feelings may be present
No role for antidepressants	Improvement with antidepressants
Family history of dementia	Family history of depression
Vague onset	Accurate onset
Brain atrophy on CT scan	Little evidence of brain atrophy on CT scan

dementia also increases exponentially with age from the age of 60. For dementia of all types, the overall incidence is about one new case per year for every hundred persons aged 65 years and over (26). Regarding the incidence of dementia, gender is not a significant factor (27).

Of all patients with dementia, 50 to 60 percent have the most common type of dementia is of the Alzheimer's type (Alzheimer's disease). There is a relative excess of Alzheimer's disease among women, and vascular dementia among men.

The second most common type of dementia is vascular dementia, which is causally related to cerebrovascular diseases. Hypertension predisposes a person to this vascular dementia. This type of dementia accounts for 15 to 30 percent of all dementia cases. Approximately 10 to 15 percent of patients have coexisting vascular dementia and dementia of the Alzheimer's type.

Risk factors for dementia are increasing age, family history, and female sex. History of head injury is a substantial risk factor, although some studies have not supported this finding (28). High education is thought to be associated with less risk for developing dementia. The evidence for depression being a risk factor for dementia remains inconsistent (29).

Management of Dementia

A structured approach to manage dementia includes treating the cause and comorbid psychiatric as well as physical illness(es) when possible, and ensuring consistent community support for the patients and carers.

Drugs aim to improve cognitive deficits, psychiatric symptoms and behavioural disturbances. The main class of medications for cognitive problems is anticholinesterase inhibitors. These include tacrine, donepezil, rivastigmine and galantamine. Tacrine is not popular now, mainly because of its toxic effect on the liver. Donepezil and galantamine are reversible inhibitors of acetylcholinesterase. Donepezil has a half-life of 72 hours. The half-life of rivastigmine and galantamine is about 7 to 8 hours. These medications are effective for mild to moderate Alzheimer's disease, as well as in mixed (vascular and Alzheimer's disease) and Lewy body dementia (30).

Pharmacological treatment of other problems include antipsychotics (for psychoses and behavioural issues), antidepressants and B-blockers. Because of various side effects, benzodiazepines should be avoided if possible. Atypical antipsychotics are now preferred in this group of patients (31), because of extrapyramidal side- effects, postural hypotension and tardive dyskinesia caused by typical antipsychotics. There is, however, concern about the use of antipsychotics (32), as there is an increased risk of stroke (33). Even though risperidone and olanzapine have become known about this issue, all antipsychotics pose this risk. There is, further concern that antipsychotics (evidence for quetiapine) can worsen the cognitive functions (34) which are already compromised in dementia, and also precipitate parkinsonian syndrome, especially in Lewy body dementia (35).

Psychological therapies include reality orientation, reminiscence therapy, validation therapy, memory therapy and resolution therapy. Reality orientation helps the patient to preserve the existing skills and focuses on the deficits of dementia, e.g., disorientation and short-term memory impairment. It is one of the best psychological treatments (36). Reminiscence therapy, in which patients are encouraged to remember the past events (at which they are good as compared to recent memory), is also helpful. There is evidence that starting with reality orientation and subsequently initiating reminiscence after some progress, is more beneficial (37). Validation therapy targets the emotional needs of patients with dementia. Memory therapy utilises simple aids to help the patients with mild dementia. Resolution therapy complements reality orientation. It has been developed on the same assumption on which validation therapy is based, ie, there is meaning underlying the confused talk and behaviour of patients (38). Environmental and social management is essential and imperative. It includes home assessments, home care, and admissions in residential and nursing care. The role of social services in the management of dementia patients cannot be overstated.

Prognosis

This depends on the underlying cause and severity of dementia at the time of diagnosis. People with dementia have a lower survival rate compared to matched control group. The mortality rate in AD is about 3–5 times more than matched group. Females with dementia have a higher survival rate than men with dementia. Factors associated with a lower survival rate: being male, psychotic features and physical illness. In AD, average duration of illness from onset of symptoms to death is 2–8 years. Vascular dementia and dementia of Lewy bodies have a poorer survival rate than AD.

Alzheimer's Dementia (AD)

Alzheimer's dementia is common in old age people. Symptoms usually start in an insidious way. Patients may start neglecting their self- care and wandering may occur. The clinical presentation changes as the illness progresses. In the early stage there is a deterioration of cognitive functions, increased tendency to get fatigued, transient depressive symptoms, and exaggeration of pre-existing personality traits. Focal neurological signs are uncommon. In the middle stage, there is praxia, agnosia and dysphasia. 5–10% of patients develop epilepsy and 50% develop incontinence, memory loss for past as well as recent events. About 25–35% develop depression, 25% develop behavioural problems, and 15% develop delusions and hallucinations. In the final stage, there is aphasia and premorbid personality is replaced by fatuous behaviour and there is gross euphoria. Neurological signs e.g., muscle rigidity, difficulty in walking, unsteadiness and double incontinence occurs.

There are several pathological changes in AD. There is cortical atrophy, neuronal loss, senile plaques, extracellular argyrophilic bodies and neurofibrillary tangles: Other histological findings include amyloid deposits around blood vessels, Hirano bodies, granulovascular degeneration of neurons and severe degeneration in the olfactory nucleus.

Aetiology could be multifactorial. According to the cholinergic hypothesis, AD results from a selective loss in colinergic neurones. This results in decreased acetylcholine levels. Positive correlation between loss in cholinergic neurones and severity of dementia.

Environmental factors include head injury, aluminium toxicity, and high cholesterol level. The evidence for aluminium, however, remains inconclusive (39).

Genetic aetiology is responsible for the familial type of AD. The risk to first-degree relatives is estimated to range from 24% to 50%. Early onset familial AD shows an autosomal dominant mode of inheritance with age-related penetrance.

Immunoglobulins have been identified in the amyloid of the plaques. Abnormalities in certain serum protein fractions, similar to those that occur in amyloidosis, have been identified in AD. Unusual HLA subtypes have been found in AD. There is an increased incidence of auto-immune disorders in relatives of patients with AD, especially thyroiditis and Grave's disease.

Risk Factors of Alzheimer's disease can be broadly divided into environmental and genetic factors. Environmental factors include old age, being female, history of head trauma and cerebrovascular disorders, poor education, chemical exposure, left-handedness, and malnutrition. Genetic factors include family history of AD, family history of Parkinson's disease, and family history of Down's syndrome.

Vascular Dementia (VD)

Vascular dementia was formerly known as arteriosclerosis dementia. It is the second most common dementia after Alzheimer's dementia. It accounts for 20–25% of dementias. It includes multi-infarct dementia, (when it is clear that multiple small infarcts are responsible for the problems) and Binswanger's disease (progressive small vessel disease). It is more common in males.

Onset of VD is abrupt, with stepwise deterioration. It may start after a succession of acute cerebrovascular accidents, but, less commonly, after a single major stroke. The sudden onset of a deficit is highly suggestive of vascular dementia. The impairment of cognitive functions is uneven. Insight and personality are intact. Epilepsy develops in 20% of the patients. Associated features include hypertension, carotid bruit, emotional lability, disinhibition, slurred speech and focal neurological signs. Hemiparesis, hemianopia or pseudobulbar palsy are typical features of vascular dementia and are unusual in degenerative dementias (40).

Risk factors of vascular dementia include stroke, hypertension, diabetes, elevated level of low-density lipids, smoking, alcohol abuse, psychological stress, poor education, and exposure to pesticides, liquid plastic and rubbers. The progress of vascular dementia is poor, and may be worse than Alzheimer's disease (41). VD may coexist with AD. The Hachinski score is a scoring system that helps to distinguish between vascular dementia and Alzheimer's dementia. A score above six suggests vascular dementia.

Lewy Body Dementia (LBD)

This type of dementia may be commoner than VD in hospital-based samples. Lewy bodies are present in Parkinson's disease but also occur in the cerebral cortex in dementia. Main features are fluctuating cognition with marked variation in attention and alertness, visual hallucinations, delusions, Parkinsonian signs, repeated falls, orthostatic hypertension, and neuroleptic sensitivity. Depression is present in about 40% of patients. Although survival time is similar to Alzheimer's disease, some patients do not survive for more than one to two years because of the accelerated progression of the illness. Although anti-parkinsonian medication improves motor symptoms, they can cause confusion and hallucinations.

Frontotemporal Dementia (FTD)

It is responsible for about 10% of the cases of dementia. Incidence is equal in men and women. Patients have focal frontal and/or temporal lobe atrophy. Clinical features include, non-fluent aphasia, early loss of insight, disinhibition, distractibility, impulsivity, hyperorality, perseveration, depression, anxiety, apathy, hypochondriasis, stereotype speech and echolalia. There are physical signs, like early primitive reflexes, incontinence, rigidity, tremors, and low and labile blood pressure. Spatial orientation is well-preserved, even at the late stage of the illness.

Pick's Disease

Some writers regard Pick's disease as a form of frontotemporal dementia. In this type of dementia, the onset is slow with steady deterioration. There is a slower time course as compared with Alzheimer's type. Personality deterioration occurs early with frontal lobe syndrome of disinhibition, and coarsening of social behaviour. There is characteristic knife- blade atrophy due to neuronal loss in the frontal and temporal lobes. Pick's cells are present in neurones, and there is also fibrous gliosis. Senile plaques and neurofibrillary tangles are absent.

Other types of dementias are dementia in CJD, dementia in Huntington's disease, dementia in Parkinson's disease, dementia in AIDS and alcohol-related dementias.

Parkinson's Disease (PD)

Parkinson's disease is an idiopathic movement disorder resulting from the progressive loss of neurones in the midbrain substantia nigra, locus coeruleus, and other brainstem dopaminergic groups.

Onset usually occurs later in life after age 40, and gradually progresses to the full-blown disease, which is characterised by bradykinesia, resting tremor, pill-rolling tremor, masklike facies, cogwheel rigidity, and shuffling gait. Intellectual impairment is common, and 40% to 80% of the patients become demented. Depression is very common and can be considered an organic mood disorder. Bradykinesia, rigidity and resting tremor are the classic clinical features of PD. Other findings may include decreased rate of blinking, a mask-like face, a soft monotonous voice, stooped posture, and walking with small steps. Cognitive changes may also occur, with secondary depression or dementia or untoward reactions to pharmacotherapy appearing in some patients. Depression is seen in a third to a half of patients with diagnosable disease.

Early symptoms of PD consist of voice changes, sleep disturbances, and wetting of the pillow with saliva during sleep. The late symptoms and signs of PD include the classic triad already mentioned-tremors, rigidity and bradykinesia plus postural changes and micrographia. While there is no cure for PD, treatment is directed toward relieving the tremor and rigidity.

Drug therapy: Anticholinergic drugs like Benzitropine, Mesylate, Dopaminergic agents

Amantadine hydrochloride, Sinemet, Brom-ocriptine, Mesylate

Monoamine Oxidase Type B Inhibitor

Drug-Induced Psychosis

The clinical features of drug-induced psychosis in patients with PD are well-defined. Visual hallucinations are the most common, and it has been recently estimated that approximately 30% of treatment patients are affected. Some patients with psychotic symptoms secondary to dopaminergic medications do not require antipsychotic therapy.

Huntington's Disease

The dominantly inherited disorder, which causes a combination of progressive motor, cognitive, psychiatric and behavioural dysfunction, results from an abnormality in the in the IT-15 gene chromosome 4. Huntington's disease occurs with a prevalence of approximation 6 per 100,000 with wide regional variation. The sexes are affected equally. Onset can occur at any age, but most commonly in young or middle adulthood. The disorder exhibits 'anticipation', that is the age of onset tends to decrease through generations, especially with paternal transmission.

Clinical Features

Chorea, involuntary fidgety movements of the face and limbs is the characteristic motor disorder. As the disease progresses, other extrapyramidal features, including rigidity, dystonia and bradykinesia, can develop, with associated dysphagia, dysarthria and pyramidal signs. Epilepsy can occur. Cognitive dysfunction goes hand in hand with motor disorder. The dementia is predominantly, 'subcortical', with the impairment of attention, executive function, speed of processing, and memory. Psychiatric symptoms and behavioural change are common: depression, apathy and aggressivity occur very commonly, with psychosis, obsessional behaviour and suicide in a significant minority.

The epicentre of the pathology lies in the striatum, the caudate and the putamen. The diagnosis can now be made with confidence by DNA analysis. Counselling by a clinical geneticist is mandatory before presymptomatic testing and should also be considered in other circumstances. Patients may seek treatment for the chorea but this is usually best avoided given the psychological and extrapyramidal side effects of the agents required—antipsychotics, dopamine depleters such as tetrabenazine or benzodiazepines.

Depression

Depression is quite common in elderly people although the presentation is different than in the younger population. Elderly people are more prone to develop excessive physical preoccupation in the form of hypochondriasis, rather than consulting the doctor for depressive symptoms. Neurotic disorders, OCD, hypochondriasis and hysteria are rare as primary disorders among the elderly. When these symptoms do occur for the first time in an older person they are usually secondary to depression. Pharmacological treatment is the same as that for younger depressed people except that lower doses have to be used and consideration must be given to the possibility of other concomitant medical problems in the elderly population. ECT is sometimes helpful for severely depressed elderly patients. As mentioned earlier in this chapter, elderly people are over-represented in the suicide statistic and a careful risk assessment is needed.

The common signs and symptoms of depressive disorders include reduced energy and concentration, sleep problems (especially early morning awakening and multiple awakenings), decreased appetite, weight loss, and somatic complaints. The presenting symptoms may be different in older depressed patients from those seen in younger adults because of an increased emphasis on somatic complaints in older persons. Older persons are particularly vulnerable to major depressive episodes with melancholic features, characterised by depression, hypochondriasis, low self-esteem, feelings of worthlessness, and self-accusatory trends (especially about sex and sinfulness) with paranoid and suicidal ideation.

Cognitive impairment in depressed geriatric patients is referred to as the dementia syndrome of depression (pseudodementia), which can be confused easily with true dementia. In true dementia, intellectual performance usually is global, and impairment is consistently poor; in pseudodementia, deficits in attention and concentration are variable. Compared with patients who have true dementia, patients with pseudodementia are less likely to have language impairment and to confabulate.

Anxiety Disorders

The anxiety disorders include panic disorder, phobias, Obsessive-Compulsive Disorder (OCD), generalised anxiety disorder, acute stress disorder, and Post-Traumatic Stress Disorder (PTSD). Anxiety disorders begin in early or middle adulthood, but some appear for the first time after age 60. An initial onset of panic disorder in older persons is rare, but can occur. The ECA study determined that the 1–month prevalence of anxiety disorders in persons aged 65 and older is 5.5 percent. By far, the most common disorders are phobias (4 to 8 percent). The rate for panic disorder is 1 percent. The signs and symptoms of phobia in older adults are less severe than those that occur in younger persons, but the affects are equally, if not more, debilitating for older patients.

Somatoform disorders, characterised by physical symptoms resembling medical diseases, are relevant to geriatric psychiatry because somatic complaints are common among older adults. Hypochondriasis is common in persons over 60 years of age, although the peak incidence is in those between 40 to 50 years of age. The disorder is usually chronic, and the prognosis is guarded. Repeated physical examinations help reassure patients that they do not have a fatal illness, but invasive and high-risk diagnostic procedures should be avoided unless medically indicated. Telling patients that their symptoms are imaginary is counterproductive and usually engenders resentment. Clinicians should acknowledge that the complaint is real, that the pain is really there and perceived as such by the patient, and that a psychological or pharmacological approach to the problem is indicated.

Alcohol Abuse

Older adults with alcohol dependence usually give a history of excessive drinking that began in young or middle adulthood. They usually are medically ill, primarily with liver disease, and are either divorced, widowed, or are men who never married. Many have arrest records and are numbered among homeless persons. A large number have a chronic dementing illness, such as Wernicke's encephalopathy and Korsakoff's syndrome. Of nursing home patients, 20 percent have alcohol dependence.

Delusional Disorder

The age of onset of delusional disorder usually is between ages 40 and 55, but it can occur at any time during the geriatric period. Delusions can take many forms; the most common are persecutory. Patients believe that they are being spied on, followed, poisoned, or harassed in some way. Persons with delusional disorder may become violent toward their supposed persecutors. Some persons lock themselves in their rooms and live reclusive lives. Somatic delusions, in which persons believe they have a fatal illness, also can occur in older persons.

Late-Onset Schizophrenia

Kraepelin first applied the term paraphrenia to a disorder involving the relatively late-onset of delusions and hallucinations. In late-onset schizophrenia, the schizophrenic symptoms appear after 45 years of age. Harris and Jeste estimated that the onset of psychoses occurs in 13% of all hospitalised schizophrenic patients in their fifties, 7% in their sixties, and only 3% after 70 years of age. A late-life onset of psychosis accounts for up to 10% of the admissions to psychiatric hospitals of patients older than 60 (35). Most studies of such late-onset disorders have shown there is a twofold to tenfold higher proportion of women than men affected by them.

Late-onset schizophrenia is often characterised by bizarre delusions that have a predominantly persecutory flavour. Auditory hallucinations are the second-most predominant psychotic symptom, and Schneiderian first-rank symptoms are also common. In contrast, a thought disorder and negative symptoms are rare. Another geriatric psychotic disorder is late-life delusional disorder, which is characterised by delusions with an erotomanic, grandiose, jealous, or somatic content.

A significant number of patients with late-onset schizophrenia show symptomatic improvement in response to antipsychotic treatment. Studies of the course of late-onset schizophrenia have generally found it to be chronic.

Schizophrenia usually begins in late adolescence or young adulthood and persists throughout life. Although first episodes diagnosed after age 65 are rare, a late-onset type beginning after age 45 has been described. Women are more likely to have a late-onset of schizophrenia than men. Another difference between early-onset and late-onset schizophrenia is the greater prevalence of paranoid schizophrenia in the late-onset type. About 20 percent of persons with schizophrenia show no active symptoms by age 65; 80 percent show varying degrees of impairment. Psychopathology becomes less marked as patients age.

The residual type of schizophrenia occurs in about 30 percent of persons with schizophrenia. Its signs and symptoms include emotional blunting, social withdrawal, eccentric behaviour, and illogical thinking. Delusions and hallucinations are uncommon. Since most persons with residual schizophrenia cannot care for themselves, long-term hospitalisation is required. Older persons with schizophrenic symptoms respond well to antipsychotic drugs. Medication must be administered judiciously, and lower-than-usual dosages are often effective for older adults.

REFERENCES

1. Gelder, M., Harrison, P. and Cowen, P. (2006). *Shorter Oxford textbook of psychiatry*. Oxford: University Press.
2. Sadock, B. and Sadock, V. (2007). *Kaplan's and Sadock's synopsis of psychiatry* (10th Edition). Philadelphia: Lippincott Williams and Wilkins.
3. Bleuler, E. (1916) *Textbook of psychiatry*, translation by Brill, A. A. (1951). New York: macmillan
4. Stuss, D. T. and Benson, D. F. (1986). *The frontal lobes*. New York: Raven.
5. Jacobson, R., Ebrahim, I. and Kopelman, M. (2007). Organic psychiatric disorders. In G. Stein and G. Wilkinson (Eds.), *Seminars in general adult psychiatry* (pp. 488–525). London: Royal College of Psychiatrists.
6. Gummit, R. J. (1995). *The epilepsy handbook*: The practical management of seizures. New York: Raven.
7. Atre-Vaitya, N. (1997). Epilepsy. In L. Thomas, H. Jobe, M. Gaviria and A. Kovilparambil (Eds.), *Clinical neuropsychiatry* (pp. 207–221). Massachusetts: Blackwell Science.
8. Neppe, V. M. and Tucker, G. J. (1992). Neuropsychiatric aspects of seizure disorders. In S. C. Yudofsky, R. E. Hales (Eds.), *The American Psychiatric Press handbook of neuropsychiatry* (2nd Edition). Washington DC: American Psychiatric Press.
9. Trimble, M. R. (1991). *The psychoses of epilepsy*. New York: Raven.
10. Pond, D. A. (1957). Psychiatric aspects of epilepsy. *Journal of Research and Education in Indian Medicine*, 49, 1441–1451.
11. Gloor, P. (1991). Neurobiological substances of ictal behavioural changes. *Advances in Neurology*, 55.
12. Jacobson, R., Ebrahim, I. and Kopelman, M. (2007). Organic psychiatric disorders. In G. Stein and G. Wilkinson (Eds.), *Seminars in general adult psychiatry* (pp. 488–525). London: Royal College of Psychiatrists.
13. Atre-Vaitya, N. (1997). Epilepsy. In L. Thomas, H. Jobe, M. Gaviria and A. Kovilparambil (Eds.), *Clinical neuropsychiatry* (pp. 207–221). Massachusetts: Blackwell Science.
14. Jacobson, R., Ebrahim, I. and Kopelman, M. (2007). Organic psychiatric disorders, In G. Stein and G. Wilkinson (Eds.), *Seminars in general adult psychiatry* (pp. 488–525). London: Royal College of Psychiatrists.
15. Young, J., Murty, L., Westby, M., Akunne, A. and Mahony, R. (2010). Diagnosis, prevention, and management of delirium; summary of NICE guidance. *British Medical Journal*, 247–249.
16. Inouye, S. K., van Dyck, C. H., Alessi, C. A., Balkin, S., Siegal, A. P. and Horwitz, R. I. (1990). Clarifying confusion: The confusion assessment method. A new method for detection of delirium. *Annals of Internal Medicine*, 113, 941–948.
17. Ely, E. W., Inouye, S. K., Bernard, G. R., Gordon, S., Francis, J., May, L., et al. (2001). Delirium in mechanically ventilated patients: validity and reliability of the confusion assessment method for the intensive care unit (CAM-ICU). *The Journal of the Medical Association*, 286, 2703–2710.
18. Lindesay, J., Rockwood, K. and Rolfson, D. (2002). The epidemiology of delirium. In J. Lindesay, K. Rockwood and A. Mcdonald (Eds.), *Delirium in old age* (pp. 27–50). Oxford: Oxford University Press.
19. American Psychiatric Association.(2013). *Diagnostic and statistical manual of mental disorders* (5th Edition). Arlington, VA: American Psychiatric Publishing.
20. Gelder, M., Harrison, P. and Cowen, P. (2006).The misuse of alcohol and drugs. In P. Cowen, P. Harrison and T. Burns

(Eds.), *Shorter Oxford textbook of psychiatry* (pp. 321–357). Oxford: Oxford University Press.

21. Sadock, B. and Sadock, V. (2007). *Kaplan's and Sadock's synopsis of psychiatry* (10th Edition). Philadelphia: Lippincott Williams and Wilkins.
22. Bowie, P. and Takriti, Y. (2004). Epidemiology of dementia, In S. Curran and J. P. Wattis (Eds.), *Practical management of dementia* (pp. 9–21). Oxon: Radcliffe Medical Press Ltd.
23. Butler, R. and Pitt, B. (1998). Assessment, In R. Butler and B. Pitt (Eds.), *Seminars in old age psychiatry* (pp. 1–15). London: The Royal College of Psychiatrists.
24. Cacabelos, R. (1997). *Dementia in clinical neuropsychiatry*. Massachusetts: Blackwell Science.
25. Prince, M. (2002). Epidemiology. In R. Jacoby and C. Oppenheimer (Eds.) *Psychiatry in the elderly* (pp. 80–101). Oxford: Oxford University Press.
26. Henderson, S. (2000). Epidemiology of psychiatric disorders: Geriatric psychiatry. In B. Saddock B and V. Saddock (Eds.), *Kaplan and Saddock's Comprehensive textbook of psychiatry* (pp. 2980–3184). Philadelphia: Lippincott Williams and Wilkins.
27. Geo, S., Hendrie, H. C., Hall, K., et al. (1998). The relationships between age, sex, and the incidence of dementia and Alzheimer disease: a meta analysis. *Archives of General Psychiatry*, 55, 809–815.
28. Mortimer, J. A., van Duijin, C. M., Chandra, V., et al. (1991). Head Trauma as a risk factor for Alzheimers's disease: a collaborative re- analysis of case-control studies. EURODEM Risk Factors Research Group. *International Journal of Epidemiology*, 20(2), 28–35.
29. Katzman, R. (1993). Education and the prevalence of dementia and Alzheimer's disease. *Neurology*, 43, 13–20.
30. Ellis, A. (2004). M in The role of memory clinic, In S. Curran and J. P. Watts (Eds.), *Practical management of dementia* (pp. 161–177). Oxon: Redcliffe Medical Press.
31. Liperoti, R., Mor, V., Lapane, K., et al. (2003). The use of atypical antipsychotics in nursing homes. *Journal of Clinical Psychiatry*, 64, 1106– 1112.
32. Gelder, M., Harrison, P. and Cowen, P. (2006). The misuse of alcohol and drugs. In P. Cowen, P. Harrison and T. Burns (Eds.), *Shorter Oxford textbook of psychiatry* (pp. 495–515). Oxford: Oxford University Press.
33. Gill, S. S., Rochon, P. A., Hermann, N., et al. (2005). Atypical antipsychotic drugs and risk of ischaemic stroke: population based retrospective cohort study. *British Medical Journal*, 299, 958– 960.
34. McShane, R., Keene, J., Gedling, K., et al. (1997). Do neuroleptic drugs hasten cognitive decline in dementia? Prospective study with necropsy follow-up. *British Medical Journal*, 314, 266–270.
35. McKieth, I., Mintzer, J., Aarsland, D., et al. (2004). Dementia with Lewy Bodies. *Lancet Neurology*, 3, 19–28.
36. Holden, U. P. and Woods, R. T. (1988). *Reality orientation*: Psychological approaches top the confused elderly (2nd Edition). Edinburgh: Churchill Livingstone.
37. Baines, S., Saxby, P. and Ehlert, T. K. (1987). Reality orientation and reminiscence therapy: a controlled cross-over study of elderly confused people. *British Journal of Psychiatry*, 151, 222–231.
38. Twining, C. (1998). Psychological treatments, In R. Butler and B. Pitt (Eds.), *Seminars in old age psychiatry* (pp. 265–278). London: The Royal College of Psychiatrists.
39. Doll, R. (1993). Review: Alzheimer disease and environmental aluminium. *Age and Ageing*, 22, 138–153.
40. Brown, J. and Rossor, M. (1998). Vascular and other dementias, In Rob Butler and Brice Pitt (Eds.), *Seminars in old age psychiatry* (pp. 73–86). London: The Royal College of Psychiatrists.
41. Brown, J. and Rossor, M. (1998). Vascular and other dementias, In Rob Butler and Brice Pitt (Eds.), *Seminars in old age psychiatry* (pp. 73–86). London: The Royal College of Psychiatrists.

Child and Adolescent Psychiatry

CHAPTER 12

In contrast to adult psychiatric disorders, diagnostic assessments, procedures and formulations in childhood and adolescent disorders are based on information gathered from a wider sources including family members especially parents and further information is also sought from schools. Again in comparison to adult patients, children very rarely present themselves for consultation. They are usually brought by parents or other close relatives, who are worried about the child's behaviour or development.

In many cases, the child's behaviour is causing stress to parents, other family members, teachers or classmates. However, in some cases, the child's problem may actually be problem of the parents or the other family members. Because children's development is so intimately associated with the quality of care provided by their parents, failure of proper parenting plays a significant role in the psychiatric problems of children. Recent literature suggests that although parent psychopathology is strongly associated with offspring psychiatric disorder (1), it is a non-specific predictor associated with a substantial proportion of offspring disorders (2).

As children would generally be not able to adequately elaborate on their issues, information from parents as well as other people such as teachers is crucial and essential. Apart from the child psychiatrist, the child and the family may need the help of various other professionals from psychological, social services, and educational services. One other conspicuous difference between adult and child psychiatry, is that in the latter medication have a limited place. Treatment is focused more on working with the family and coordinating services from other agencies mentioned above.

In child psychiatry, there are two important aspects to be dealt with. One is the early identification of any psychiatric or emotional problem or the presence of any intellectual or developmental deficit and the other is providing assistance to parents and teachers for the provision of adequate environment for the healthy emotional and intellectual development of the child. Hence, child psychiatry is very closely interlinked with paediatrics as well as general psychiatry.

Assessment

Assessment in child psychiatry is a sophisticated, complex, challenging and multi-faceted process. It involves the important and crucial skill of engageing the child and the family successfully. Most children will be anxious or reluctant, and one needs a very empathic and delicate approach to obtain the desired information. As both verbal, as well as non-verbal information is helpful, the interviewer should have the ability to synthesise and utilise this. Apart from psychiatrists, it may be necessary for psychologists, social workers, nurses, paediatricians, and occupational therapists to undertake and share comprehensive assessments. The need and extent of involvement of other professionals, apart from the psychiatrist, will differ and depend on the problems of each individual child.

Assessment in Child Psychiatry Comprises the Following Steps

a. Interview with the child
b. Interview with the parents
c. In order to accurately assess the child's psychiatric problems, it is essential to have information about the child's relationship and functioning within the family and school, etc. Establishing contact with the school teachers and other individuals involved in the care of the child and obtaining further information is, therefore, very important.
d. Detailed physical examination should be done if needed, in order to identify or exclude any medical illness. Moreover, assessment of the level of intellectual functioning is desirable as it might be necessary to arrange psychological testing.

Interview with the Child

The initial assessment should evaluate the child's developmental progress in various domains, the presence of psychopathology and any potential risks. It is very important to structure the interview according to the age of the child. Children under 12 years of age should always, initially, be seen in the company of their parents, in order to avoid triggering anxiety and apprehension in the child, which is an invariable accompaniment of a situation with which the child may be unfamiliar.

It is always helpful to obtain initial information from parents before interviewing the child. In a child above 12 years of age, it is advisable to see the child first, before calling in the parents, so that one can establish a therapeutic working relationship. At the start of the interview, one should not question the child, immediately about the presenting problems or specific complaints for which he has been referred either by the family physicians or teachers. It is always helpful to talk about things that the in which the child is interested, as the child will feel more at ease if the interviewer asks, in a friendly manner, questions about his school, his classmates, his teachers and games which the child likes to play at school. These general questions will provide a lot of information besides reducing anxiety and apprehension in the child. This also gives the interviewer an opportunity to observe the child, not only the outward appearance but also his manner of responding to questions, the level of comprehension as well as the general knowledge that the child may or may not possess. Once the child feels relaxed, the interviewer starts with the probing questions in an indirect manner, which does not have the connotation of accusation. For example, if a child is brought by the parents with the problem of stealing, it is pointless to ask the child, 'Do you steal?', because the response is bound to be, 'No!'. It is better to make a generalised statement like, 'At times some children are tempted to take things which don't belong to them. Have you ever felt like this?'. This approach makes the child more comfortable in the interview situation and he may be able to verbalise his feelings more freely. Younger children can express themselves more freely with toys, play material and colouring materials. It is imperative to assess the child's view of the problem and to focus on cultivating the child's engagement in the process.

Interview with the Parents

Before embarking on taking a very structured history, it is more helpful to let the parents talk about the reasons for bringing the child to the psychiatric services. Many times, the actual problem with the child may be totally different from what the parents express and this provides a valuable insight into the disturbed parent-child relationship. Later, a detailed developmental and medical history of the child is essential. Family history and history of any psychiatric or medical problem in the siblings are also very relevant. Interpersonal relationships within the family also need exploration, and observation should also be made as to how parents relate to each other, and to the child during the interview situation.

Establishing Contact with the School Teachers

It is always helpful to get information about the academic achievements and social interaction of the child from teachers but this should be done with prior permission from the child and the parents. Some families are very reluctant to accept that there is a psychological problem and may not want to involve the teachers or the academic institution, so they may need detailed explanation and assurance.

Detailed Physical and Psychological Examinations

Although a routine physical examination is not routinely done during the first psychiatric consultation, it ought to be considered as its importance and that of relevant medical investigations cannot be overemphasized. A psychiatrist should be able to examine the basic physical or neurological systems but if indicated the opinion of a paediatrician should be sought. Before performing the physical examination, permission from the parents should be sought, and the child should be explained the reasons for this.

The diagnostic instruments used for children and adolescents are much the same as those used for adults. These include intelligence tests, checklists, rating scales, achievement tests, neuropsychological tests and projective tests. The clinician should arrive at a tentative diagnosis with the help of the structured interview and his observation of the behaviour patterns of the child or adolescent, before embarking on the battery of tests.

Classification of Child and Adolescent Disorders

Classifying and categorising psychiatric disturbances in children and adolescents is very complex because of the varying developmental levels, influences of external environment, presence or absence of adequate stimulation, individual behaviour patterns and the presence of any concomitant medical illness. There are similarities in ICD-10 and DSM-5 classifications, as they both focus on clinical-descriptive approach to diagnosis.

Attention Deficit Hyperactivity Disorder (ADHD)

In ICD-10, this disorder is called hyperactivity disorder. This is the most common psychiatric disorder among school-age children. Children with this disorder can experience considerable social, academic and psychological impairment. They are rejected by peers and adults and treated in a negative fashion (3).

The characteristic features are marked restlessness, and a marked pattern of inattentiveness and impulsiveness that interferes with functioning or development. Hyperactivity is more than just overactivity. There is restlessness which is coupled with inconsistent attention. There is excitable, impulsive and disinhibited behaviour. Children with ADHD dislike delays and are very impatient. They have difficulty sustaining focus and attending to instructions in academic and social situations. They frequently lose possessions like books and notebooks. They repeatedly get up and wander about, have difficulty persisting with any one task, change their activities frequently, interrupt others, shout out their replies, do not wait their turn in games, and are easily distracted. The most obvious abnormality is not in the amount but in the control of activity. As mentioned above these children are also likely to be very impulsive. They have an inability to delay gratification, they act hastily without due consideration to consequences and hence engage in risky behaviours (e.g., running across the street without looking carefully for the potential traffic).

Some children are restless and impulsive but reasonably attentive, while others can be predominantly inattentive and comparatively less hyperactive. For ADHD to be present, the pattern of being inattentive, restless, excitable, impulsive and impatient must be excessive. It must be persistent over time and be pervasive (the hyperactivity must present in more than one situation, e.g., at home and at school), and should interfere with the child's ordinary functioning and development. Pervasiveness across situations is a key requirement of ICD- 10 and DSM-5 definitions. Both classificatory systems place emphasis on inattentiveness and overactivity as the most important features for diagnostic purposes. Moreover, both ICD-10 and DSM-5 require at least six months of symptoms. In contrast to ICD-10 (which specifies that the onset of symptoms should be before the age of 6 years), DSM-5 diagnostic criteria requires that several symptoms should be present before the age of 12 years. Though hyperactivity generally dates back to the preschool years, referral is often delayed until the early school years. This is the period when the child's inattentiveness, learning problems and disruptiveness become increasingly troublesome. A hyperactivity diagnosis is not made when restlessness and poor restlessness and poor concentration are due to a mood disorder, an anxiety disorder, or schizophrenia.

While assessing symptoms, attention is primarily assessed from how long the child persists when engaged in a range of tasks including playing alone, reading, drawing or playing with a friend. Motor activity is assessed by taking into account how long the child can stay seated during the previously mentioned tasks, what proportion of the time they are fidgeting, and how often they run off on family outings or at the supermarket.

Common associated features include defiant aggressive and antisocial behaviours, problems with social relationships, IQ under 100 in many but not all children, specific learning problems, clumsiness and neurodevelopment immaturities and a history of specific developmental delay, for example, in language acquisition. Differential diagnoses include oppositional defiant disorder, intermittent explosive disorder, stereotypic movement disorder, autism spectrum disorder, Tourette's disorder, specific learning disorder, intellectual disability, reactive attachment disorder, anxiety disorders, depressive disorders, bipolar disorder, disruptive mood dysregulation disorder, substance use disorders, personality disorders, psychotic disorders, medication-induced symptoms of ADHD and neurocognitive disorders. The most common comorbid disorders with ADHD are oppositional defiant disorder and conduct disorder. Significant comorbidity exists with ADHD and mood and anxiety disorders. There is a controversial suggestion of association of ADHD in prepubertal children, with over 90% of those meeting criteria for bipolar disorder also meeting criteria for ADHD. However, follow-up studies indicate that ADHD plus bipolar disorder is infrequent. The overlap between ADHD and Tourette's disorder is well-established.

Aetiology

Family, adoption and twin studies suggest that genetic factors make a major contribution. Although children with epilepsy and cerebral palsy show higher rates of this syndrome, and rates are even higher with an associated intellectual disability, most children with hyperactivity have no neurological symptoms or signs.

There is some evidence that hyperactivity can be triggered by adverse reactions to the presence of various additives and naturally occurring substances in specific foods and drinks (4). Temperament seems to play a role as children who have been active from the first few months are likely to remain so during their childhood years. Psychosocial factors also influence hyperactivity, as indicated by the link between social deprivation and institutional rearing.

Epidemiology

Prevalence rates differ widely between the different countries, in UK being 0.5–1% while in North America prevalence is 3–5%. The main reasons for the discrepancy being differences in parents' and teachers' perceptions of behaviour and differences in diagnostic practice (5).

The diagnosis of ADHD is recently becoming more common in Mediterranean countries. The male to female ratio is around 3:1 (6). It is more common in younger children. Hyperactivity is linked with deprivation. It is a little more common in inner cities, very poor rural areas, in families of low socio-economic status, and among children reared in institutions.

Treatment

Psychoeducational

The first steps in treatment are psychoeducational. Many people believe that this disorder is caused by inadequate parenting even though the evidence is that they are initially caused by genetic and biological mechanisms with psychosocial factors maintaining or escalating initial manifestations (7). Information and advice is very important. The nature of the disorder needs to be explained to the child, the family and the school. They need to be reassured that hyperactivity is neither the parents' nor the child's fault.

Behavioural and Cognitive Management

Behavioural parent training is the most commonly prescribed psychological intervention. It has been observed that parents of the affected children use over controlling and inadequate strategies (8). Parent-training programmes are based on social learning theory and apart from using direct instructions, utilise modelling and role-playing techniques to reinforce positive behaviour and reduce the use of punitive strategies. This helps in manageing defiant and inappropriate behaviour of the child effectively (9). Cognitive behaviour therapy is often useful. It helps children in enhancing self-control by teaching them self-instructional strategies. And may be the only treatment needed for the mildest cases. Social skills training targets the child's problems with peers and adults, typically in a group setting (10).

Pharmacological

Although psychopharmacology is the mainstay of treatment for children suffering from severe ADHD, it should not be the only intervention since medication provides temporary relief from hyperactivity symptoms and is not curative. Medication, however, allows invaluable opportunity during which the child's disruptive behaviour and inattentiveness is minimised or controlled and positive influences (e.g., good parenting and good teaching, etc.) on development can be perceived by the child. In other words, for the duration of its action, medication creates a near normality situation, so that the child can enjoy more normal peer relationships and can pay attention to what is being taught by parents and teachers.

Atomoxetine is licensed in the UK for children as well as adults. In children over 6 years, the usual dose is 40 mg to 80 mg daily. For adults, weighing over 70 kg, the usual dose range is 40 mg to 100 mg daily. It can be increased to 120 mg daily (unlicensed dose) again under the direction of a specialist. For those adults and children over 6 years of age and weighing under 70 kg, the initial starting dose is 500 micrograms/ kg daily for 7 days and then increased gradually according to response. The usual maintenance dose is 1.8 mg/kg daily.

Other stimulants are more commonly used than atomoxetine. Methylphenidate is more popular, although there is evidence that dexamphetamine may be marginally more effective (11). There is not much evidence to the claim that methylphenidate is a little less likely to reduce growth than dexamphetamine. Nevertheless, for most clinicians, methylphenidate remains the first choice probably because it lacks the street reputation of an amphetamine. Two-thirds of children with ADHD will respond (12). Most clinicians are reluctant to prescribe stimulants below the age of 5 years. This is partly because the diagnosis of ADHD is not reliable in these children. It is advisable to use dexamphetamine rather than methylphenidate, in children with poorly controlled epilepsy, as it raises the seizure threshold (13). Although it is an established practice to monitor weight and height every six months, follow-up studies have shown that growth retardation is not common in most children (14). It is still advisable that caution is exercised in prescribing stimulants to children who already have growth retardation. Since most children exhibit hyperactivity symptoms at school, it is also recommended that to start medication on the weekend or during school holidays so that parents can see the benefits and are reassured (15). Methylphenidate and dexamphetamine do not have a tolerance issue and once started can be given, if needed, for years. Common initial side effects include appetite suppression, headache, stomach ache, dysphoria and jitteriness. They generally disappear gradually and spontaneously, or can be managed by reduction in dose. Appetite suppression or difficulty in getting to sleep can usually be overcome by adjusting timing or dosage. Methylphenidate's clinical effect results in about three hours. Five mg after breakfast and after lunch is the usual initiating dose and regimen. Another 5 mg is added as a mid-afternoon dose if needed. The impact of dose increase is usually evident after two days or so. The maximum daily dose is 50 mg. It is recommended that the daily dose should be decided after a step-wise increase in dose according to the response, rather than applying 'mg/kg approach' (16). As stimulants can cause tachycardia and also increase systolic blood pressure, great caution is needed in the presence of congenital heart disease, coarctation, Marfan's syndrome or secondary hypertension.

There can be adverse reactions with MAOIs. There is no substantial evidence for the belief that if one stimulant is ineffective, then the other would work. Combination or alternative pharmacological strategies are recommended instead. Clonidine (25μg-250μg) can be added and prescribed as an evening dose. It is helpful for overactivity and insomnia but does not have much role on inattention. It should not be withdrawn suddenly. Guancifine can also be used instead of clonidine. Risperidone in low doses can also be added to a stimulant but this option has not been vigorously evaluated. Tricyclics can be considered as alternatives to stimulants. Imipramine (25 mg to 75 mg/day) has been often and successfully used, but has tolerability issues (e.g., antimuscarinic effects). Bupropion is also an option for stimulant refractory or intolerant patients. Clonidine and tricyclic antidepressants can produce cardiac dysrhythmias, baseline and intermittent ECGs should be done.

In some children, dietary interventions are helpful to a modest extent when specific foods are excluded from their diets. When the diet may is restricted to a small amount of meat, a single vegetable and one fruit for some weeks, it may result in improvement in some children. Other foods can then be reintroduced one by one and consequently, if a particular food is found to precipitate relapse, it can then be removed.

Course and Outcome

Children suffering from mild forms of ADHD have a reasonable outcome, although the symptom of restlessness might still persist. Overactivity in preschool children tends to predict conduct disorder in middle childhood (17). Those with severe hyperactivity, show impaired cognitive test performance and poor scholastic achievement during adolescence. A considerable number develop antisocial behaviour during adulthood and have a higher risk of substance abuse, and disturbance in occupational and social functioning (18). The negative critical responses of parents, teachers and peers to a child's hyperactivity may worsen the symptoms and adversely influence the prognosis.

Conduct Disorders

Conduct disorders are characterised by a repetitive and persistent pattern of dissocial, aggressive or defiant conduct by children and adolescents. Such behaviour, when at its most extreme, amounts to major violations of age appropriate social expectations. Features of conduct disorder can also be symptomatic of other psychiatric conditions, in which case the underlying diagnosis should be given the primary importance. Conduct disorders usually manifest in early childhood, persist through adolescence, and sometimes progress into adulthood. Assessment of conduct disorders should include precise details of the child's antisocial behaviour, any triggering factors and various other aspects of the child's emotional and family life.

The symptoms are clustered in four areas: aggression to people and animals, destruction of property, deceitfulness and theft, and serious violations of rules. Examples of behaviours on which the diagnosis is based include the following: excessive levels of fighting or bullying, cruelty to animals or other people, severe destructiveness to property, fire setting, stealing, repeated lying, truancy from school and running away from home, staying out all night despite parental prohibitions, unusually frequent and severe temper tantrums, defiant provocative behaviour and persistent severe disobedience.

There are substantial differences between DSM-5 and ICD-10 regarding conduct disorders. ICD-10 subtypes of conduct disorders are: conduct disorder confined to family context; unsocialised conduct disorder; socialised conduct disorder; oppositional defiant disorder; other conduct disorder; conduct disorder unspecified. In the conduct disorder confined to family context, there is dissocial or aggressive behaviour, in which the disruptive and abnormal behaviour is entirely or almost entirely confined to the home. Unsocialised conduct disorder is characterised by the combination of persistent dissocial or aggressive behaviour, with a significant pervasive abnormality in the individual's relationships with other children. Socialised conduct disorder is diagnosed when the persistent dissocial or aggressive behaviour occurs in individuals who are generally well integrated into their peer group.

ICD-10 only requires one major behaviour to have been present in a repetitive and persistent pattern in the past six months; isolated dissocial acts are excluded. A list of 23 behaviours is given, but unlike DSM-5, there is some weighting of criteria as seven behaviours of greater severity need to have been present only once in order for the criteria to be fulfiled. Examples include forced sexual activity, use of weapons, and physical cruelty to someone. Hyperkinetic disorder, mood disorder, pervasive developmental disorder, and schizophrenia are excluded.

DSM-5 has a separate category for oppositional defiant disorder and subdivides conduct disorder into three sub-types, based on the age at onset of the disorder. These are childhood onset and adolescent onset conduct disorder, and an unspecified onset subtype, when there is insufficient information to determine age at onset.

The diagnostic criteria A of DSM-5 has fifteen symptoms, three of which have to be present for the last 12 months, and one of these have to be present for the past six months. There is no differential weighting of the various antisocial behaviours listed.

a. A repetitive and persistent pattern of behaviour in which either the basic rights of others, or major age-appropriate societal norms or rules are violated, as manifested by the presence of three (or more) of the following criteria in the past 12 months, with at least one criterion present in the past six months.

Aggression to people and animals

1. Often bullies, threatens, or intimidates
2. Often initiates physical fights
3. Has used a weapon that can cause serious physical harm to others (e.g., broken bottle, bat, knife, gun, etc.)
4. Has been physically cruel to others
5. Has been physically cruel to animals
6. Has stolen while confronting a victim (e.g., mugging, armed robbery, extortion)
7. Has forced someone into sexual activity
8. Destruction of property
9. Has deliberately engaged in fire setting with the intention of causing serious damage
10. Has deliberately destroyed others' property (other than by fire setting)

Deceitfulness or theft

1. Has broken into someone's house, building or car
2. Often lies to obtain goods or favours to avoid obligations (i.e. 'cons' others)
3. Has stolen items of non-trivial value without confronting a victim (e.g., shoplifting, but without breaking and entering)

Serious violation of rules

1. Often stays out at night despite parental prohibitions, beginning before 13 years of age
2. Has run away from home overnight at least twice (or once without returning for a lengthy period)
3. Often truant from school, beginning before the age of 13 years

b. The behaviour in disturbance causes clinically significant impairment in social, academic, or occupational functioning.

c. If the individual is aged 18 years or older, criteria are not met for antisocial personality disorder (19).

Epidemiology

According to the Isle of Wight study, the one year prevalence rate was about 3%, but in London, it was at least 6% (20). The male to female ratio is between 5:1 and 3:1, depending on the age range studied, but at all ages boys predominate. Only around adolescence the difference between boys and girls begins to close, as the disorder increases in girls. The peak age of onset is in late childhood and early adolescence.

Aetiology

Conduct disorder is a heterogenous disorder. It is generally believed that genetic liability is triggered by environmental factors (21). Some other factors (e.g., poor coping skills) act as mediators between these two. The risk-resilience model for conduct disorders (22) proposes that it is the interaction between gradual accumulation of risk factors and absence or weakening of protective factors, that lead to conduct disorders. Familial aggregation supports the idea of genetic contribution.

Studies have shown that medical conditions like epilepsy and other cerebral function disorders increase the risk of conduct and other emotional disorders (23).

Psychological factors include learning disabilities, problems with attention span, poor academic performance, and lack of appropriate skills to cope with conflict, and inability to restrain when stressed. Social risk factors are poor parenting and family functioning, marital conflicts, drug abuse environment, and poor and crowded housing.

There is considerable evidence that children who are already at risk for developing conduct disorders and view media violence are at higher risk. One study demonstrated that violence on television contributes to enhancing violence among boys (24). Protective factors include good social skills, good relationship with parents, areas of competence outside school and high intelligence.

Course and Outcome

Early onset disturbances of conduct are more frequently persisting as compared to those individuals in which conflicting behaviours begin later rather than earlier. The latter group is less likely to progress to covert and overt delinquent acts, or to have a persistent disorder into adulthood (25). 40% of children with conduct disorder develop antisocial personality disorder (26). Many others continue to have difficulties in various domains of life e.g., interpersonal relationships.

Treatment

The various treatment for conduct disorders have modest success. However, combining various interventions can have synergistic effect and improvement. Multimodal approaches that target various aspects of conduct disorder show more improvement. Moreover, it has been demonstrated that in order to maintain improvement, long-term intervention is helpful (27). Treatments have to be targeted according to the different developmental needs of children, and there is no intervention that is beneficial across all ages.

Although conduct disorder is rarely present in preschool children, early and preventive intervention is helpful. Identifying the temperamental traits of children, parental support and education (e.g., how to handle temper tantrums) is beneficial. At school age, the inadequate social skills of the child should be addressed, and support for enhancing academic achievements given. Efficacy of Multisystemic Therapy (MST) has been demonstrated (28). MST involves the patient, family, peers, school and other social network variables that are associated with identified problems (29). Family therapy is also recommended and treatment of any comorbidity is essential. As inconsistent and punitive attitudes of some parents play a role in the development of disruptive behaviours of children, parent management training may be helpful.

For adolescents, psychoeducational support, family interventions, help with social skills, conflict resolution, and anger management, are helpful. There is some evidence, but no definite data, about lithium, carbamazepine, and SSRIs in controlling aggressive behaviour in children with conduct disorders.

Oppositional Defiant Disorder

This is characterised by the presence of markedly defiant, disobedient, provocative and disruptive behaviour. There is a recurrent pattern of angry or irritable mood. Children with this disorder are resentful, are annoyed easily, lose their temper quickly and provoke arguments with adults. They make conscious efforts to irritate or annoy others. This sort of behaviour does not occur in normal children of similar age and cultural context. In this disorder, there is a marked absence of more severe dissocial or aggressive acts, that violate the law or the rights of others.

The symptoms of this disorder may be confined to only one setting e.g., at home. The oppositional defiant disorder often preceeds the development of conduct disorder, especially for those with childhood-onset type of conduct disorder. DSM-5 specifies at least six months duration of these symptoms for diagnosis.

This disorder characteristically occurs in children below the age of 9 or 10 years and rarely starts later than early adolescence. It is more prevalent in boys than in girls before puberty and the sex ratio appears to be equal after puberty. The prevalence is around 3.3%. It is important to differentiate the disorder from the normal and adaptive oppositional behaviour of children at specific developmental stages. The normal oppositional behaviour differs in frequency and intensity and is more or less seen in other children of similar ages.

The main treatment of this disorder is family intervention. Careful assessment of family interactions is done and parents and the child are trained in management skills. Parents are discouraged to indulge in harsh or punitive behaviour. Behaviour therapy focuses on selectively reinforcing and appreciating desirable behaviour of the child and ignoring or not reinforcing inappropriate behaviour.

Anxiety Disorders

Anxiety is very common in childhood and it can be quite difficult to differentiate between normal anxiety and anxiety disorders in childhood. Children understandably feel anxious in new situations such as joining nursery or school or when their families socialise and visit new people or when friends are visiting. However, when anxiety is out of proportion, irrational and persisting, that's when the child and the family needs professional help.

DSM-5 includes separation anxiety disorder and selective mutism under anxiety disorders, but reactive attachment disorder is mentioned under the chapter 'Trauma and Stress-Related Disorders'.

1CD-10 classifies anxiety disorders as emotional disorders with onset specific to childhood. They include separation anxiety disorder of childhood, phobic anxiety disorder of childhood, social anxiety disorder of childhood, post-traumatic disorder, and obsessive-compulsive disorder. It also has a category of sibling rivalry disorder. Anxiety disorders are quite common in childhood (30). Surveys of anxiety disorders have suggested the prevalence around 6–9 percent among 7–11 years old children (31).

Generalised Anxiety Disorder (GAD)

Children and adolescents with GAD have worries that are out of proportion, diffused, and not specific to any particular situation. They are frightened in multiple settings and expect negative outcomes from their activities. Their worry may be about trivial matters about the past, present or future. Children can worry about school work, their appearance, money problems, to such an extent that there is interference with everyday functioning. Worry may be accompanied by headaches and stomach aches, etc. GAD, in contrast to other anxiety disorders, is more likely to occur with other psychopathology. The rate of GAD in school- age children is estimated to be approximately 3 percent. A child with GAD has a 60 percent chance of also having separation anxiety disorder or a social phobia.

Management is along the lines of cognitive–behavioural techniques. Cognitive Behaviour Therapy (CBT) has been well-tested. It is based on the notion that distorted cognitions are responsible for the unreasonable anxiety and CBT aims to replace negative beliefs with more neutral, positive or realistic thoughts. Although medication has no strong evidence for GAD in children, Selective Serotonin Reuptake Inhibitors (SSRIs) may be helpful in some cases. Although some concerns have been raised about increased suicidal ideation in children using SSRIs, there are no conclusive studies to substantiate this.

Separation Anxiety Disorder

This disorder affects about 3–4% of 7–11 years old children (32) and is slightly more common in females. The onset is usually before the age of 6 years. This disorder increases the risk of developing agoraphobia in adult life. Children have unreasonable anxiety at separation from parents or other caregivers, and this interferes with the child's well-being functioning. Children typically try to resist activities that will result in separation from caregivers.

Children who suffer from this disorder, often refuse to attend school, are seemingly ill in the morning when they are due to leave for school. Anxiety may manifest in physical symptoms such as headaches, vomiting and stomach ache, etc. Children are reluctant to attend school camps, are worried that some harm may come to their parents while they are separated from them and may also have vivid fantasies about this preoccupation, and have difficulty when their parents go out of the house and may require consistent assurance by the parents. The key symptom in making the diagnosis is the child's irrational fear that some harm may come to the parents or he or she may be abandoned by the parents.

This disorder should be suspected in any child who misses school excessively, although non- attendance at school could be due to many other possible reasons. The onset of this disorder is often triggered by a traumatic event or a fearful experience, but it can also emerge out of blue. It is not uncommon for one of the parents to have an anxiety disorder or an anxious and overprotective personality.

Separation anxiety disorder becomes less intense and may disappear during adulthood. Specific questions to elicit symptoms of separation anxiety disorder are based on the Diagnostic Interview Schedule for Children (33). Examples are:

- Have you worried a lot recently about something bad happening to your mother or father like having an illness or accident?
- Have you worried a lot that your mother or father may go away and never come back?
- Have you had to be dragged or forced to go to school?

Management includes involving the family, minimising the stressors, encourageing the child to express his or her fears, and behavioural techniques (like systemic desensitisation, exposure and response prevention) for a quick return to school before the problem becomes chronic and entrenched. The daily school attendance may start off on a partial basis. Parents need to understand that it is essential to expose their child to anxiety-invoking situations, and that parents need to be consistent in dealing with this issue. School staff also need to be involved in the process of returning to school. There is very little evidence of the role of medication although sometimes small doses of anxiolytics may be indicated and helpful in severe anxiety.

Panic and Phobic Anxiety Disorder

The essential and key feature of panic disorder is the repeated experience of unprovoked spontaneous panic attacks, which may lead to restricting the child's independent activities. Panic disorder is diagnosed when there is no association of anxiety with any specific situation. A panic attack is manifested by a period of intense fear, terror, and discomfort accompanied by feelings of impending doom or disaster. The symptoms develop suddenly and are manifested by way of palpitations, accelerated heart rate, sweating, trembling, occasional feeling of chest pain or discomfort, breathlessness, choking, feeling of dizziness, nausea or abdominal pain and fear of death.

A prevalence of the panic disorder has been reported as less than 1% in one study (34). Background factors include genetic and constitutional factors, shy and inhibited temperament, overprotective parents, specific frightful experiences and life events, dysfunctional cognitive appraisal of stressful events, and social adversity (35).

There are only case studies regarding medication for panic disorder in children, which show that tricyclic antidepressants and benzodiazepines may be helpful (36).

Minor fears are common in children but severe phobias are unusual in middle childhood. Specific phobias in adults correspond to phobic anxiety disorder in children. In phobic disorder there is a remarkable and unreasonable fear of a specific object. When there is avoidance behaviour and interference with functioning, because of a specific fear, diagnosis of specific phobia is made. Fears may be connected with sleep, darkness, closed and open spaces, heights, animals and thunderstorms. Children develop anticipatory anxiety for the phobic situation. Behavioural techniques, mentioned above for separation anxiety disorders, are employed to treat phobic anxiety disorder.

Social Anxiety Disorder

This usually starts before the age of 6 years. Children having this disorder have marked fear and anxiety about strangers which adversely affects the social and peer relationships, as they continue to avoid them. It has been demonstrated that these children have inhibited temperament during infancy (37).

Social anxiety is centred around a fear of scrutiny by other people in comparatively small groups, leading to avoidance of social situations. They may be discrete i.e. restricted to eating in public, to public speaking, etc., or diffuse, involving almost all social situations outside the family circle. Direct eye contact may be particularly stressful. They may present as a complaint of blushing, hand tremor, nausea or urgency of micturition. Treatment is based on behavioural methods.

Sibling Rivalry Disorder

Although it is normal for a child to feel emotionally upset or jealous at the birth of a sibling, as the mother would be giving more attention to the newborn, this jealousy becomes a disorder if this jealousy and rivalry persists and results in family or social problem.

If this disorder becomes severe there may be a risk of physical harm to the newborn child. On the other hand, child with this disorder may start exhibiting regressed behaviour e.g., loose bladder or bowel control, and there may be frequent temper tantrums and sleep problems. Parents need advice to give appropriate and consistent attention to the child so that he or she feels reassured and valued.

Post-Traumatic Stress Disorder (PTSD)

DSM-5, as well as ICD-10, acknowledge that Post-Traumatic Stress Disorder (PTSD) can occur in children, as a result of significant stressors. DSM-5 criteria for PTSD differ significantly from the DSM-IV criteria. DSM-5 classifies PTSD under a new chapter 'Trauma and Stress-Related Disorders'. The diagnostic thresholds have also been lowered for children and adolescents. Furthermore, separate criteria has been added for children under 6 years or younger.

PTSD is caused by an unusual and extreme stress, such as witnessing an accident or murder, being kidnapped, being raped or tortured, or exposure to natural or man-made disaster, e.g. war, earthquakes or floods. Children can also develop PTSD after witnessing domestic violence. The clinical symptoms resemble PTSD occurring in adult life, and include flashbacks, nightmares, increased arousal, marked anxiety, and disturbed sleep. PTSD differs from other anxiety disorders in that the patient reports far more frequent re-experiencing of the traumatic event.

Symptoms usually begin within the first three months after the trauma. The term 'delayed expression' is used in DSM-5 recognising that there may be a delay of months or even years before the diagnostic criteria is met. Symptoms include disturbance by intrusive and repeated images and thoughts about the event. Sleep disturbances, nightmares and separation difficulties are common. They also experience concentration and memory problems. There may be reluctance to participate in new activities in school-age children as well as in pursuing developmental opportunities. Although children might also experience emotional numbness, most writers agree that it is very difficult to elicit evidence of emotional numbness in children (38).

Regarding the prevalence of PTSD, one study reported a lifetime rate of 1% (39), whereas another reported a much higher rate of 7.8% (40). Treatment is similar to that given to adults, with the exception of the cautious use of medication. There are however very few Randomised Controlled Trials (RCT) in children. Group treatments as well as individual treatments are employed. Cognitive techniques like challenging maladaptive thoughts, and guided mastery to control distressing feelings can be helpful. Relaxation and other anxiety reducing techniques are also employed. Eye Movement Desensitisation and Reprocessing (EMDR) technique is also used in children. Again there are no RCTs, but some authors have reported success with this therapy (41).

Obsessive-Compulsive Disorder

Obsessive-compulsive Disorder (OCD) is more common in children and adolescents than it used to be recognised. The prevalence rate of this disorder is now said to be 0.5–2% in adolescents. Although prevalence is lower in prepubertal children, it can occur in children aged seven years. Rates rise exponentially with age (42). OCD is equally common in boys and girls but is more common in prepubertal boys. The onset can be gradual or sudden (43). In general, the symptoms of OCD resemble very closely to those present in adults, and include a wide variety of obsessive thoughts and compulsive rituals (44).

The essential symptomatology of obsessive-compulsive disorder comprises repeated, recurrent and intrusive thoughts, and actions on which the child has no control. These thoughts and actions are termed as obsessions and compulsions respectively.

Because the child recognises the obsessive thoughts and compulsive rituals as absurd, they are kept secret from parents, other caregivers or teachers for long periods.

Children with OCD show evidence of both obsessions and compulsion but rituals are more common than obsessional thoughts. The child may become preoccupied with contamination and start spending a long time washing, and/or rearranging things in the bedroom in a certain order. The child may attempt to deny or minimise the ritualistic behaviours. Obsessional thoughts are usually elicited by direct questioning. There is associated anxiety that may be marked, and specific fears and depression are also common. These obsessions and compulsions lead to impaired social and academic functioning and can be extremely stressful for the child as well as the family.

The involvement of the family is crucial in the management, and treatment begins with family education about the disorder. Teachers may also be helpful with the child's behavioural programme. The treatment outcome of obsessive-compulsive disorder is best when medication is combined with cognitive behaviour therapy. Behavioural approaches, like exposure and response prevention, have shown considerable improvement (45).

Clomipramine has been recommended in adolescents (46) and fluoxetine has also shown some evidence for efficacy (47). If there is no satisfactory response with one Selective Serotonin Reuptake Inhibitor (SSRI) for about 10–12 weeks, another SSRI may be tried. A low initial dose with slow upward titration is recommended in children. Although there are no RCTs regarding augmentation strategies in children, some success has been reported with clonazepam and buspirone.

Mood Disorders

These disorders, also referred to as affective disorders, include depressive as well as bipolar disorders. Mood disorders, though not commonly recognised by family and clinicians, are not only prevalent in children and adolescents but are also, a cause of serious disturbance in behaviour and social functioning.

Depressive Disorders

Depressive disorder is not an uncommon problem in adolescents and adolescent depressive disorder shows significant continuity into adult life. Depressed young people also make suicidal attempts and studies have shown that depression is one of the strongest predictors of a subsequent suicidal attempt, even when the association with other risk factors was controlled (48). Prevalence rates for depressive disorders are 0.5%-2.5% in pre-adolescence, and are higher during adolescence, about 2% to 8% (49). When all kinds of depressive disorder are included, then the prevalence can be as high as 10% (50).

The rates are different in males and females as the age increases. Age trends in depression are stronger in girls than in boys. Before puberty rates of depressive disorders are higher in boys. In mid-teens, girls outnumber boys by about 2 to 1 (51).

DSM-5 diagnostic criteria for depressive disorder in children is same as for adults, and in ICD-10 as well, there are no symptom modifications for children or adolescents. Both DSM-5 and ICD-10 divide depressive disorder into mild, moderate and severe categories. ICD-10, however, defines severity by the symptoms, whereas in DSM-5, severity is defined in terms of symptoms and functional impairment. Both classifications, distinguish between psychotic and non-psychotic form of severe or major depressive disorder.

A major depressive episode has at least five symptoms, and presents for at least two weeks. Shorter periods may be acceptable for diagnosis, if symptoms are unusually severe and of rapid onset. Either a depressed mood or a loss of pleasure or interest is compulsory for diagnosis. However, in children and adolescents, the mood can be irritable. There also has to be a deterioration in functioning level. The development level of children influences the presentation of depressive symptoms and children present the symptoms in a variable manner. Symptoms may include low mood, diminished interest in activities which were a source of pleasure before, weight loss or sometimes weight gain, insomnia, irritability, agitation, poor concentration, guilt feelings or ideas of worthlessness, non-compliance with expected norms of behaviour at home and at school, and a decline in social and academic functioning. Clinically unexplained physical complaints, e.g., headaches, abdominal pain and a general state of lethargy are commonly seen in children suffering from a depressive illness. On the other hand, at times, impulsive and destructive behaviour, uncontrolled and unprovoked aggression and a lack of interest in pleasurable activities should alert the family and the clinician as to the presence of a major mood disturbance.

Many children who present with depressive disorder also have another psychiatric disorder. The most common comorbid conditions are conduct disorder and anxiety disorders. Studies have suggested that anxiety tends to precede depression (52).

Management

It is important that the child resumes the normal and required level of functioning as soon as possible. It is also imperative to keep in mind the medical causes of depression, (e.g., infectious mononucleosis, influenza, hepatitis, hypothyroidism and Cushing's disease) and medications that can cause depressive symptoms (e.g., corticosteroids).

The treatment strategy needs to include medication, psychotherapy as well as psychosocial interventions. Cognitive behaviour therapy, which targets the maladaptive cognitive beliefs and strives to improve self-esteem and problem-solving abilities is quite effective. Interpersonal therapy as well as family-focused psychoeducational therapy are other valuable options. Regarding psychopharmacotherapy, although there are various classes of antidepressant medication available, Selective Serotonin Reuptake Inhibitors (SSRIs) being the first choice. Although safer in overdose as compared to tricyclic antidepressants because of reduced cardiovascular toxicity, they are not free from side effects and may also have withdrawal problems. Common side effects are insomnia, gastrointestinal symptoms, and behavioural activation. It should also be remembered that as SSRIs have significant effects upon the hepatic cytochrome P450 oxidase system, there is a potential for adverse drug reactions when they are combined with other medications. It is preferable that children are given as low effective doses as possible.

Bipolar Affective Disorder

Bipolar disorder is rare before puberty. Among adolescents, a bipolar disorder occurs equally in both genders, and about 20–40 percent of adolescents who initially suffer from major depressive disorder, develop bipolar disorder within a period of five years. Bipolar disorder may be preceded by a comorbid conduct disorder (53). The diagnostic criteria for bipolar disorder in children is the same as that for adults. ICD-10 requires at least two episodes of elevated and depressed mood, while only one hypomanic or manic episode is the requirement of DSM-5 (depressive episode is not required).

Mania is characterised by elation of mood (irritability can be a conspicuous feature instead), feeling over energetic, increased sexual libido, overactivity, decreased need for sleep, over spending, overtalkativeness with flight of ideas, and easy distractability, with short attention span. There is significant disruption in occupational or social functioning. Mood congruent delusions and other psychotic symptoms may be present but are not essential for the diagnosis.

Hypomania is a lesser form of mania, with a lesser degree of mood elevation and various other symptoms. It needs to be remembered that mild forms of mania or hypomania, can be easily confused with conduct disorder and attention deficit disorder (54), and mania with psychotic symptoms can be difficult to differentiate from schizophrenia (55).

Treatment strategies are the same as for the management of the bipolar disorder in adults, and consists primarily of medication. There is some evidence that lithium can be effective in children and adolescents (56), but as lithium has a narrow therapeutic window and significant side effects, cautious use is recommended. Anticonvulsants can be helpful for the treatment and prophylaxis of bipolar disorder in the young when it is rapid cycling (57). Psychosocial strategies including family counselling and education are helpful.

Suicide and Self-Harm in Children

Suicide under the age of 12 years is very rare (58). However, suicide is the fourth common cause of death in the adolescent group in the UK and the suicide rate in young males continues to rise (59). For completed suicides, the male to female ratio is about 4:1 (60). Recently, there is also an increase in suicide rates among young girls in the UK from ethnic minorities. It needs to be borne in mind that in many countries the rates of suicides in young population are escalating because of the stressful socio-economic conditions.

Attempted suicide is much more common than suicide. In the 10–14 year age group it is rare but in 15–19 year olds it occurs about 500 per 10000 per year (61). According to one study the male to female ratio of attempted suicide is 1:6 (62). It is worth mentioning that sometimes a completed suicide may not have been the clear intention and plan (sometimes things may have gone wrong accidentally), whereas those children who have attempted suicide, might have made a genuine attempt.

There is excess in the lower socio-economic class. Children who attempt suicide have some common background features. These include having parents with mental health disorders (especially depressive and personality disorders), parents who have marital problems and are not having adequate communication with their children. 50% of children who attempt suicide have depressive disorder. Some have antisocial problems, and it is has also been observed that having medical problems and association with children who have already made self-harm attempts, also increases the risk of self-harm. Another risk factor is substance abuse.

Effort should be made to ascertain the reasons for the suicide attempt. In case these remain obscure, sexual abuse should be considered as a possible cause. Overdose with paracetamol is one of the commonest way, but sometimes psychotropic medication is used. Other method of self-harm is wrist cutting. All suicidal behaviour or gestures should be taken seriously and a thorough assessment carried out, as a substantial number of children will make further attempt(s). Five useful screening questions are (63):

- Have you had problems for longer than a month?
- Were you alone at the house at the time?
- Did you plan the overdose for more than three hours?
- Are you feeling hopeless about the future?
- Were you feeling sad for most of the time before the overdose?

Treatment for any psychiatric disorder is mandatory and family therapy is desirable if there are problems within the family.

Schizophrenia

Schizophrenia is a very serious and enduring mental illness. There is considerable evidence to support the view that schizophrenia presenting in childhood and adolescence shows continuity with the adult form of the disorder at the levels of symptoms, clinical course and underlying neurobiology (64).

In children and adolescents, the gradual and insidious onset is characterised by deterioration in social and academic functioning, before the appearance of psychotic symptoms (65). Onset in children and adolescents is also characterised by negative symptoms, incoherence of thought, disorganised behaviour, hallucinations in different modalities and fewer systematised or persecutory delusions (66). Schizophrenia is very rare before the age of 10 years. But its incidence rises rapidly through adolescence. It most commonly presents in adolescence or early adulthood, the peak ages of onset ranging from 15 to 30 years. The prevalence rate in late adolescence is 3 per 10, 000. In this group, boys are more commonly affected than girls (67).

The diagnostic criteria in children is the same as for adults. According to DSM-5, the disturbances have to be present for at least 6 months. The 6-month period must include at least 1 month of symptoms. Schizoaffective disorder and mood disorders with psychotic symptoms have to be ruled out. It also has to be ensured that the symptoms are not due to the direct affect of a medical condition or substance abuse.

Depressive and anxiety symptoms may precede the onset of schizophrenia. Characteristic features are thought disorder, bizarre and mood-incongruent delusions, hallucinations, significant deterioration in functioning and behavioural disturbances. Children tend to have less complex delusions. It is important to differentiate the thought disorder of psychosis, from that of either developmental delay or language disorders (68). Mannerisms and stereotypies usually occur at a later stage.

Negative symptoms include, paucity of speech, poverty of thought content, apathy, avolition, and flat affect. When the onset is not acute, the child's behaviour may be dismissed as just being lazy, anxious or withdrawn. More commonly, the child may show some degree of developmental delay (69). Children who develop schizophrenia have higher rate of developmental abnormalities and many researchers regard this enduring mental illness as a developmental disorder (70).

Treatment strategies are the same as for adults. However special attention and consideration has to be given to the educational needs of children and the family situation (71). When prescribing traditional antipsychotics, it needs to be emphasised that there is greater risk of extrapyramidal symptoms and treatment resistance in younger patients. Cognitive remediation has shown to be beneficial in the areas of memory and social functioning. Problem-solving and social skills training are also helpful.

Personality Disorders

DSM-5 defines a personality disorder as an enduring pattern of inner experience and behaviour that deviates markedly from the expectations of the individual's cultural background, is pervasive and inflexible, has an onset in adolescence or early adulthood, is stable over time, and leads to distress or impairment. This pattern is manifested in two or more areas: cognition, affectivity, interpersonal functioning and impulse control. When assessing personality functioning, it is important to take into account the social background.

Although some children may exhibit early signs of enduring personality characteristics that are disturbing, many clinicians are rightly and understandably not keen to label them as personality disorders. According to ICD- 10, it is unlikely that the diagnosis of personality disorders will be appropriate before the age of 16 or 17 years. Although DSM-5 also has some reservations about diagnosing personality disorders in children, and states that for a personality disorder to be diagnosed in an individual younger than 18 years, the features must have been present for at 1 year. However, one exception to this is antisocial personality disorder, which cannot be diagnosed in individuals younger than 18 years. DSM-5 also recognises that by definition, personality disorder requires an onset no later than early adulthood, individuals may not come to clinical attention until relatively late in life.

Most of the studies of personality disorders have been on borderline personality disorder. There have been no studies published of treatment effectiveness. CBT and dialectical behaviour therapy have shown improvement in some patients.

Tic disorders

Tics are repetitive and rapid muscle contractions or sounds that are usually out of voluntary control. Tics are classified as simple or complex tics or as motor or vocal tics. Simple motor tics are experienced in one or small group of muscle (e.g., eye blinking or facial grimace) and are further subdivided into clonic, tonic or dystonic types. Complex motor tics involve several muscles as in hopping movements, bending knees or sometimes obscene gesturing.

Vocal tics are also subdivided into simple vocal tics (sniffing or grunting, etc.), or complex vocal tics (e.g., patient may use comprehensible phrases like, 'go to hell'). Like almost all involuntary movements, anxiety worsens the tics.

For diagnostic purposes, tics disorders are classified into four categories: transient tics disorder, chronic motor or vocal tics disorder, Tourette's disorder, and tic disorder not otherwise specified. For Tourette's and chronic tics disorder, the duration criteria is at least 12 months and that the symptoms have been present before the age of 18 years. For transient tics disorder the duration criteria is more than four weeks but less than one year. For all types of tics disorders there has to be a marked distress or impaired functioning. In some children, the tics last only for few weeks and in 80–90 percent of cases improve within 5 years.

Tourette's Disorder

This is one of the tics disorders. Tic disorders comprise four categories: Tourette's disorder, persistent (chronic) motor or vocal tic disorder, provisional tic disorder, and the other specified and unspecified tic disorders. Diagnosis of any tic disorder is based on the presence of motor and/ or vocal tics, duration of tic symptoms, age at onset and absence of any known cause such as another medical conditions or substance use. A tic is a sudden, rapid, recurrent, nonrhythmic motor movement or vocalization.

According to DSM-5, the diagnostic criteria for Tourette's disorder specifies that onset should be before the age of 18 years, both multiple motor and one or more vocal tics have been present at some time during the illness, although not necessarily concurrently and the tics have persisted for more than a year since the onset of first tic although they may wax and wane in frequency. Although there may be distress or functional impairment, it is not a requirement for the diagnosis. Usually, prodromal behavioural symptoms like attention difficulties, hyperactivity, and poor tolerance frustration occur. The average age of onset of tics is 7 years, but they may occur much early. The onset is associated with emotional disturbance.

The tics usually begin in the face and neck and later involve other muscles. Grimacing, puckering the forehead, raising eyebrows, blinking eyelids, winking, wrinkling the nose, twitching mouth, biting the lips, extruding the tongue, nodding, jerking or shaking the head, twisting the neck sideways, head rolling, jerking the hands or arms, plucking fingers or writhing fingers, clenching fists, shrugging shoulders, shaking a foot, knee or toe, jumping and making sucking or smacking sounds are the commonest forms (72). About a third of patients exhibit coprolalia (involuntary utterances of obscenities). Echolalia and echopraxia occurs between 10 to 40 percent of cases.

Tourette's disorder affects roughly 3–10 per 10,000 children or adolescents (73). The disorder is three to four times more common in boys. It is ten times more prevalent in children and adolescents than in adults.

A comprehensive assessment has to be carried out including any developmental problems child's functioning at home and school, the range and severity of symptoms, and any precipitating factors or stressors. Sometimes there is also an increase in tics severity or frequency due to starting school, change of school, problems at school with peers, examination challenges, fatigue, and excitement.

Some children can suppress tics for considerable periods, especially at school. Others describe their tics as intentional but irresistible.

Common comorbid disorders like Obsessive-Compulsive Disorder (OCD) and Attention Deficit Hyperkinetic Disorder (ADHD) can dominate the clinical picture. OCD can occur in 20 to 40 percent of Tourette's disorder. On the other hand, some patients with Tourette's disorder have some symptoms of OCD but not enough to justify the diagnosis of OCD. Some clinicians distinguish OCD associated with Tourette's disorder (tic-related OCD) and OCD without comorbid Tourette's disorder. Patients with tic-related OCD, are more likely to have aggressive or sexual obsessions, as well as more hoarding, ordering, and touching compulsions (74).

In differential diagnosis, tics from other abnormal movements need to be considered. These include athetoid and choreiform movements occurring in cerebral palsy, Huntington's chorea and Sydenham's chorea. In these disorders, the movements are non-repetitive and multiple groups of muscles are affected (75). Stereotypies associated with severe intellectual disability and autistic spectrum disorders should be considered as well in the differential diagnosis. They may look like complex motor tics but it is very rare to have complex tics without some simple tics. Although the aetiology of Tourette's disorder is not known, altered dopamine function and aberrant cortico-striatal connectivity and autoimmune abnormalities are suspected (76) (77).

Treatment includes pharmacotherapy, behavioural treatments like relaxation training and habit reversal, psychotherapy, educational interventions, and family therapy. Neuroleptics like haloperidol, pimozide, and sulpiride, have been successfully used to reduce tic severity, although side effects (e.g., dystonic reactions) can be problematic. Risperidone has also been tried. Clonidine (dosage range 0.25–0.5 mg daily in single or divided doses) has also been used in severe cases with hyperactivity, but side effects like sedation and postural hypotension limit its use. Selective Serotonin Reuptake Inhibitors (SSRIs) can alleviate the associated obsessions and compulsions.

Specific Developmental Disorders of Speech and Language

According to ICD-10, these disorders have the following common features:

a. Onset is invariably during infancy or childhood.
b. An impairment or delay in the development of functions that are strongly related to biological maturation of the central nervous system.
c. A steady course that does not involve remissions and relapses that end to be characteristic of many mental disorders.

These conditions are not directly attributable to neurological or speech mechanism abnormalities, sensory impairments, mental retardation, or environmental factors. The child's language ability is impaired in various situations. As a general rule, a language delay that is sufficiently severe to fall outside the limits of two standard deviations may be regarded as abnormal. However, the level of severity in statistical terms is of less diagnostic use in older children, as there is a natural tendency towards progressive improvement. ICD-10 highlights certain other difficulties as well, like accurately diagnosing these disorders including differentiation from mental retardation or global developmental delay, and differentiation from a disorder secondary to severe deafness or to some specific neurological or other structural abnormalities. These disorders are more common in boys.

Specific Speech Articulation Disorder

In this disorder, the child's use of speech and sounds is below the appropriate level for his or her mental age, but in which there is a normal level of language skills. The diagnosis should only be made when the severity of articulation is outside the limits of normal variation for the child's mental age; non-verbal intelligence is within the normal range; expressive and receptive language skills are within the normal range; the articulation abnormalities are not directly attributable to a sensory, structural or neurological abnormality; and the mispronunciations are clearly abnormal in the context of colloquial usage in the child's subculture.

Expressive Language Disorder

In this disorder, the child's ability to use expressive spoken language is markedly below the appropriate level for his or her mental age, but in which language comprehension is within normal limits.

As a general rule, the absence of single words by the age of two years, and not be able to speak two word phrases by the age of three years is taken as a significant delay. Again, this diagnosis should only be made when the severity of the delay in the development of expressive language is outside the limits of normal variation for the child's mental age, but receptive language skills are within normal limits.

Treatment is mainly through special education.

Receptive Language Disorder

In this disorder, the child's comprehension of language is below the appropriate level for his or her mental age. In almost all cases, expressive language is markedly disturbed and abnormalities in word-sound production are common. According to ICD-10 diagnostic guidelines, the diagnosis should only be made when the severity of the delay in receptive language is outside the normal limits of variation for the child's mental age, and when the criteria for a pervasive developmental disorder are not met. Of all the varieties of specific developmental disorders of speech and language, this disorder has the highest rate of socio-emotional-behavioural disturbance. Treatment is through special education.

Acquired Aphasia with Epilepsy (Landau-Kleffner Syndrome)

In this disorder, the child having previously made normal progress in language development loses both receptive and expressive language skills but retains general intelligence. Onset of the disorder is accompanied by paroxysmal abnormalities on the EEG, and in majority of cases also by epileptic seizures. In some cases the loss of language occurs gradually over a period of some months, but in the majority it is abrupt with skills being lost within days or weeks. The aetiology remains unknown, and treatment of the seizures does not always lead to improvement in language.

Specific Developmental Disorders of Scholastic Skills

The aetiology of these disorders is not known. In these disorders, the normal patterns of acquisitions are disturbed from the early stages of development. These disorders are thought to develop from the abnormalities in cognitive processing that derive largely from some type of biological dysfunction. These are much more common in boys.

The difficulties mentioned in ICD-10 in diagnosing these disorders include the need to differentiate the disorders from normal variations in scholastic achievement, the need to take developmental course into account, the difficulty that scholastic skills have to be taught and learned and are not simply a function of biological maturation, the problem in differentiating abnormalities in an individual child, that cause reading difficulties from those that derive from or are associated with poor reading skills and finally, the continuing uncertainties over the best way of subdividing the specific developmental disorders of scholastic skills. In specific reading disorder, there is a specific and significant impairment in the development of reading skills, which is not solely accounted for by mental age, visual acuity problems or inadequate schooling. Assessment is carried out by an educational or clinical psychologist. Treatment is educational unless there are additional medical or behavioural problems requiring additional and separate intervention.

In specific spelling disorder, there is similarly a specific and significant impairment in the development of spelling skills in the absence of a history of specific reading disorder, which is not solely accounted for by low mental age, visual acuity problems, or inadequate schooling. The ability to spell orally and write out words correctly are both affected. According to ICD-10, the child's spelling performance should be significantly below the level expected on the basis of his or her age, general intelligence, and school placement, and is best assessed by means of an individually administered, standardised test of spelling.

The specific disorder of arithmetic skills, involves a specific impairment in arithmetic skills, which is not solely expected on the basis of general mental retardation or of grossly inadequate schooling. Treatment is by remedial teaching.

Other Behavioural and Emotional Disorders

In ICD-10, this umbrella heading comprises non-organic enuresis, non-organic encopresis, feeding disorder, pica, stereotyped movements, stuttering, and cluttering. In non-organic enuresis disorder, there is involuntary voiding of urine by day or night, which is abnormal in relation to the individual's mental age and which is not a consequence of a lack of bladder control due to any neurological disorder, to epileptic fits, or to any structural abnormality of the urinary tract. Secondary enuresis usually begins about the age of 5 to 7 years. It may be a single and isolated condition or it may be associated with a more widespread emotional or behavioural disorder.

In non-organic encopresis disorder, there is repeated voluntary or involuntary passage of faeces, usually of normal or near-normal consistency, in places not appropriate for that purpose. Like non-organic enuresis, this disorder may either occur as a monosymptomatic disorder, or it may form part of a wider disorder, especially an emotional disorder.

Feeding disorder generally involves the refusal of food and extreme faddiness in the presence of an adequate food supply, and a reasonably competent care giver, and the absence of organic disease. There may or may not be associated rumination (repeated regurgitation without nausea or gastrointestinal illness). Treatment is directed to the parent's management of the problem. They should be encouraged to ignore the feeding problem and refrain from offering special foods for the child. Instead the child should be offered a normal meal and then left to decide whether to eat it or not.

In pica, there is persistent eating of non-nutritive substances (e.g., soil and wood etc.). Pica can be one of the presenting symptoms of a more widespread psychiatric disorder (such as autism) or an isolated problem. This phenomenon occurs commonly in children with learning difficulties but occurs in children of normal intelligence as well. Pica usually diminishes as the child grows older.

In stereotyped movement disorders, there are voluntary, repetitive, stereotyped, non-functional (and often rhythmic) movements that do not form part of any recognised psychiatric or neurological condition. Non-injurious movements like head-rocking or body-rocking are not included here as they are not good indicators of psychopathology. ICD-10 emphasises the stereotyped self-injurious movements as repetitive head banging, face slapping and biting of hands or other parts of the body.

In stuttering (stammering), speech is characterised by frequent repetition or prolongation of sounds or words, or by frequent hesitations or pauses that disrupt the rhythmic flow of speech. There may be associated movements of the face and other parts of the body that coincide in time with the repetitions, prolongations, or pauses in the speech flow.

In cluttering, there is a rapid rate of speech with breakdown in fluency, but no repetitions or hesitations, of a severity to give rise to reduced speech intelligibility. Speech is erratic and dysrhythmic, with rapid, jerky bursts of speech, producing groups of words unrelated to the grammatical structure of the sentence.

Disorders of Social Functioning

According to ICD-10, these include somewhat heterogeneous group of disorders, which have common abnormalities in social functioning that begin during the developmental period, but that (unlike the pervasive developmental disorders) are not primarily characterised by a constitutional social incapacity or deficit that pervades all areas of functioning. These include selective mutism, reactive attachment disorder of childhood, disinhibited attachment disorder of childhood, and other childhood disorders of social functioning.

Elective Mutism

In this disorder (also called selective mutism), the child speaks in certain situations and does not in others. The child usually speaks at home but not at school, and with strangers. The onset is usually in early childhood. It occurs equally in sexes, and there is no association with social class. Some children have a history of either some speech delay or articulation problems associated with social anxiety.

According to ICD-10, the following are Required

a. A normal or near-normal level of language comprehension
b. A level of competence in language expression that is sufficient for social communication
c. Demonstrable evidence that the individual cannot and does not speak normally or almost normally in some situations

Diagnosis requires that the failure to speak is persistent over time and there is consistency and predictability with respect to the situations in which the child will speak and not speak. Children with this disorder may communicate by gestures, head movements, pulling and pushing, and sometimes by uttering monosyllabics. Associated features include personality traits like being obstinate and manipulative, over protective parents, bullying by peers, social phobia and intellectual disability.

The prevalence is 1 per 1000 (78). Pervasive developmental disorders, schizophrenia, specific developmental disorders of speech and language and transient mutism as part of separation anxiety in young children, have to be excluded.

Behavioural methods (e.g., +ive reinforcement schedules) are the treatment of choice. It is important to involve the teachers and classroom assistants. Social skills training and family therapy are helpful. Low doses of SSRIs have been used in some serious cases.

Reactive Attachment Disorder

Attachment to parents and other key caregivers is of immense importance for the children's development. Psychosocial maladjustment or problems can subsequently result if this attachment is not secure. The disorder probably occurs because of parental neglect or abuse.

According to DSM-5, this disorder is characterised by a pattern of markedly disturbed and developmentally inappropriate attachment behaviours, in which a child rarely or minimally turn preferentially to an attachment figure for comfort, support, protection and nurturance. The essential feature is absent or grossly underdeveloped attachment between the child and caregiving adults. Children with this disorder have the capacity to form selective attachment. The child is hypervigilant and fearful, and there is a lack of responsiveness to comforting. The child may appear sad, and exhibit withdrawal reactions such as huddling on the floor. Social play is restricted or disturbed by negative emotional responses. This disorder may also be accompanied by a failure to thrive physically and by impaired physical growth. DSM-5 diagnostic criteria specify that the onset should be before the age of five, the child not being autistic and has a developmental age of mental age of at least nine months.

The key aim is to positively enhance the child's caregiving environment. Social services have an important role. Although attachment-based interventions have been developed to improve severe relationships difficulties, their success so far is modest and their benefit in attachment disorders is not established (79).

Disinhibited Attachment Disorder

This disorder usually manifests around the age of two years (according to ICD-10 criteria, it has to be present before the age of five years), and comprises a particular pattern of abnormal social functioning. It is characterised by clinging, and later diffuse, non-selectively focused attachment behaviour. Usually, there is difficulty in forming close relationships with peers, although the child approaches other children and adults in an inappropriately friendly manner. Associated features include overactivity, short attention span, emotional lability, poor tolerance of frustration, and aggressive behaviour (80). It tends to persist in spite of marked changes in environmental circumstances.

It occurs much more conspicuously in children reared in institutions from infancy and is thought to be in part because of the lack of selective attachments, which are consequent to frequent changes in caregivers. There may be a history of recent abuse. Management consists of providing support to the child's caregivers to improve their ability to promote healthy development, communication skills, and relationships with peers.

School Refusal

School refusal is an irrational fear to attend school, where the child refuses to go to school. It is not a diagnosis but a presenting complaint. It can, however, be the manifestation of an underlying psychiatric disorder. It needs to be differentiated from truancy, when the child secretly avoids attending the school. School refusal is equally common in boys and girls and there is no association with any particular socio-economic class. The onset is usually insidious but can start abrupt sometimes. Problems at school are sometimes the reason, but most children are of average intelligence and academic ability. Family size is not associated with more prevalence but youngest children are over-represented. There may be clear triggers like a move to a new school, significant event(s) at home or an illness.

School refusal peaks at three stages: on starting school, after school transfer and in early teens. 5 years, 11 years, and 14–15 years are the most common ages for presentation.

The child may present with complaints of headache, stomach ache, nausea, and limb pains, and either refuses to go to school or returns back shortly. The child may express dislike of a particular teacher or may complain of being bullied at school. These complaints are typically absent during weekends or holidays. Associated features are inconsistent parental behaviour or attitude, and over-emotional involvement of one parent (predominantly the mother). School refusal occurs in less than 1% in the community (81). Severe school refusal occurs in less than 1 per 1000 children aged 10–11 years, but is more common in 14 year olds (82).

Involving an educational psychologist in the management of school refusal is very important. Behavioural approaches are effective. If the problem develops suddenly, then a rapid return to school is recommended, whereas a gradual approach (desensitisation) is more effective for chronic cases. Psychoeducation for the parents and family therapy are also helpful. Liaison with school staff is of paramount importance.

Child Abuse

Child abuse is an umbrella term for emotional abuse, neglect, physical abuse, and sexual abuse. In emotional abuse, children can be subjected to hostility, not given due attention and love and various undesirable ways resulting in lowering their self-esteem and self-confidence. Neglect is another mode of child abuse where the child is not given appropriate medical or physical care. Physical abuse includes non-accidental injury, non-organic failure to thrive and Munchausen syndrome by proxy. The commonest non-accidental injuries clinically presented are multiple bruising, burns, abrasions, bites, bone fractures, and retinal haemorrhage. Parents may bring the child with the complaint of the child crying constantly or not feeling well and the injury may only be revealed on examination.

It needs to be borne in mind that there are still cultural differences regarding parental views and attitudes as to what constitutes a normal range of physically hitting or smacking a child. There has, however, been an increasing awareness in many countries (e.g., the UK) that physically abusing a child even with the sincere intention of parents or teachers to discipline a child, is not acceptable. Legislation, forbidding the use of physical punishment at school or home, has also been introduced in many countries.

In non–organic failure to thrive, the weight gain is considerably less than expected and no medical cause is found. It is usually because of deficient diet given by the parent(s). The child starts to put on more weight when in hospital or when placed with foster parents.

Munchausen Syndrome by Proxy

In Munchausen syndrome by proxy (also known as factitious illness by proxy or illness induction syndrome), a parent (predominantly the mother), who has fabricated or induced the illness presents the child for medical consultation. In some cases the father may also be responsible (83). Even when there is some medical cause for the complaint, the presentation and picture put forward by the mother is grossly exaggerated (84).

Children are usually of pre-school age. Fabrication methods include false reporting of symptoms, falsification of specimens or charts, poisoning, smothering, and withholding food or medicines. Some mothers report epileptic fits, others put their own blood in the child's urine or faeces samples. The child may be given hypnotic or diuretic medication by the mother (85). Usually the child is brought repeatedly to the A&E department with a request for investigation(s). When the mother is not present the presenting signs and symptoms alleviate and even disappear. Typically the parent(s) deny any knowledge of the illness. Non- accidental injuries and non-organic failure to thrive can often coexist (86).

Considerable diagnostic difficulties can consequently occur and the child is subjected to intensive investigations. However, once there is suspicion of this syndrome, further investigations should be terminated. Child should be examined and assessed in the absence of mother who is usually very reluctant to leave the child. Once the diagnosis is confirmed, the parents should be confronted, social services be involved, and the child's safety issues be discussed at length.

Sexual Abuse

The term sexual abuse refers to encourageing or forcing children in sexual activities which they do not fully understand, and to which they are unable to give an informed consent. A more formal definition of child sexual abuse is: 'the involvement of dependent, developmentally immature children and adolescents in sexual activities they do not truly comprehend, to which they are unable to give informed consent, or that violate the social taboos of family roles' (87).

The offender is usually male. The majority of children know their abuser before commencement of the abuse. Active sexual abuse is often preceded by a gradual or insidious process in which the abuser identifies a particular child and develops a close relationship with the child. This is termed 'grooming'. Much sexual abuse takes place within the family and step-fathers are over-represented among abusers (88). The same abuser may abuse children both within and outside the family, including biological as well as step-children.

Sexual abuse includes penetrative acts (e.g., vaginal, anal or oral penetration) or non-penetrative acts (e.g., deliberate exposure of child to pornography or adult gentalia, subjecting the child to sexual stimulation, or persuading the child to stimulate the adult for masturbation, and fondling, etc.). In some children sexual abuse is a single episode but majority of children are abused more than once or on a long-term basis.

Some of the maintaining factors for ongoing sexual abuse are secrecy, helplessness, entrapment, threats by the abuser, neglect or refusal by the mother to help in spite of being aware of the child abuse by her husband or partner, and in certain cultures non-disclosure by the child or other family members to protect family honour. Children are more likely to report abuse when the offender is a stranger. Many children do not report the sexual abuse at the time of occurrence and others do not report at all. The prevalence of sexual abuse is not known because of under reporting. However, rates of reporting have been increasing over the past few decades. The annual incidence is about 2 per 1000 children per year (89).

Children from all social classes can be sexually abused and some authors believe there is no leaning towards lower socio-economic status (90). One study, however, demonstrates that there is slightly greater likelihood of children from lower social class (91). However, the association with lower social class is greater for physical abuse rather than sexual abuse. Girl victims are about four times as common as boy victims (92). Population based studies have shown no ethnic differences in the rates of child sexual abuse (93).

The adverse consequences of sexual abuse are predominantly psychological (94), and is a significant risk factor for the development of psychopathology in childhood and psychiatric disorders in adult life. Sexual abuse can, in the long-term, result in psychiatric disorders (e.g., borderline personality disorders, substance misuse, post-traumatic stress disorder, disassociation and depressive disorders), behavioural disturbances (e.g., relationship difficulties, promiscuity and sex crimes) and also neurobiological dysregulations such as increased level of cortisol (95). It is very important to realise that it is unusual for children to lie or fantasise about sexual abuse and their reporting should be taken seriously unless proven otherwise. Changes in child's behaviour, refusal to communicate, emotional withdrawal, aggressive behaviour, falling academic performance, running away from home, suicidal attempts, recurrent urinary infections, sexually transmitted diseases and anorexia nervosa should raise suspicions and anxieties about the possibility of sexual abuse (96).

Whenever sexual abuse is suspected or presented, multi-disciplinary professional approach is essential. The main aims are to ascertain if sexual abuse has occurred, the type of abuse and the extent of abuse. The child's needs will include, immediate and long-term protection from sexual abuse, and help and support for the effects of the abuse. One very important decision is about separating the child from the family (97). Families usually have a tendency to either deny or minimise the seriousness of the situation. Some mothers may require help with their own childhood sexual abuse or current mental health issues. There is evidence that cognitive therapy is helpful for sexually abused children having psychiatric problems (98). Some adults who are previously unaware of having been sexually abused, suddenly recall the abuse. This may occur spontaneously or during a psychotherapeutic session. It has also been suggested that sometimes these memories are not accurate and have been induced by questions or suggestions from the therapists (99). This phenomenon has been called the false memory syndrome.

Pervasive Developmental Disorders

Pervasive developmental disorders is the name given to a group of disorders that are characterised by delay and deviance in the development of social, communication and other skills. They include Asperger's disorder, Rett's disorder, autistic disorder, and childhood disintegrative disorder.

Autistic Disorder

Some clinicians are of the view that the term 'pervasive developmental disorder' is misleading for autistic disorder as the deficits are not fully pervasive. Autistic disorder is also known as childhood autism and infantile autism. Although important for all childhood disorders, a detailed history and comprehensive medical and developmental examination is even more desirable before the diagnosis of autistic disorder is made. This is because of the considerable potential for misdiagnosis. In this disorder, there is significant and sustained delay and deviance in three critical areas of development: social interaction and ability to share interests and emotions; the use of language and communication; and patterns of behaviour which are restricted or stereotyped. There is, however, a marked range of symptoms expression in autistic disorder. At one extreme the children are almost entirely mute and remain withdrawn from any kind of social interaction. Those children who are on a higher functioning level, may socially interact but are not able to sustain this. It is important to bear in mind that over the course of illness, the behavioural features change. For diagnostic purposes, the onset of illness and the core psychopathology has to be present prior to or by the age of three years. The disorder is very rarely recognised in the first year, and a majority of the parents parents nevertheless feel and complain that the development was never entirely normal. Unlike normally developing children, an autistic child will not develop an interest in social interaction and social environment. There may be no engagement with normal games of infancy, and the child may lack the usual play skills.

Some children when they grow may passively accept social interaction but do not seek this themselves and their style of interaction may be 'odd'. There is poor eye contact and lack of empathy. About 50 percent of children with autistic disorder do not speak at all, and parents may report the delay in language development as the most frequent complaint. About 25% of children develop some language which then either stops developing further or is lost. Speech often has a highly pedantic quality (100).

When a child with autistic disorder speaks, the style is less flexible, monotonous and robot-like. Echolalia (repetition of speech of others) and pronoun reversal ('you' instead of 'I') are conspicuous parts of the speech which may be nonreciprocal, that is, language that is not meant as communication. The language of others is interpreted extremely literally and the child usually fails to understand humour or sarcasm.

The activities are remarkably restricted and the child has considerable difficulty in adjusting to any change in the routines, time and environment. A minor rearrangement of furniture, for example, can result in huge distress and a temper tantrum. Interest is developed in peculiar and repetitive activities such as, collecting certain items and arranging them in a certain rigid order. The attachment to objects differs from transitional objects in the sense that the objects chosen are hard instead of soft (a teddy bear, etc.). The child may also develop stereotypical movements like hand flapping, finger twiddling, body rocking, tiptoe walking or assuming odd postures. Echopraxia (copying of other people's movements) may be present.

Intellectual disability is one of the most common comorbidity and about 80 percent of children suffer with this. About 30 percent suffer from mild to moderate intellectual disability and about 45 percent from severe to profound intellectual disability. Only about 5% have an IQ over 100 (101). There may also be executive function deficits as some children may find it difficult to organize information and plan ahead (102). On the other hand, a small number of autistic children may have unusual abilities that involve complex mathematical skills or rote memory (103).

Autistic children can have hypersensitivity and hyposensitivity to sensory stimuli. Some children can be acutely sensitive to noise, while some may not notice and respond to minor sounds. Erratic sleeping and eating patterns cause significant distress to families. Other features include mood disturbances, self-injurious behaviour and aggression against others. Epilepsy develops in 10–35 percent of autistic children and they may have minor physical anomalies like, ear malformations.

Differential Diagnoses

These include developmental or acquired language disorders, neurogenerative disorders with progressive dementia, childhood integrative disorder, childhood schizophrenia, Rett syndrome, Asperger disorder (which is regarded by some clinicians and researchers as a minor version of autistic disorder), Fragile X syndrome, developmental language disorder, deafness, and generalised intellectual disability without autistic disorder.

Epidemiology

Prevalence rates range from 0.7 to 21.1 per 10,000. This variability is because of methodological issues like sample sizes, syndrome definition, and aspects of screening. There is higher incidence in boys than girls, with an average ratio of 3.5 or 4.0 to 1. This ratio varies, however, as a function of intellectual functioning. Some studies have reported ratios of up to 6 (or more) to 1 in individuals with autism without learning difficulty, whereas reported ratios within the moderately to severely intellectual disability range have been as low as 1.5 to 1. Females are under represented in the non-intellectual disability, but the reason for this is not known (104). The current studies do not support the earlier impression that autism is associated with upper social class (105).

Aetiology

Regarding aetiology, there are various theories including psychosocial and biological. The previous speculation that mothers who are unresponsive to the child's emotional needs may be responsible for this disorder, has now been abandoned. There are similarly no established biological abnormalities detected so far.

Genetic factors contribute to this disorder as there is a 2 to 3 percent recurrence of autism amongst siblings, which is 50 to 100 times the rate of autism in the general population. Siblings of autistic children also have a higher than expected rate of language delay (106). Neuroanatomical abnormalities, immunological factors, and disturbances in neurochemistry have also been implicated but the findings have been inconsistent. In addition, some medical conditions like Fragile X syndrome and tuberous sclerosis, have also been associated with autistic disorder.

Treatment

The main goals of treatment are to reduce disruptive behaviours and to enhance language acquisition. Communication and self-help skills are encouraged and taught. These children usually need intensive and structured education, speech therapy and behaviour therapy.

As with all medications, the potential benefits and adverse effects should be taken into account. Psychopharmacology has a very limited role, but brief courses of medication may sometimes be useful to reduce the associated behavioural problems (107) although SSRIs, clonidine, naltrexone, and antipsychotics may be sometimes helpful. SSRIs may improve depressive and anxiety symptoms, self-injury, and obsessional or repetitive behaviour. Clonidine may have a beneficial, although modest, effect on activity levels. It may, however, cause sedation and hypotension. Naltrexone may also mildly decrease self-injurious tendencies and activity levels. Small doses of antipsychotics may help in reducing agitation and stereotypic behaviour. Epileptic drugs are needed if associated epilepsy is present. Stimulants may help with associated hyperactivity.

Prognosis

Autistic disorder is usually a life long disability and most individuals are unable to live independently. Only about 10% of adults with full autistic syndrome are working and some may have friends and families. One good predictor of improvement is the IQ of the child and whether speech was present at five years of age (108).

Asperger's Disorder

This is a disorder of uncertain nosological validity (109). It is characterised by the same kind of qualitative abnormalities of reciprocal social interaction that typify autism, together with a lack of empathy and a restricted, stereotypic, and repetitive repertoire of interests and activities. There is a preoccupation with special interests and the child may obtain and accumulate extensive information in a mechanical way (110). In other words, the abnormalities in Asperger's syndrome are qualitatively similar to those seen in autistic disorder, but to a lesser extreme. This disorder, however, differs from autistic disorder primarily in that it lacks clinically significant delays in spoken or receptive language, cognitive development, self-help skills and interest in the environment.

The condition has sometimes been considered as a schizoid personality or autistic psychopathy (111). Most individuals are of normal general intelligence but it is common for them to be markedly clumsy and have partial insight into their difficulties. There is a strong tendency for the abnormalities to persist into adolescence and adult life and it seems that they represent individual characteristics that are not greatly affected by environmental influences. Psychotic episodes occasionally occur in early adult life.

Diagnosis is based on the combination of a lack of any clinically significant general delay in language or cognitive development plus, as with autism, the presence of qualitative deficiencies in reciprocal social interaction and restricted, repetitive, stereotyped patterns of behaviour, interests and actives. There may or may not be problems in communication similar to those associated with autism, but significant language retardation would rule out the diagnosis. Differentiating Asperger's syndrome from autistic disorder is not very difficult but it becomes challenging when the autistic child does not have any learning difficulties Asperger's syndrome differs in that the onset is usually later and the outcome is more positive.

According to ICD-10, if the child meets the criteria for autistic disorder, this should take precedence over the diagnosis of Asperger's syndrome.

Epidemiology

The prevalence is 3–4 per 1000 children (112). It is more prevalent in males than females with a reported ratio of 9 to 1. Parents of these children may exhibit some sort of social or language difficulties themselves.

Aetiology

Aetiology remains unknown but it is generally believed that genetic factors are important. In some families, both autistic disorder and Asperger's syndrome may occur which possibly suggest similar aetiological factors.

Treatment

There is no medical treatment. The main focus of treatment is supportive and symptomatic, and in many ways overlaps with the treatment strategies for autistic disorder without intellectual disability. As people with Asperger's syndrome usually do well academically, they understandably encounter difficulties in accessing educational interventions from authorities who are initially unable to appreciate the depth of their problems.

Acquisition of self-sufficiency skills in all areas of functioning, and problem-solving strategies for troublesome situations like urgent social demands or novel situations, are extremely important.

Communication therapy would aim at training the patients non-verbal behaviour including the use of gaze for social interaction and monitoring of voice inflection. Similarly helping them to find appropriate jobs (e.g., those jobs which do not have much social and time pressure, etc.) is part of the management.

Rett's Syndrome

This is an X-linked dominant progressive neurodevelopmental disorder, only reported in girls. There is a characteristic onset, course, and pattern of symptomatology. Typically, after an apparently normal or near-normal early development of the child, there is a developmental plateau, followed by partial or complete loss of acquired hand skills and speech, and slowing in head growth. Loss of acquired fine motor manipulative skills are particularly characteristic.

The onset is between 5 months and 48 months (usually between 6 months and 12 months). Midline hand-wringing sterotypes, with the arms flexed in front of the chest or chin, stereotypic wetting of the hands with saliva, lack of proper food chewing, episodes of hyperventilation, almost always a failure to gain bowel and bladder control and often excessive drooling and protrusion of the tongue occur. This is accompanied by loss, partial loss or lack of development of language. Social and play development are arrested in the first 2 or 3 years, but social interest tends to be maintained. During middle childhood, trunk ataxia and apraxia, tend to develop and sometimes there are choreoathetoid movements. Complications include contractures and kyphoscoliosis, due to the abnormal posture and immobility (113). Kyphoscoliosis compromises the respiratory function often severely. Severe mental handicap invariably results. Fits frequently develop during the early or middle childhood. Occasionally there is a history of sleep disturbances.

The course of the disorder, in terms of progressive motor deterioration, confirms the diagnosis. There is an absence of any psychological causation for the symptoms. Estimates of the prevalence of Rett's disorder range from 1 in 15,000 to 1 in 22,000 females. The precise aetiology of this disorder is not known, although a neurobiological basis is thought to be the cause.

Autistic disorder, childhood integrative disorder and Asperger's syndrome need to be considered in the differential diagnosis, although diagnosis of Rett's disorder in most cases is not difficult in older individuals. As preschool children with Rett's disorder may show difficulty with social skills, it may be confused with autistic disorder. Rett's disorder can be differentiated from autistic disorder because of its distinctive pattern of developmental loss and characteristic clinical features. In childhood disintegrative disorder, the onset of symptoms is typically later than that of Rett's disorder. Moreover, the period of normal development is much longer in childhood disintegrative disorder (which also usually affects males). In contrast to Rett's disorder, the cognitive and language skills do not deteriorate in Asperger's syndrome.

Regarding the prognosis of Rett's disorder, it needs to be emphasised that it is a progressive neurodegenerative disorder, affected individuals are usually in wheelchairs by their late teens, and there is an increased risk of sudden death. There is no specific treatment including pharmacological. Special education, behaviour modification, and physical and respiratory therapy may be useful in alleviating some symptoms.

Childhood Disintegrative Disorder

Previously known as Heller's syndrome, the childhood disintegrative disorder is a rare condition and carries a poor prognosis. This is a pervasive developmental disorder (other than Rett's syndrome) that is defined by a period of normal development over the first two years, and by a definite loss, over the course of a few months, of previously acquired skills in at least several areas of development. There is, in addition, the onset of characteristic abnormalities of social, communicative, and behavioural functioning. Often there is a prodromic period of vague illness; the child becomes restive, irritable, anxious, and overactive. This is followed by impoverishment and then loss of speech and language, accompanied by behavioural disintegration. Receptive and expressive language are lost, often with a loss of coordination and bowel or bladder function (114).

In some cases, the loss of skills is persistently progressive (usually when the disorder is associated with a progressive diagnosable neurological condition), but more often the decline over a period of some months is followed by a plateau and then a limited improvement. The prognosis is usually very poor, and most individuals are left with severe mental retardation. Diagnosis is based on an apparent normal development up to the age of at least two years, followed by a definite loss of previously acquired skills; this is accompanied by qualitatively abnormal social functioning.

In some respects, the syndrome resembles dementia in adult life, but it differs in three key respects: there is usually no evidence of any identifiable organic disease or damage (although organic brain dysfunction of some type is usually inferred); the loss of skills may be followed by a degree of recovery; and the impairment in socialisation and communication has deviant qualities typical of autism rather than intellectual decline.

In most cases, the child's development and behaviour deteriorate significantly to a lower level of functioning. Some children may show recovery of some skills and few make a good recovery. There is no specific pharmacological treatment. Special education and behavioural treatments are helpful to develop some of the lost skills.

REFERENCES

1. Beidel, D. C. and Turner, S. M. (1997). At risk for anxiety: I. Psychopathology in the offspring of anxious parents. *Journal of the American Academy of Child and Adolescent Psychiatry*, 36, 918–24.
2. McLaughlin, K., et al. (2012). Parent psychopa- thology and offspring mental disorders: result from the WHO World Mental Health Surveys. *British Journal of Psychiatry*, 200, 290–299.
3. Barkley, R. A., Karlsson, J., Pollard, S. and Murphy, J. V. (1985). Developmental changes in the mother-child interactions of hyperactive boys: Effects of two dose level of Ritalin. *Journal of Child Psychology and Psychiatry*, 26, 705–715.
4. Feingold, B. F. (1975). Hyperkinesis and learning difficulties linked to artificial food and colours, *American Journal of Nursing*, 75, 797–803.
5. Graham, P., Turk, J. and Verhulst, F. (1999). Neurodevelopmental and neuropsychiatric disorders. In P. Graham, J. Turk and F. Verhulst (Eds.), *Child psychiatry. A developmental approach* (3rd Edition). Oxford: Oxford University Press.
6. Szatmari P, Offord, D. R. and Boyle, M. H. (1989). Ontario Child Health Study: prevalence of attention deficit disorder with hyperactivity. *Journal of Child Psychology and Psychiatry*, 30, 65– 99.
7. Hinshaw, S. P. (1994). *Attention deficits and hyperactivity in children*. Thousand Oaks, CA: Sage.
8. Mash, E. J. and Johnston, C. (1990). Determinants of parenting stress: Illustration from families of hyperactive children and families of physically abused children. *Journal of Clinical Psychology*, 19, 313–328.
9. Cunningham, C. E., Davis, J. R., Bremner, R., Dunn, K. W. and Rzasa, T. (1993). Coping modelling problem-solving versus mastery modelling: effects on adherence, in-session process, and skill acquisition in residential parent-training program. *Journal of Consulting and Clinical Psychology*, 61, 871–877.
10. Schachar, R, and Tannock, R. (2002) Syndromes of hyperactivity and attention deficit. In M. Rutter and E. Taylor (Eds.), *Child and adolescent psychiatry*. Oxford: Blackwell Publishing.
11. Greenhill, L. L., Abikoff, H. B., Arnold, L. E., et al. (1996). Medication Treatment strategies in the MTA study: relevance to clinicians and research. *Journal of the American Academy of Child and Adolescent Psychiatry*, 34, 1304–1313.
12. Elia, J., Borcherding, B. G., Rapoport, J. L. and Keysor, C. S. (1991). Methylphenidate and dextroamphetamine treatments of hyperactivity: Are there true non-responders? *Psychiatry Research*, 36, 141–155.
13. Taylor, E. (1994). Physical treatments. In M. Rutter, E. Taylor and L. A. Hersov (Eds.), *Child and adolescent psychiatry*. Oxford: Blackwell Scientific.
14. Barklay, R. A., Karlson, J., Strzlecli, E. and Murphy, J. V. (1984). The effects of age and dosing of Ritalin on the mother-child interactions of hyperactive children. *Journal of Consulting and Clinical Psychology*, 52, 750–758.
15. Hill, P. (1999). The hyperactive child. In M. Lader and D. Naber (Eds.), *Difficult clinical problems in psychiatry*. London: Martin Dunitz.
16. Rapport, M. D. and Denney, C. (1997). Titrating methylphenidate in children with attention deficit/ hyperactivity disorder: Is body mass predictive of clinical response? *Journal of the American Academy of Child and Adolescent Psychiatry*, 36, 523–530.
17. Richman, N., Stevenson, J. and Graham, P. (1982). *Preschool to school: A behavioural study*. London: Academic Press.
18. Barkley, R. A., Anastopoulos, A. D., Guevremont, D. C. and Fletcher, K. E. (1991). Adolescents with behavioural adjustment, academic functioning, and treatment utilization. *Journal of Child Psychology and Psychiatry*, 30, 379– 390.
19. American Psychiatric Association(2013). *Diagnostic and statistical manual of mental disorders* (5th Edition). Arlington, VA: American Psychiatric Publishing.
20. Rutter, M., Cox, A., Tupling, C., Berger, M. and Yule, W. (1975). Attainment and adjustment in two geographical areas. 1. Prevalence of psychiatric disorders. *British Journal of Psychiatry*, 126, 493–509.
21. Cadoret, R., Yates, W., Troughton, E., et al. (1995). Genetic environmental interaction in the genesis of aggressivity and conduct disorders. *Archives of General Psychiatry*, 52, 916–924.
22. Steiner, H. (2000). Disruptive Behaviour Disorders. In B. Saddock and V. Saddock (Eds.), *Kaplan and Saddock's Comprehensive Textbook of Psychiatry*. Philadelphia: Lippincott Williams and Wilkins.
23. Howe, G., Feinstein, C., Reiss, D., Molock, S. and Berger, K. (1993). Adolescent adjustment to chronic physical disorders, 1: Comparing neurological and non-neurological conditions. *Journal of Child Psychology and Psychiatry*, 34, 1153–1171.
24. Huesmann, L. R. (1986). Psychological processes promoting the relation between exposure to media violence and aggressive behaviour by the viewer. *Journal of Social Issues*, 42, 125–139.
25. Loeber, R., Wung, P., Kenan, K., et al. (1993). Developmental pathways in disruptive child behaviour. *Development and Psychopathology*, 5, 103–134.
26. Robins, L. N. (1966). *Deviant children grown up*.Baltimore: Williams and Wilkins.
27. Kazdin, A. (1997). Psychosocial treatments for conduct disorder in children. *Journal of Child Psychology and Psychiatry*, 38, 161–178.
28. Henggeler, S. W., Rowland, M. D., Halliday- Boykins, C., et al. (2003). One year follow–up of multisytemic therapy as an alternative to the hospitalisation of youths in psychiatric crises. *Journal of the American Academy of Child and Adolescent Psychiatry*, 42, 543–551.
29. Mcardle, P. (2005). Conduct disorders. In S. Gowers (Ed.), *College seminar series in child and adolescent psychiatry* (2nd Edition). London: Royal College of Psychiatrists.
30. Anderson, J. (1994). Epidemiological Issues.In T. Ollendeck, N. King and W. Yule (Eds.), *International Handbook of phobic and anxiety disorders in children and adolescents*. New York: Plenum.
31. Bird, H. R. (1996). Epidemiology in childhood disorders in a cross-cultural context. *Journal of Child Psychology and Psychiatry*, 37, 35–49.
32. Benjamin, R. S., Costello, E. J. and Warren, M. (1990). Anxiety disorders in a paediatric sample. *Journal of Anxiety Disorders*, 4, 293–316.
33. Shaffer, D., Schwab-Stone, M., Fisher, P., et al. (1993). The Diagnostic Interview Schedule for Children-Revised Version (DISC-R): 1 Preparation, field–testing, inter-rater reliability, and acceptability. *Journal of the American Academy of Child and Adolescent Psychiatry*, 32, 643–650.
34. Verhulst, F. C., Van der Ende, J., Fernand, R. F. and Schulman J. L. (1997). The prevalence of DSM-III-R diagnosis in a national sample of Dutch adolescents. *Archives of General Psychiatry*, 54(94), 329–336.

35. Graham, P., Turk, J. and Verhulst, F. (1999).Development and developmental psychopathology. In P. Graham, J. Turk and F. Verhulst (Eds.), *Child psychiatry. A developmental approach*(3rd Edition). Oxford: Oxford University Press.

36. Allen, A., Leonard, H. and Swedo, S. (1995).Current knowledge of medication for the treatment of childhood anxiety disorders.*Journal of the American Academy of Child and Adolescent Psychiatry*, 34, 976–986.

37. Schwartz, C. E., Snidman, N. and Kagan, J. (1999). Adolescent social anxiety as an outcome of inhibited temperament in childhood. Journal of the *American Academy of Child and Adolescent Psychiatry*, 38, 1008–1015

38. Frederick, C. J. (1985). Children traumatized by catastrophic situations. In S. Eth and R. Pynoos (Eds.), *Post-traumatic Stress Disorder in children*. Washington DC: American Psychiatric Press.

39. Helzer, J. E., Robins, L. N. and McEvoy,L.(1987). Post-traumatic stress disorder in the general population: findings of the Epidemiological Catchment Area survey. *New England Journal of Medicine*, 317, 1630–1634.

40. Kessler, R. C., Sonnega, A., Bromet, E., Hughes,M.and Nelson, C. B. (1995). Post-traumatic stress disorder in the National Comorbidity Survey. *Archives of General Psychiatry*, 52, 1048– 1060.

41. Tinker, R. H and Wilson, S. A. (1999). *Through the eyes of a child: EMDR with children*. New York: Norton.

42. Heyman, I., Fombonne, E., Simmons, H., et al. (2001). Prevalence of obsessive-compulsive disorder in the British nation wide survey child mental health. *British Journal of Psychiatry*, 179, 324–329.

43. Rapoport, J. L. (1986). Childhood obsessive-compulsive disorders.*Journal of Child Psychology and Psychiatry*, 27, 289–295.

44. Maina, G., Albert, U., Bogetto, F. and Ravizza,L.(1999). Obsessive-compulsive syndromes in older adolescents. *Acta Psychiatrica Scandinavia*, 100, 447–450.

45. Shafran, R. (1998). Cognitive behaviour therapy for childhood obsessive disorder. In P. J. Graham (Ed.), *Cognitive Behaviour Therapy for children and families*. Cambridge: Cambridge University Press.

46. Deveaugh-Geiss, J., Maroz, G., Biederman, J., et al. (1992). Clomipramine hydrochloride in childhood and adolescent obsessive- compulsive-disorder—a multi centre trial. Journal of the *American Academy of Child and Adolescent Psychiatry*, 31, 45–49.

47. Riddle, M. A., Scahill, L., King, R., et al. (1992).Double blind cross-over trial of fluoxetine and placebo in children and adolescents with obsessive-compulsive disorder.*Journal of the American Academy of Child and Adolescent Psychiatry*, 31, 1050–1056.

48. Lewinsohn, P. M., Rohde, P. and Seeley, J. R. (1994). Psychosocial risk factors for future adolescent suicide attempts. *Journal of Consulting and Clinical Psychology*, 62, 297–305.

49. Harrington, R. (1994). Affective Disorders. In M. Rutter, E. Taylor and L. Hersolv (Eds.), *Child and adolescent psychiatry*. London: Blackwell Science.

50. Angold, A., Costello, E. J. and Worthman, C. M.(1998). Puberty and depression. The roles of age, pubertal status, and pubertal timing. *Psychological Medicine*, 28, 51–61.

51. Angold, A. and Rutter, M. (1992). Effects of age and pubertal status on depression in a large clinical sample. *Development and Psychopathology*, 4, 5–28.

52. Kovacs, M., Gatsonis, C., Paulaskas, S. and Richards, C. (1989). Depressive disorders in childhood. IV. A longitudinal study of comorbidity with and risk of anxiety disorders. *Archives of General Psychiatry*, 46, 776–782.

53. Quackenbush, D., Kutcher, S., Robertson, H., Boulos, C. and Chaban, P. (1996). Premorbid and postmorbid school functioning in bipolar adolescents:Description and suggested academic interventions. *Canadian Journal of Psychiatry*, 41, 16–22.

54. Kovacs, M. and Pollock, M. (1995). Bipolar disorder and comorbid conduct disorder in childhood and adolescence. *Journal of the American Academy of Child and Adolescent Psychiatry*, 34, 715–723.

55. Carlson, G. A., Fennig, S. and Bromet, E. J. (1994). The confusion between bipolar disorder and schizophrenia in youth: where does it stand in the 1990s? *Journal of the American Academy of Child and Adolescent Psychiatry*, 33, 453–460.

56. Geller, B., Cooper, T. B., Sun, K., et al. (1998). Double-blind and placebo controlled study of lithium for adolescent bipolar disorders with secondary substance dependency. *Journal of the American Academy of Child and Adolescent Psychiatry*, 37, 171–178.

57. Ryan, N. D., Bhatara, V. S. and Perel, J. M. (1999). Mood stabilisers in children and adolescents.*Journal of the American Academy of Child and Adolescent Psychiatry*, 38, 529-536.

58. Graham, P., Turk, J. and Verhulst, F. (1999).Development and developmental psychopathology. In P. Graham, J. Turk and F. Verhulst (Eds.), *Child psychiatry. A developmental approach*(3rd Edition). Oxford: Oxford University Press.

59. Fombonne, E. (1998). Suicidal behaviours in vulnerable adolescents: Time trends and their correlates. *British Journal of Psychiatry*, 173, 154– 159.

60. Office of Population Censuses and Surveys. (1998). *Mortality statistics. Cause*: England and Wales. London: HMSO.

61. Graham, P., Turk, J. and Verhulst, F. (1999). Neurodevelopmental and neuropsychiatric disorders. In P. Graham, J. Turk and F. Verhulst (Eds.), *Child psychiatry. A developmental approach* (3rd Edition). Oxford: Oxford University Press.

62. Cotgrove, A. (1995). Depression and self-harm. In S. Gowers (Ed.), *College seminar series in child and adolescent psychiatry* (2nd Edition). London: Royal College of Psychiatrists.

63. Kingsbury, S. (1996). Pathos: a screening instrument for adolescent overdose: A research note. *Journal of Child and Adolescent Psychiatry*, 37, 609–686.

64. Hollis, C. (2002). Schizophrenia and Allied Disorders. In M. Rutter and E. Taylor (Eds.), *Child and adolescent psychiatry*. Oxford: Blackwell Publishing.

65. Werry, J. S., Mcclellan, J. M., Andrews, L. and, Ham, M. (1994). Clinical features and outcome of child and adolescent schizophrenia. *Schizophrenia Bulletin*, 20, 619–630.

66. Werry, J. S., Mcclellan, J. M., Andrews, L. and, Ham, M. (1994). Clinical features and outcome of child and adolescent schizophrenia. *Schizophrenia Bulletin*, 20, 619–630.

67. Graham, P., Turk, J. and Verhulst, F. (1999).Adolescence and psychiatric disorders often beginning in adolescence. In P. Graham, J. Turk and F. Verhulst (Eds.), *Child psychiatry. A developmental approach* (3rd Edition). Oxford: Oxford University Press.

68. McClellan, J. M. (2000). Early onset schizo- phrenia. In B. Saddock and V. Saddock (Eds.), *Kaplan and Saddock's*

comprehensive textbook of psychiatry. Philadelphia: Lippincott Williams and Wilkins.

69. Zeitlin, H. (1986). *The Natural History of Psychiatric Disorder in Childhood*. Maudsley Monographs. London: Oxford University Press.
70. Murray, R. M. (1994). Neurodevelopmental schizophrenia: The rediscovery of dementia praecox. *British Journal of Psychiatry Supplement*, 6–12.
71. Graham, P., Turk, J. and Verhulst, F. (1999).Adolescence and psychiatric disorders often beginning in adolescence. In P. Graham, J. Turk and F. Verhulst (Eds.), *Child psychiatry. A developmental approach* (3rd Edition). Oxford: Oxford University Press.
72. McCraken, J. (2000). Tic disorders. In B. Saddock and V. Saddock (Eds.), *Kaplan and Saddock's comprehensive textbook of psychiatry*.Philadelphia: Lippincott Williams and Wilkins.
73. Goodman, R. and Scott, S. (2005). *Child Psychiatry*. Oxford: Blackwell Publishing.
74. McCraken, J. (2000). Tic disorders. In B. Saddock and V. Saddock (Eds.), *Kaplan and Saddock's comprehensive textbook of psychiatry*. Philadelphia: Lippincott Williams and Wilkins.
75. Graham, P., Turk, J. and Verhulst, F. (1999). Neurodevelopment and neuropsychiatric disorders. In P. Graham, J. Turk and F. Verhulst (Eds.), Child psychiatry. A developmental approach (3rd Edition). Oxford: Oxford University Press.
76. Pringsheim, T., Davenport, W. J., Lang, A., et al. (2003). Tics. *Current Opinion in Neurology*, 16, 523–527.
77. Hoekstra, P. J., Kallenberg, C. G., Korf, J., et al. (2002). Is Tourette's syndrome an autoimmune disease? *Molecular Psychiatry* 7, 437–445.
78. Kolvin, I and Fundudis, T. (1981). Elective mute children: psychological development and background factors. *Journal of Child Psychology and Psychiatry*, 22, 219–232.
79. Goodman, R. and Scott S. (2005). *Child psychiatry*. Oxford: Blackwell Publishing.
80. Graham, P., Turk, J. and Verhulst, F. (1999).Development and developmental psychopathology. In P. Graham, J. Turk and F. Verhulst (Eds.), *Child psychiatry. A developmental approach*. (3rd Edition). Oxford: Oxford University Press.
81. Last, C. G. and Francis, G. (1988). School phobia. In B. Lahey and A. Kazdin (Eds.), *Advances in clinical child psychology*. New York: Plenum.
82. Rutter, M., Graham, P., Chadwick, O. and Yule,W. (1976). Adolescent turmoil: Fact or fiction? *Journal of Child Psychology and Psychiatry* 17, 35– 56.
83. Meadow, R. (1988). Munchausen syndrome by proxy perpetrated by men. *Archives of Disease in Childhood*, 78, 210–216.
84. Meadow, R. (1982). Munchausen syndrome by proxy. *Archives of Disease in Childhood*, 60, 385– 393.
85. Graham, P., Turk, J. and Verhulst, F. (1999).Maltreatment in the family. In P. Graham, J. Turk and F. Verhulst (Eds.), *Child psychiatry. A developmental approach* (3rd Edition). Oxford: Oxford University Press.
86. Goodman, R. and Scott S. (2005). *Child Psychiatry*. Oxford: Blackwell Publishing.
87. Schechter, M. and Roberge, L. (1976). Child sexual abuse. In R. Helfer and C. Kempe (Eds.), *Child abuse and neglect*: The family and the community. Cambridge: Ballinger
88. Russel D. E. H. (1984). The prevalence and seriousness of incestuous abuse: stepfathers versus biological fathers. *Child Abuse and Neglect*, 8, 15–22.
89. Jones, D. P. H. (2000). Child Abuse and Neglect. In M. G. Gelder, J. J. Lopez-Ibor Jr and N. C. Andreasen (Eds.), *The new Oxford textbook psychiatry*. Oxford: Oxford University Press.
90. Earnshaw, S. (1995). Disorders of parenting.In S. G. Gowers (Ed.), *Seminars in child and adolescent psychiatry*. London: Royal College of Psychiatrists.
91. Goodman, R. and Scott S. (2005). *Child psychiatry*. Oxford: Blackwell Publishing.
92. Badgley, R., Allard, H., McCormich, N., et al. (1984). *Sexual offenses against children*. Ottawa: Canadian Government Publishing Centre.
93. Korbin, J. (1997). Culture and child maltreatment. In M. Helfer, R. Kempe and R. Krugman (Eds.), *The battered child*. Chicago: University of Chicago Press.
94. Glaser, D. (2000). Sexual Abuse. In M. Rutter and E. Taylor (Eds.), *Child and adolescent psychiatry*. Oxford: Blackwell Publishing.
95. Putnam, F. W. (2003). Ten year research update review: Child sexual abuse. *Journal of the American Academy of Child and Adolescent Psychiatry*, 42, 269–278.
96. Graham, P., Turk, J. and Verhulst, F. (1999).Maltreatment in the family. In P. Graham, J. Turk and F. Verhulst (Eds.), *Child psychiatry. A developmental approach* (3rd Edition). Oxford: Oxford University Press.
97. Gelder, M., Harrison, P. and Cowen, P. (2006). Child Psychiatry. In P. Harrison, P. Cowen and T. Burns (Eds.), *Shorter Oxford textbook of psychiatry*. Oxford: Oxford University Press.
98. Ramachandani, P. and Jones, D. P. H. (2003). Treating psychological symptoms in sexually abused children: from research findings to service provision. *British Journal of Psychiatry*, 183, 484–490.
99. Gelder, M., Harrison, P. and Cowen, P. (2006). Reactions to stressful experiences. In P. Harrison, P. Cowen and T. Burns (Eds.), *Shorter Oxford textbook of psychiatry*. Oxford: Oxford University Press.
100. Ghaziuddin, M. and Gerstein, L. (1996). Pedantic speaking style differentiates Asperger syndrome from highly functioning autism. *Journal of Autism and Developmental Disorders*, 26, 585–595.
101. Wing, L. and Gould, J. (1979). Severe impairments of social interaction and associated abnormalities in children: epidemiology and classification. *Journal of Autism and Developmental Disorders*, 9, 11–29.
102. Bishop, D. (1993). Autism, executive functions and theory of mind: a neuropsychological perspective. *Journal of Child Psychology and Psychiatry*, 34, 279–293.
103. O'Connor, N and Hermelin, B. (1984). Idiot savant claendrical calculations. *Psychological Medicine*, 14, 801–806.
104. Volkmar, F. R., Klin, A. (2000). Pervasive developmental disorder. In B. Saddock and V. Saddock (Eds.), *Kaplan and Saddock's comprehensive textbook of psychiatry*. Philadelphia: Lippincott Williams and Wilkins.
105. Volkmar, F. R., Klin, A. (2000). Pervasive developmental disorder. In B. Saddock and V. Saddock (Eds.), *Kaplan and Saddock's comprehensive textbook of psychiatry*. Philadelphia: Lippincott Williams and Wilkins.
106. Bailey, A., Phillips, W. and Rutter, M. (1996). Autism: towards an integration of clinical,genetic, neuropsychological, and neurobiological perspectives. *Journal of Child Psychology and Psychiatry*, 37, 89–126.

107. Gilman, J. T. and Tuchman, R. F. (1995). Autism and associated behavioural disorders; pharmacotherapeutic intervention. *Annals of Pharmacotherapy*, 29, 47–56.

108. Goodman, R. and Scott, S. (2005). *Child psychiatry*. Oxford: Blackwell Publishing.

109. Gilchrist, A., Green, J., Cox, A., et al. (2001). Development and current functioning in adolescents with Asperger syndrome: a comparative study. *Journal of Child Psychology and Psychiatry and Allied Disciples*, 42, 227–240.

110. Tantum, D. (1988). Asperger's syndrome: An annotation. *Journal of Child Psychology and Psychiatry*, 29, 245–255.

111. Wolff, S. (1991). 'Schizoid' personality in childhood and adult life I: The vagaries of diagnostic labelling. *British Journal of Psychiatry*, 159, 615–620.

112. Ehlers, S. and Gillberg, C. (1993). The epidemiology of Asperger syndrome: a total population study. *Journal of Child Psychology and Psychiatry*, 34, 1327–1350.

113. Hagberg, B. (1993). Rett syndrome- clinical and biological aspects. *Clinics in developmental medicine*. Cambridge: Cambridge University Press.

114. Volkmar, F. R. and Rutter, M. (1995). Childhood disintegrative disorder: Result of the DSM-IV autism field trial. *Journal of the American Academy of Child and Adolescent Psychiatry*, 34, 1092–1095.

CHAPTER

13 Intellectual Disability

In this chapter, psychiatric aspects of intellectual disability are discussed. Dual disability is the term used to refer to the overlap between psychiatric disorders and intellectual disability. The terms intellectual disability, learning disability or learning difficulty have been the preferred terms instead of the previous terms like mental handicap, mental retardation, or mental subnormality. DSM-5 uses the term intellectual disability. The term mental retardation is replaced in ICD-11, with intellectual developmental disorders to indicate that these are disorders that involve impaired brain functioning.

Intellectual disability is characterised by impairment of development of skills, which have an adverse impact on various domains of intelligence, including cognitive, language, motor, and social. The deficits in abilities as well as in behaviours required for social and personal sufficiency, is known as adaptive functioning.

The diagnosis of intellectual disability refers to the reduced level of a person's intellectual and adaptive functioning, with the resultant decreased ability to meet the routine and daily demands of life. It is important to bear in mind that intellectual disability is not a unitary concept but instead refers to a broad behavioural syndrome, which have a wide range of causes, manifestations, and variable outcomes. Persons diagnosed as having intellectual disability, therefore, represent a wide spectrum of abilities, clinical presentations and behavioural patterns (1).

Although intellectual disability has a higher incidence of psychiatric disorders as compared to the general population, the psychiatric disorders seen in persons with intellectual disability are the same as those in the general population (2). This fact, however, presents with unique diagnostic and treatment challenges. One particular difficulty in classifying people with an intellectual disability is that they may show severe impairments in one particular area (e.g., language), or may have a particular area of higher skill (e.g., in simple visuo-spatial tasks) against a background of severe intellectual disability (3). ICD-10, therefore, recommends that the diagnostic category be chosen based on global assessments of ability and not on any single area of specific impairment or skill (4).

Epidemiology

In a study done in 1929, the total prevalence of intellectual disability was 27 per 1000, and the prevalence of moderate and severe intellectuall disability was 3.7 per 1000 (5). Subsequent studies done in different countries have come up with similar findings (6). In one recent study, the prevalence of mild mental intellectual disability was 0.37 to 0.59%, whereas the prevalence of moderate, severe and profound intellectual disability was 0.3 to 0.4% (7). Intellectual disability is 9 times more common in class 5 as compared to class 1 (8).

Regarding the prevalence of psychiatric disorders among severe intellectual disability patients, many studies have found that about half have psychiatric disorder, with the highest rates among the most profound learning disabilities patients (9). Among patients with severe intellectual disability, hyperactivity, stereotypies, and self-injury are especially frequent (10).

Classification

An assessment of both social adaptation and Intelligence Quotient (IQ) are necessary to determine the level of intellectual disability. Due to problems of cross cultural validity, the IQ levels should be used as a guide and should not be applied rigidly. According to ICD-10, the categories of intellectual disability (based on IQ) should be considered arbitrary divisions of complex continuum.

ICD-10 also recommends that the IQ should be ascertained from standardised, individually administered intelligence tests for which the local cultural norms have been determined, and the test selected should be appropriate to the individual's level of functioning and additional specific handicapping conditions (11). In ICD-10 mild mental retardation is defined as having an IQ from 50 to 69, moderate mental retardation having an IQ from 35 to 49, severe mental retardation having an IQ from 20 to 34, and profound mental retardation having an IQ below 20.

In DSM-5, the various levels of severity are defined on the basis of adaptive functioning and not IQ scores. The reason behind this is that the levels of required support is according to the adaptive functioning. It is, moreover, felt that in the lower end of IQ range, the IQ measures are less valid (12).

Mild intellectual Disability (1Q 50–70)

85 percent of people with intellectual disability have a mild intellectual disability. These children are not easily detected in the early years of life, as their appearance is unremarkable and there are minimal sensory or motor deficits. Similarly, they have nearly normal language abilities and they exhibit appropriate social behaviour during the pre-school years.

As they get older, however, such cognitive deficits as poor ability to abstract, may distinguish them. In most cases, they can achieve some educational and vocational success (unskilled or semi-skilled manual labour) in a supportive environment. Nearly 60% of children with mild intellectual disability will present with behavioural problems by the age of 21 year (13).

Moderate Intellectual Disability (IQ 35–49)

People in this group account for about 10 percent of those with intellectual disability (14). They usually have obvious neurological deficits and suffer from various syndromes associated with intellectual disability. They are unable to benefit from formal education and schooling but can be trained in special training centres in various self-help, social and occupational skills. Their academic achievement is usually limited to the middle-elementary school. Moderate intellectual disability is likely to be diagnosed at a younger age than mild intellectual disability. Their social isolation increases gradually. Their receptive language skills are better than the expressive skills. Children with moderate intellectual disability are usually aware of their difficulties and handicaps, and obviously feel frustrated by their limitations. They continue to require a relatively high level of supervision (e.g., with accommodation issues). If their tasks are carefully structured and supervised, they may have the potential to become competent (to a certain extent) at occupational tasks.

Severe Intellectual Disability (IQ 20–34)

This group constitutes about 3–4 percent of intellectual disability patients. Severe intellectual disability is 25 percent more common in males than females, mostly due to X-linked conditions. Severe intellectual disability is generally obvious in the preschool years. Children usually have gross physical abnormalities, and suffer from a marked degree of motor impairment or other associated deficits, indicating the presence of clinical significant damage to, or maldevelopment of the central nervous system (15).

They are incapable of leading an independent life and are unable to guard themselves against exploitation. Such individuals need constant supervision and a very clear structure to their lives. By adolescence, if language is poor, non-verbal forms of communication may have evolved; the inability to articulate fully may reinforce the physical means of communicating. Behavioural approaches can help promote some self-care, although they generally need extensive supervision.

Profound Intellectual Disability (IQ Below 20)

Children with profound intellectual disability are a highly vulnerable group as they are severely limited in their ability to understand or comply with simple requests. Their communication and motor skills are markedly affected and they require constant supervision in the daily basic needs. Even in adulthood, nursing care is needed. This group comprises about 1–2 percent of people with intellectual disability, and an organic aetiology can be identified in most cases.

Challenging Behaviour

Challenging behaviour is formally defined as the behaviour of such an intensity, frequency and duration that the physical safety of the person or others is in serious jeopardy, or a behaviour which is likely to seriously limit or deny access to the use of ordinary facilities (16). Around 20 percent of intellectual disability children and adolescents, and 15 percent of adults with intellectual disability present with some sort of challenging behaviour (17).

Mental illness is one of the many causes and contributory factors for challenging behaviour. Behavioural problems in people with intellectual disability arise from an interplay of two types of factors: those which are independent of the environment (e.g., functional mental illness) and ones that are dependent on the environment (e.g., failed communication attempts). Some authors believe that unmet universal emotional needs are also a cause of behavioural disturbances (18).

Intellectual Disability and Forensic Problems

There is a higher rate of criminal behaviour in people with mild intellectual disability as compared to the general population. The common offenses are arson and sexual (usually exhibitionism). The aetiology is multi-factorial.

Aetiology of Intellectual Disabilities

There are many causes of intellectual disability, but in about 50% of cases, the aetiology remains uncertain. The prevalence of diagnosable causes of mental retardation varies with the degree of the disability. When the intellectual disability is severe, a prenatal cause can be identified in 59 to 73% of patients, but in mild disability such a cause can be identified in only 23 to 43% of patients (19). One study found that most cases of intellectual disability (especially mild intellectual disability) are not due to a single cause, but due to an interaction of both inherited and environmental factors (20). Other studies have supported this finding. In more than 50% of severe intellectual disabilities, physical factors, especially prenatal causes, are responsible (21). In developing countries (e.g., Pakistan), post-natal causes (e.g., hypothyroidism, trauma, and infection) remain quite important and frequent, in contrast to developed countries in which genetic and perinatal causes are comparatively more common than post-natal causes (22).

Prenatal: Genetic disorders

Chromosomal aberrations

Trisomy 21, Trisomy 13, Cri du chat syndromes

Malformations due to microdeletions

Angelman's and Prader-Willi syndromes, William's syndrome, Rubinstein-Taybi syndrome

Monogenic mutations

Tuberous sclerosis, metabolic disorders, Fragile X syndrome

Multifactorial intellectual disability

Familial intellectual disability

Malformations: Cause unknown

Malformations of the CNS

Holoprosencephaly, lissencephaly, neural tube defects

Multiple malformation syndromes

De Lange's syndrome, Sotos' syndrome

Prenatal: Disorders due to External Causes

Maternal infections

Rubella and HIV, cytomegalovirus and Toxoplasmosis

Toxins

Fetal alcohol syndrome, fetal hydantoin syndrome

Toxaemia, placental insufficiency

Intrauterine growth retardation, prematurity

Other

Radiation, trauma

Perinatal causes

Infections

Meningitis, herpes

Delivery problems Asphyxia, trauma

Other causes

Hypoglycaemia, hyperbilirubinaemia

Post-Natal Causes

Infections

Meningitis, encephalitis

Toxins

Lead poisoning

Other CNS disorders

Cerebrovascular accidents, tumours, traumas

Some Specific Disorders

Down Syndrome

Down syndrome is one of the common examples of a genetic condition that is not inherited. Nearly all cases result from an extra full or partial chromosome. It is a frequent cause of moderate to severe intellectual disability, and only a minority of children with Down syndrome have an IQ above 50. It occurs in 1 in every 600–1000 newborns, but because of increased detection of this condition by amniocentesis (and subsequent termination of pregnancy), the incidence has decreased. Although the increasing age of the mother increases the risk of having a baby with Down syndrome, 80% of babies with Down syndrome are born to mothers under 35 years of age (23).

There are three types of chromosomal aberrations. Patients with trisomy 21 (three chromosome 21, instead of the usual two) represent the overwhelming majority (about 94% of total cases). They have 47 chromosomes, with an extra chromosome 21. Secondly, non- disjunction occurring after fertilisation in any cell division results in mosaicism, a condition in which both normal and trisomic cells are found in various tissues. In some cases, translocation occurs. This is a fusion of two chromosomes, usually 21 and 15, resulting in a total of 46 chromosomes, despite the presence of an extra chromosome 21.

Physical characteristics of Down syndrome include, slanted eyes, epicanthal folds, flat nose, small mouth with furrowed tongue, flattened occiput, stubby hands, fingers and single transverse palmar crease. Associated medical conditions are cardiac anomalies (especially septal defects), gastrointestinal abnormalities, and impaired hearing. Children with Down syndrome are placid, cheerful, and cooperative and adapt easily at home, but when they reach adolescence, the picture changes, as they experience various emotional difficulties, behaviour disorders, and (rarely) psychotic disorders. Language function is relatively weak, but children usually retain as interpersonal cooperation and conformity with social conventions. There is association between Down syndrome and Alzheimer's type dementia, and about 40% of patients over the age of 40 years develop dementia (24). Many patients do not live beyond the age of 40, although life expectancy is now increasing.

Fragile X Syndrome

Fragile X syndrome is the most common cause of inherited intellectual disability, affecting 1 in 4000 males (25). It is believed to occur in about 1 of every 1,000 males and 1 of every 2,000 females (26). The intellectual disability ranges from mild to severe. However, not all affected people exhibit low intelligence (27).

The syndrome results from a mutation on the X chromosome at what is known as the fragile site (Xq27.3). The typical phenotype includes an elongated face, prominent ears, high arched palate, short stature, flat feet, hyperextensible joints, and post-pubertal macroorchidism. Facial features are less marked in females and children. About 20% children do not have many physical signs except conspicuous ears. 20% of affected males also have epilepsy (28). There is a high rate of ADHD, and pervasive developmental disorders, such as autism. Female carriers are often less impaired than males. A link, although not very strong, has been proposed with autism.

Prader-Willi Syndrome

Prader-Willi syndrome is thought to result from a small deletion involving chromosome 15, usually occurring randomly. The estimated prevalence is 1 in 10,000–25,000.

Persons with the syndrome exhibit intellectual disability, hyperphagia, strabismus, obesity, hypogonadism, small stature, hypotonia, and small hands and feet. In addition, temper tantrums, impulsivity, mood fluctuations, stubbornness, aggression, skin picking, repetitive speech, as well as obsessive and ritualistic behaviours have been reported (29). Children with this syndrome often have oppositional and defiant behaviour.

Cat's Cry (Cri-du-chat) Syndrome

This syndrome involves loss of the whole or part of the long arm of chromosome 5. Children have severe intellectual disability, and many have microcephaly, low-set ears, oblique palpebral fissures, hypertelorism, and micrognathia. The characteristic cat-like cry (caused by laryngeal abnormalities) gradually changes and disappears with increasing age (30).

Phenylketonuria (PKU)

PKU is the commonest inborn error of metabolism. In this autosomal recessive disorder, there is an absence or inactivity of the liver enzyme phenylalanine hydroxylase. Because of this, phenylalanine (an essential amino acid) is not converted to paratyrosine. It occurs in about 1 of every 10,000 to 15,000 live births. Most patients have severe intellectual disability, but some may have borderline or even normal intelligence. Children with PKU are hyperactive, exhibit erratic and unpredictable behaviour, and have serious communication problems. They also have an association with epilepsy, have temper tantrums and often display bizarre movements of their bodies and upper extremities.

Guthrie test is widely used to make early detection, as a subsequent low-phenylalanine diet can have significant prognostic implications. However, omission of phenylalanine from the diet, can cause anaemia, hypoglycaemia, oedema, and even death.

Children who receive a diagnosis before the age of three months and are placed on an optimal dietary regimen may have normal intelligence (31), but a similar dietary regimen does not have a positive impact on the intelligence level of older children and adolescents.

Other Disorders

It is beyond the scope of this book to discuss all the disorders.

Some other important disorders are: Tuberous sclerosis, Angelman syndrome, Sturge-Weber syndrome, Rett's disorder, Neurofibromatosis, Lesch-Nyhan syndrome, Adrenoleukodystrophy and Maple Syrup urine disease.

Psychiatric Disorders

Schizophrenia

When IQ is less than 45, it is difficult to diagnose schizophrenia with certainty. One author has stated that diagnosis of schizophrenia is not possible with an IQ of less than 40 (32). The lifetime risk is 3% in those with intellectual disability, in contrast to 1% in the general population (33).

People with an intellectual disability exhibit less psychopathology, especially persecutory delusions and formal thought disorder (34). Similarly, thought echo, delusional perception, passivity phenomenon and thought withdrawal is also less common. However, this apparent finding may be due to the difficulty the patient has in describing these experiences (35).

Although about 90% of patients have auditory hallucinations, they can occur in all modalities. The content of hallucinations may be simple. In severe intellectual disability patients, paranoid symptoms and catatonia are conspicuous. Atypical symptoms reported include disturbed and aggressive behaviour, bizarre rituals and hysterical behaviour (36). In addition, there may be sleep disturbance and fearfulness.

Treatment of schizophrenia remains the same as in those patients

Without intellectual disability. However, the withdrawal of medication from people with an intellectual disability needs to be done slowly (37). Apart from other atypical antipsychotics, clozapine has also been tried in this population, although there may be practical difficulties to follow the mandatory guideline (e.g., blood monitoring).

Mood Disorder

In contrast to schizophrenia, the rate of depressive disorder in people with an intellectual disability is similar to that in the general population (38). The rate of suicide is much less in those suffering from moderate to severe intellectual disability. Impaired social functioning and intelligence influence the clinical presentation, and the depressive disorder usually presents with a deterioration in social skills (39). People with a mild intellectual disability almost show the same symptoms as the general population, but tearfulness may be more conspicuous. Those with severe intellectual disability present with more somatic symptoms and their behavioural correlates (e.g., sleep and appetite changes and social withdrawal). SSRIs are the preferred antidepressants, as tricyclics are more notorious at lowering the epilepsy threshold.

Bipolar affective disorder is comparatively easier to diagnose than schizophrenia (40). During the manic phase, irritability, aggression, overactivity and reduced sleep can be conspicuous. Lithium, carbamazepine, and valproic acid, have all been successfully used. The side effects, however, need to be monitored more carefully in people with intellectual disabilities.

Other Psychiatric Disorders

Various other psychiatric disorders including generalised anxiety disorder, obsessive-compulsive disorder, phobic disorders, and personality disorders, also occur in people with intellectual disability. Small doses of SSRIs and benzodiazepines (like temazepam) are commonly used.

Intellectual Disability and Epilepsy

Epilepsy commonly occurs in the population with intellectual disability, and the prevalence rate increases with the severity of brain damage and the degree of intellectual disability (41). Anti-epileptic medications have proven to be effective in many cases.

Assessment and Management

It is important to bear in mind that intellectual disability patients have complex, multiple and changing needs (42). A multidisciplinary approach is therefore not only appropriate but essential. The key aims should be to help them to integrate into the general community (e.g., use of normal community services and facilities) as much that is possible, to treat co morbid medical or psychiatric problems, enhance the skills and strengths, to assist in building up their relationships, and provide appropriate occupation and accommodation.

One goal is also to discover the specific cause, as it enables genetic counselling for the family, and may indicate specific treatment for the child e.g., special diets for certain enzyme defects. Even if no specific cause is found, a detailed psychological, medical, and social assessment would be pivotal in making decisions for the management.

Severe cases of intellectual disability are usually obvious from a very early age, because of the apparent developmental delays and physical abnormalities present. Mild cases may remain undetected until learning difficulties become apparent, especially at school. Presence of any communication problem or sensory impairment should be looked into, and it is important to consider deafness and emotional disturbance as the possibilities.

A very comprehensive physical and psychological assessment needs to be carried out in all cases of intellectual disability. Assessment should include a very detailed medical history (with particular attention to the mother's pregnancy, labour, and delivery problems), family history (including a family history of intellectual disability and psychiatric issues), a physical and neurological examination and mental state examination. Chromosome studies and testing of blood and urine for abnormal metabolites is very important. The patient's verbal abilities should be kept in mind, and leading questions should be avoided because there is high chance that suggestibility will influence the child's answers. When interviewing the patient, the interviewer's attitude and manner of communication has a significant bearing on the amount and quality of information obtained. Although there should be directiveness and structure to the interviewer's questions, communication with intellectual disabilities children should be on the appropriate level. It is a good idea to explore and ascertain the patient's understanding of his or her own limitations as well as strengths.

A mental state examination has to be preferably done in a simple, flexible and informal manner, taking into account the level of understanding and communication difficulties of each person. The information obtained from the patients and the relatives can be supplemented by the help of various formal tests. Some commonly used rating scales are: The Adaptive Behaviour Schedule (43), The Aberrant Behaviour Checklist (44) and Behaviour Disturbance Scale (45), Diagnostic Assessment for the Severely Handicapped (46), Psychopathology Instrument for Mentally Retarded Adults (47) and The Psychiatric Assessment Development Schedule for Adults with Disabilities (48).

Drug Treatment

Antipsychotics, mood stabilising medication, antidepressants and anxiolytics are widely used in intellectual disability patients. However, as these patients tend to be very sensitive to the effect of medication, small doses should be initiated and increased cautiously and gradually, if needed.

Role of Psychologists and Psychotherapies

Psychologists have an important role in assessing their patient's intelligence, deficits or skills. They help to plan individual behavioural treatment. Although there is a role of psychotherapies in the management of intellectual disability patients, it is limited because of problems with comprehension and language. Behaviour therapy is used to shape and enhance social behaviours and to minimise aggressive and destructive behaviours. Cognitive therapy is helpful in minimising erroneous beliefs. Relaxation exercises are also useful. Desirable behaviour or the acquisition of skills is given positive reinforcement and similarly, unwanted behaviour is discouraged.

Family and Social Interventions

Social and educational support are important aspects of management. Family education can enhance realistic expectations of parents, and can, in addition, give the parents the basic information regarding causes and treatment plans. As people with intellectual disability commonly feel socially isolated, improving the quantity and quality of social competence should be an essential part of their care. Children with mild intellectual disabilities should be educated in ordinary schools whenever possible. Sheltered accommodation, community homes, and hostels provided by the local authority are frequently used, but those with 'challenging behaviour' or acute psychiatric disorders would probably require hospital admission.

REFERENCES

1. Ludwik, S., Szymanski, L. S. and Wilska, M. (2006). Childhood disorders: Mental retardation. In J. Kay and A. Tasman (Eds.), *Essentials of psychiatry* (pp. 289–297). Chichester: John Wiley and Sons Ltd.
2. World Health Organisation. (1992). *ICD-10 Classification of mental and behavioural disorders–* clinical description and diagnostic guidelines. Geneva: WHO.
3. World Health Organisation. (1992). *ICD-10 Classification of mental and behavioural disorders–* clinical description and diagnostic guidelines. Geneva: WHO.
4. World Health Organisation. (1992). *ICD-10 Classification of mental and behavioural disorders–* clinical description and diagnostic guidelines. Geneva: WHO.
5. Lewis, E. O. (1929). *Report on an investigation into the incidence of mental deficiency in six areas*. London: HMSO.
6. Gelder, M., Harrison, P. and Cowen, P. (2006).The misuse of alcohol and drugs. In P. Cowen,P. Harrison and T. Burns (Eds.), *Shorter Oxford textbook of psychiatry* (pp. 429–469). Oxford: Oxford University Press.
7. McLaren, J. and Bryson, S. E. (1987). Review of recent epidemiological studies of mental retardation: prevalence, associated disorders, and aetiology. *American Journal of Mental Retardation*, 92, 243–254.
8. Fraser, W. I. (1997). The psychiatry of intellectual disability. In R. Murray, P. Hill and P. Mcguffin (Eds.), *The essentials of postgraduate psychiatry*, (3rd Edition, pp. 425–429). Cambridge: Cambridge University Press.
9. Scott, S. (1994). Mental retardation. In M. Rutter, E Taylor and L. Hersov (Eds.), *Child and adolescent psychiatry:* Modern approaches (pp. 616– 646). Oxford: Blackwell Scientific Publications.
10. Deb, S., Thomas, M. and Bright, C. (2001). Mental disorder in adults with intellectual disability; 2. The rate of behaviour disorder among a community based population aged between 16–64 years. *Journal of Intellectual Disability Research*, 45, 495–505.
11. World Health Organisation. (1992). *ICD-10 Classification of mental and behavioural disorders–* clinical description and diagnostic guidelines. Geneva: WHO.
12. American Psychiatric Association.(2013). *Diagnostic and statistical manual of mental disorders* (5th Edition). Arlington, VA: American Psychiatric Publishing
13. Koller, H., Richardsons, S. A., Katz, M. and Mclaren, J. (1983). Behavioural disturbance since childhood among a 5-year birth cohort of all mentally retarded young adults in a city. American *Journal of Mental Deficiency*, 87, 386–389.
14. Gelder, M., Harrison, P. and Cowen, P. (2006). The misuse of alcohol and drugs. In P. Cowen,P. Harrison and T. Burns (Eds.), *Shorter Oxford textbook of psychiatry* (pp. 429–469). Oxford: Oxford University Press.
15. World Health Organisation. (1992). *ICD-10 Classification of mental and behavioural disorders* clinical description and diagnostic guidelines. Geneva: WHO.
16. Emerson, E., Barret, S., Bell, C., et al. (1987). *Developing services for people with severe learning difficulties and challenging behaviours*. University of Kent: Institute of Social and Applied Psychology.
17. Deb, S., Thomas, M. and Bright, C. (2001). Mental disorder in adults with intellectual disability; 2. The rate of behaviour disorder among a community based population aged between 16–64 years. *Journal of Intellectual Disability Research*, 45, 495–505.
18. Baumeister, A. A. (1989). Causes of severe maladaptive behaviour in persons with severe mental retardation: *A review of hypothesis*. Bethesda, USA: National Institute of Health.
19. Ludwik, S., Szymanski, L. S. and Wilska, M. (2006). Childhood disorders: mental retardation. In J. Kay and A. Tasman (Eds.), *Essentials of psychiatry* (pp. 289–297). Chichester: John Wiley and Sons Ltd.
20. Penrose, L. (1938). *A clinical and genetic study of 1280 cases of mental deficiency*., London: HMSO.
21. Broman, S., Nichols, P. L., Shaughnessy, P., et al. (1987). *Retardation in young children*: A development study of cognitive deficit. Hillsdale: Lawrence Erlbaum.
22. Gelder, M., Harrison, P. and Cowen, P. (2006). The misuse of alcohol and drugs. In P. Cowen, P. Harrison and T. Burns (Eds.), *Shorter Oxford textbook of psychiatry* (pp. 429–469). Oxford: Oxford University Press.
23. Muir, W. J. and McKechanie, A. G. (2010). Intellectual disability. In E. C. Johnstone, D. C. Owens, S. Lawrie, A. A. M. Mcintosh and M. Sharpe (Eds.), *Companion to psychiatric studies* (8th Edition, pp. 541–594). Edinburgh: Churchill Livingstone.
24. Muir, W. J. and McKechanie, A. G. (2010). Intellectual disability. In E. C. Johnstone, D. C. Owens, S. Lawrie, A. A. M. Mcintosh and M. Sharpe (Eds.), *Companion to psychiatric studies* (8th Edition, pp. 541–594). Edinburgh: Churchill Livingstone.
25. Pembrey, M. E., Barnicoat, A. J., Carmichael, B., Bobrow, M., and Turner, G. (2001). An assessment of screening strategies for Fragile X syndrome in the UK. *Health Technology Assessment*, 5, 1–95.
26. Ludwik, S., Szymanski, L. S. and Wilska, M. (2006). Childhood disorders: mental retardation. In J. Kay and A. Tasman (Eds.), *Essentials of psychiatry* (pp. 289–297). Chichester: John Wiley and Sons Ltd.
27. Fryers, T. and Russell, O. (2003). Applied epidemiology. In W. Fraser and M. Kerr (Eds.), *Seminars in the psychiatry of intellectual disability* (2nd Edition, pp. 16–48). London: Royal College of Psychiatrists.
28. Fryers, T. and Russell, O. (2003). Applied epidemiology. In W. Fraser and M. Kerr (Eds.), *Seminars in the psychiatry of intellectual disability* (2nd Edition, pp. 16–48). London: Royal College of Psychiatrists.
29. Milner, K. M., Craig, E. E., Thompson, R. J., Veltman, M. W., Thomas, N. S., Roberts, S., et al. (2005). Prader–Willi syndrome: Intellectual abilities and behavioural features by genetic subtype. *Journal of Child Psychology and Psychiatry*, 46, 1089–1096.
30. Sadock, B. J. and Sadock, V. A. (2007). *Kaplan and Sadock's Synopsis of psychiatry*: Behavioural sciences/ clinical psychiatry (10th Edition). Philadelphia: Lippincott Williams and Wilkins.
31. Sadock, B. J. and Sadock, V. A. (2007). *Kaplan and Sadock's Synopsis of psychiatry*: Behavioural sciences/ clinical psychiatry (10th Edition). Philadelphia: Lippincott Williams and Wilkins.
32. Reid, A. H. (1983). Psychiatry of mental handicap: a review. *Journal of the Royal Society of Medicine*, 76, 587–589.
33. Turner, T. H. (1989). Schizophrenia and mental handicap: an historical review, with implications for further research. *Psychological Medicine*, 19, 301–314.
34. Meadows, G., Turner, T., Campbell, L., et al. (1991). Assessing schizophrenia in adults with mental retardation: a comparative study. *British Journal of Psychiatry*, 158, 103–105.

35. Muir, W. J. and McKechanie, A. G. (2010). Intellectual disability. In E. C. Johnstone, D. C. Owens, S. Lawrie, A. A. M. Mcintosh and M. Sharpe (Eds.), *Companion to psychiatric studies* (8th Edition, pp. 541–594). Edinburgh: Churchill Livingstone.
36. Turner, T. H. (1989). Schizophrenia and mental handicap: an historical review, with implications for further research. *Psychological Medicine*, 19, 301–314.
37. Muir, W. J. and McKechanie, A. G. (2010). Intellectual disability. In E. C. Johnstone, D. C. Owens, S. Lawrie, A. A. M. Mcintosh and M. Sharpe (Eds.), *Companion to psychiatric studies* (8th Edition, pp. 541–594). Edinburgh: Churchill Livingstone.
38. Deb, S., Thomas, M. and Bright, C. (2001). Mental disorder in adults with intellectual disability; 2. The rate of behaviour disorder among a community based population aged between 16–64 years. *Journal of Intellectual Disability Research*, 45, 495–505.
39. Sovner, R. and Hurley, A. D. (1983). Do the mentally retarded suffer from affective illness? *Archives of General Psychiatry*, 40, 262–266.
40. Fraser, W. I. (1997). The Psychiatry of Intellectual disability. In R. Murray, P. Hill and P. Mcguffin (Eds.), *The essentials of postgraduate psychiatry* (3rd Edition, pp. 429–425). Cambridge: Cambridge University Press.
41. Corbett, J. A., Harris, R. and Robinson, R. G. (1975). *Epidemiological issues in mental retardation and developmental disabilities*, Vol VII. New York: Brunner Mazel.
42. Holland, A. (2008). The psychiatry of intellectual disability. In R. M. Murray, K. S. Kendler, P. Mcguffin, S. Wessley and D. G. Castle (Eds.), *Essential psychiatry* (4th Edition, pp. 283–294). Cambridge: Cambridge University press.
43. Nihira, K., Foster, R., Shelhaas, M. and Lelland, H. (1974). *AAMD Adaptive behaviour scale.* Washington DC: American Association on Mental Deficiency.
44. Aman, M. G., Sing, N. N., Stewart, A. W. and Field, C. J. (1985). The Aberrant Behaviour Checklist: A behaviour rating scale for the assessment of treatment effects. *American Journal of Mental Deficiency*, 89, 485–491.
45. Leudar, I., Fraser, W. and Jeeves, M. A. (1987). Theoretical problems and practical solutions to behaviour disorders in retarded people. *Health Bulletin*, 45, 347–355.
46. Matson, J. L., Gardner, W. I., Coe, D. A. and Sovner, R. (1991). A scale for evaluating emotional disorders in severely and profoundly mentally retarded persons. *British Journal of Psychiatry*, 159, 404–409.
47. Senatore, V., Matson, J. L. and Kazdin, A. E. (1985). An inventory to assess psychopathology of mentally retarded adults. *American Journal of Mental Defiency*, 89, 459–466.
48. Moss, S. C., Goldberg, D., Simpson, N., et al. (1993). *The psychiatric assessment schedule for adults with developmental disorders.* University of Manchester: The Hester Adrian Centre.

Forensic Psychiatry

CHAPTER 14

Psychiatry is a branch of medicine that incorporates biological, psychological, and social information and constructs for assessing and treating patients. Forensic psychiatry is different. Forensic psychiatrists are trained not only to treat psychiatric patients but in many cases are required to evaluate an individual's mental state and history in relation to the legal system. On the other hand people involved with the legal system generally do not wish to consult a psychiatrist for help with their psychiatric problems. In some cases, the expertise of forensic psychiatrists is sought to ascertain the potential risk that an individual might be posing to others.

Forensic psychiatry is, therefore, related to issues that are relevant to psychiatry and the law. It can be more formally defined as that part of psychiatry that deals with patients and problems at the interface of the legal and psychiatric systems, and its expertise requires specific skills in addition to the skills of general psychiatry and knowledge of other specialist areas of psychiatry (1). Although forensic psychiatrists are routinely involved in the assessment and treatment of mentally abnormal offenders and prepare psychiatric reports for the courts, in some cases, general psychiatrists are also required to perform these duties.

Regarding epidemiology of crimes, men seem to predominate, with one study demonstrating that 80% of crimes are committed by men in all cultures (2). As people from ethnic minorities are more likely to be poor and unemployed and have unstable accommodation, they are at higher risk of committing crimes. This is probably why they may be over-represented in the forensic patients group (3). Crime is predominantly committed by young people (males between 18–20 years). Generally, crime decreases with age, except for a small peak for women aged 40–50 years, around the time of their menopause (4). One author has highlighted the factors that influence and contribute to offending behaviour (5). These include genetic causes, particular type of personality, impulsivity traits, intelligence, family and peer influences, lower socioeconomic status, and ethnicity. Although the genetic influence has been confirmed, it has a modest effect. There is interaction of individual (e.g., impulsivity, large family size) with the social factor (deprivation because of lower socioeconomic class), to increase the risk of offending.

One study showed that alcohol and substance abuse, as well as antisocial personality disorder, are significantly associated with crime (6). As compared to general population, more psychiatric disorders are present in the prison population (7). However, this does not necessarily imply that their mental disorder was responsible for the crime. The majority of patients with psychoses are no more dangerous than general population, and only a small number of people with psychotic illnesses commit violent offences. There is no evidence that more homicide is committed by psychiatric patients (8). A very robust review found that anti social personality disorder had highest prevalence in prisons, followed by depressive disorder and psychosis in descending order (9). The same study demonstrated that about one in seven prisoners have a treatable psychiatric illness. Women in prisons have higher rates of neurotic illnesses, substance abuse and self-harm than men (10). The rates of suicides in prisons in males is higher as compared to general population (11), and is much more higher in female prisoners.

Psychiatric Disorders and Crime

Schizophrenia

Paranoid schizophrenia can sometimes lead to serious violence. Morbid jealousy on its own, or as a part of schizophrenia carries a very high risk of violence towards sexual partner. The association between delusions, hallucinations and violence, has been much debated, but the symptoms are more likely to result in violence when they cause a feeling of personal threat or when there is an intrusion of thoughts that can override self-control. High scores on the threat-control override scale are predictors of violence even when other psychotic symptoms remain constant (12).

Alcohol and Substance Abuse

Alcohol and substance use significantly increases the risk of violence and crime (13). Alcohol abuse has been implicated in various crimes, including domestic violence, child abuse, and rape. Risk of offending increases three to four times in drug users than non-drug users, being highest in crack users and lowest among marijuana users (14).

Affective Disorders and Neurosis

The role of depressive disorders in offending behaviour is controversial and probably rare (15). In one study those hospitalised with affective disorders were not at increased risk for violent crime after account was taken of substance misuse and personality disorder (16). The role of depressive disorders in offending behaviour is rare. Depressive disorder is more generally associated with the risk of suicide, rather than violence. Shoplifting has been associated with depression, particularly in middle-aged females.

Both mania and hypomania may lead to disinhibited behaviour, which may result in convictions for breach of the peace, road-traffic offences, and sexual offence. Neurotic symptoms are common in offenders. Post-traumatic stress disorder has been more often implicated.

Personality Disorders

Surveys of offender populations invariably report high rates of personality disorders. People with personality disorder who offend have frequently abused alcohol or drugs, and often have anxiety and stress-related disorders as well. Studies of sex offenders have shown high rates of personality disorders (17).

Intellectual Disabilities

Below average intelligence is a predictor of offending (18), and people with intellectual disabilities are three to four times over-represented among offenders. Individuals with mild intellectual disability show a higher rate of offending compared with peers without intellectual disability and peers with a more severe intellectual disability, who rarely commit serious offences (19). One study has shown an association between intellectual disability and arson (20).

Organic Conditions

The onset of minor offending such as shoplifting, minor sex offences and fraud at a late age may be due to dementia (e.g., Alzheimer's disease) owing to its reduction of intellectual functioning, judgement and normal inhibitions in social behaviour. Brain damage from head injury, even in the absence of significant cognitive impairment, may result in significant changes in personality, resulting in excessive aggression. In one study, organic brain disease was one of the major mental illnesses having a risk of violence (21).

Epilepsy

Contrary to what is commonly believed, there is no evidence of an association between epilepsy and crime. Epilepsy is a rare contributory factor to offending and one large meta analysis showed that the incidence of epilepsy was the same in prisons, as in the general population (22).

Risk Assessment and Management of Violence

Assessment of risk for violence of certain individuals is required by the legal system. It is also done, if indicated, in clinical psychiatric practice. Assessment is done of the risk that those individuals will cause certain types of harm under particular conditions within particular periods of time. Historically, this assessment is referred to as an assessment of dangerousness. However, since there is no agreed definition of dangerousness, this term will not be used.

The aim of assessment is to determine the presence of risk of violence and any protective factors, and to formulate an understanding of an individual case, so as to make a risk management plan. Assessment of risk of harm to others essentially entails assessing the nature, likelihood, frequency, duration, extent, and imminence of the violent act. Assessment involves gathering information from various sources including interviews, documents and rating scales. It is extremely important to ascertain that the collated information is comprehensive and reliable so that a reasonable decision can be made regarding the risk.

It is important to bear in mind that risk assessment cannot be hundred percent accurate, the risk can change over time and that the risk of violence can be minimised but not entirely eliminated. The purpose of risk assessment is to look for factors so that the risk can be reduced and appropriately managed. The prediction of violence is quite challenging and difficult. It is well-established that short-term predictions are more reliable and the clinicians are not only less capable of making long-term accurate judgements, but also over predict violence (23). Moreover, it is extremely difficult, if not impossible to make any predictions about those persons who do not have a history of violence. There are some patients who do not exhibit violence until the development of a mental illness. Even though it seems that the mental illness made these patients more violent than they otherwise would have been, the percentage of mentally unwell people who exhibit violence is not known (24).

There are three approaches to assess the risk of violence: actuarial, clinical and structured. The actuarial approach refers to any mathematical means of combining information in order to predict risk (25). It involves the collection of demographic data, history and current presentation, and subsequent weighting this information to calculate a figure that gives a predictive value to the likelihood of violence. Some researchers have strongly advocated to incorporate statistical concepts into clinical decision making (26), as they believe that this will increase the predictive power of the clinical assessment.

The second approach is the clinical approach, where the gathered information about risk factors is interpreted through the clinical experience of the clinician (27). The third way, called the structured professional judgement, attempts to combine and integrate the features of actuarial and clinical approaches, and there is evidence that this method of risk assessment is both reliable and valid (28).

There are numerous rating scales available for risk assessment. Some of them are: Violence Risk Appraisal Guide (VRAG) (29), Historical Clinical Risk-20 (HCR-20) (30), Violence Risk Scale (VRS) (31) and Sexual Offender Risk Appraisal Guide (SORAG) (32). Clinicians have to do a risk assessment of violence in the near future, especially when considering admission subsequent to an incident, or when parole is being considered. With these cases, current mental state and recent behaviour (e.g., threats, hostility, and social stressors) is more important, even though the relevance of past violence cannot be underestimated. In other cases, clinicians will be required to estimate the risk of long-term violence. Here, actuarial factors (past offences) will be comparatively more significant. In doing a risk assessment, all efforts should be made to get an extensive history and to include appraisal of all medical and social notes. The individual characteristics and environmental or situational factors must be taken into account when making predictions (33).

According to one model of violence, there is interaction between developmental factors, chronic and situational stress, and factors that might disinhibit the individual's control and behavioural regulation (34). History of a chaotic childhood, and physical or sexual abuse predisposes to future violent behaviour. A single, young male from a lower socioeconomic status has a higher risk. Having antisocial, explosive or impulsive personality traits, lack of coping skills, and an association with sub-culture prone to violence increases the risk of violent behaviour.

Ongoing stresses causing frustration is likely to contribute to violence. Some of the disinhibitory factors are drugs or alcohol abuse, intellectual disabilities, organic brain syndromes and severe mental illnesses. The significance of a clear understanding of precipitating factors that led to previous incidents, a detailed history, a meticulous interview and a thorough mental state examination, cannot be overstated.

As violent sexual offenders have a history of fantasies of violence, it is important to inquire in a subtle way, about sadistic fantasies. The following points would be helpful:

- Does he overreact to situations which threaten his self-esteem?
- Does he find violence pleasurable?
- How is the attitude towards treatment of mental illness?
- Are depressive or psychotic symptoms well-controlled?
- How does he feel about the violent incident? (Lack of guilt or remorse and an indifferent attitude should significantly heighten the concern).

When discussing the index offence, the patient should be encouraged to recount the details of how it happened, and what he was thinking, feeling and perceiving at the time. Authors have stressed the high importance of the triad of patient, circumstances and victim in the analysis of offending behaviour (35).

Regarding the management of violence, various strategies are recommended. These include admission, use of mental health legislation, medication and psychotherapy. Treatment of mental illness has to be ensured. Anticonvulsants, especially carbamazepine, have been used to control episodic behaviour disorders, and there is substantial evidence for effectiveness (36). Lithium has also been shown to reduce aggression (37). Beta blockers such as, Propranolol, have also been used. Psychotherapy and cognitive-behavioural techniques can be helpful, provided patients are not acutely unwell.

Offences

Homicide

Homicide is a general term given to all unlawful killings. Homicide is said to be murder when the offender is of sound mind and discretion (over the age of 10 years), and had malice aforethought (i.e. the intent to cause death or grievous bodily harm) (38). Manslaughter implies homicide without malice aforethought. Voluntary manslaughter includes provocation, the doctrine of diminished responsibility, and killing in the pursuance of a suicide pact. Involuntary manslaughter means that the killing was not intended and includes constructive manslaughter where the intention is to commit an unlawful or dangerous act, gross negligence, where there is disregard for the lives and safety of others, and an unlawful omission (39).

In all countries, young men are both the principal perpetrators and victims of homicide. The rates of homicide vary from country to country. In a national study conducted in the UK among all known homicides, it was found that 14% had symptoms of mental illness at the time of the homicide and the most common diagnosis was personality disorder (22%) (40). The same study found that in mentally abnormal offenders the victims were more often family members than strangers, when compared with victims of mentally normal perpetrators.

Infanticide

Under the UK's Infanticide Acts, infanticide is defined as having occurred when a woman by any wilful act caused the death of her child under the age of 12 months, but at the time of the act or omission the balance of her mind was 'disturbed by reason of her not being fully recovered from the effect of giving birth to the child or the effect of lactation consequent upon the birth of the child'. The jury can return verdict of not guilty of murder but guilty of infanticide. It may be charged at the onset, or serve as a defence to murder. In practice, defendants are sentenced leniently (41). A conviction for infanticide usually results in a sentence of a community rehabilitation (probation) order, often with a condition of psychiatric treatment (out- or in-patient).

Rape

Rape is more frequent than reported to police, and furthermore, only one-third of reported cases are proceeded by police. Rape is sexual intercourse (whether vaginal or anal) with a person who does not consent. Victims are predominantly women. Although most jurisdictions define rape in terms of lack of consent, not all jurisdictions recognise male rape, and additionally, some countries like USA define lack of consent by age (42). Post-traumatic stress disorder or sexual dysfunction may subsequently develop. When requested, the offender should be assessed in a standard way. Although mental illness is not common, personality disorders, substance misuse, and intellectual disability are usually present. Anti libidinal drugs may be used in the management of rapists, but if these drugs are to be considered, they would only be as part of an overall package of offender management (43).

Child Sexual Abuse

This is discussed in more detail in chapter 'Child and Adolescent Psychiatry'. In the UK, it is illegal to have any heterosexual activity with a person aged under 16, or homosexual activity with people aged under 18 years (44). Paedophiles (defined as those having a primary sexual interest in prepubertal children) rarely have mental illness. They may be heterosexual or homosexual, and are predominantly men.

Indecent Exposure (Exhibitionism)

Exhibitionism is the legal term for indecent exposure. It is the most common sexual offence. This is a behaviour in which the genitals are exposed inappropriately with the intention of provoking some reaction by the witness. The perpetrator gets pleasure by causing interest, admiration, disgust or fear. However, the purpose is not to progress to assault or sexual intercourse. Sexual excitement occurs in anticipation of the exposure, and orgasm occurs during or after the event. It is most common in men aged between 25 and 35 years. There is rarely a history of psychiatric disorder or other criminal behaviour. These men, however, may have substance abuse or other types of compulsive behaviour (45). The definition comprises a pattern of repetitive behaviour which does not necessarily serve erotic gratification, and is sometimes experienced as an irresistible urge (46). Although not common, females and homosexual men also indulge in indecent behaviour. Females uncover breasts or buttocks in a seductive manner and homosexual men expose genitals towards men.

Stalking

This is repeated, unwanted, and intrusive targeting of a particular victim with following and other harassment (47). There is an intense preoccupation with the victim, the perpetrator follows the victim, communicates through various means (telephone, postal or electronic mail), and/or indulges in threats. Stalking is predominantly a male activity against females.

Incest

Incest is broadly defined as sexual relations between family members forbidden by taboos, social customs and values, and the law. In a nuclear family, sexual relations between parents and child, grandchild and grandparent, and siblings are forbidden. In the extended family, similar restriction is between uncle and niece.

The most common form of incest is between daughter and father. Fathers are usually in late 30s or early 40s, when they begin to have psychological problems. They are usually of normal intelligence with no history of criminal offences or major psychiatric illnesses (48). The daughters are approaching puberty and are attractive to them. Unlike the common belief most fathers are not alcoholics. Incestuous behaviour involves other forms of sexual activities such as touching, fondling, mutual masturbation and oral-genital contact. But the legal definition of incest requires that sexual intercourse has taken place. According to another study (49), father usually initiates incestuous behaviour before the daughter is sexually mature (between 8 and 12 years). The progress to actual sexual intercourse can be gradual. In many cases, however, the incestuous behaviour continues without leading to incest. It is important to realise that incest is not rape.

Bestiality

Bestiality consists of using animals as sexual objects. It is rarely a preferred sexual activity and is usually an opportunistic act. It may occur both in men as well as women, and happens more commonly in rural areas. The Sexual Offences Act of UK states: 'it is felony for a person to commit buggery with another person or with any animal'. The maximum penalty is life imprisonment.

Offences Against Property

Arson

Fire setting is a very serious crime as it might result in a loss of lives, apart from the damage to the property. The maximum penalty of life imprisonment can be imposed. It may be committed by criminals, psychiatric patients, personality disorder patients, psychotic patients, those with intellectual disability and children and adolescents with conduct disorder (50). Another study also found that substance abuse was a common diagnosis apart from personality disorders and psychoses (51).

Psychiatric morbidity among those diagnosed with intellectual disability does not differ between men and women (52). One study (53) has attempted to conduct an analysis for the motives for arson. Motives include: financial reward (insurance claims), covering up another crime like murder, political purposes, revenge and sexual satisfaction. Arson can result because of mental illnesses like schizophrenia, mania and severe depression.

Shoplifting

This is predominantly a crime committed by women, although slightly more men than women are convicted of this crime. Regarding social class, professional and managerial groups are over-represented among shoplifters, as compared to the general population. A substantial number of female shoplifters include those who are living comfortably and even have money with them at the time of offence (54).

Although most shoplifters are not mentally unwell, people who do shoplifting may suffer from antisocial personality disorder, depressive illness, mania, schizophrenia, dementia, or intellectual disability. Substance abuse patients may steal from shops in order to fund their habit. Shoplifting may also be due to absent-mindedness, due to medical conditions such as epilepsy or hypoglycaemia, or drugs such as benzodiazepines.

Kleptomania is a rare condition. It refers to repeated failure to control an impulse to steal objects that are not required and which are later discarded. One study found additional diagnoses of anxiety disorders and eating disorders (55).

MENTAL DISORDERS AND COURT PROCEEDINGS

Psychiatric Defences

Fitness to Plead

Fitness to plead refers to an individual's mental state at the time of the trial and can change. Sometimes a mentally disordered defendant may not be able to defend him or herself, and is said to be unfit to plead. In order to make this plea successful, the defendant would have to prove that he or she is not able to understand the charges, instruct counsel, appreciate the significance of pleading, challenge a juror, examine a witness, and understand and follow court proceedings. Among these, the most important legal criteria is the ability to instruct the counsel and to understand and follow the court proceedings (56). This plea is likely to be successful only in cases such as severe mental illness or severe intellectual disability. If the individual is found unfit to plead, then there is a provision for a trial of the facts, resulting then in discretionary sentencing, including detention in hospital, a guardianship order, a supervision and treatment order or absolute discharge.

Legal Insanity (Not Guilty by Reason of Insanity)

The special defence of insanity exists because it is recognised that offences can be committed directly because of psychotic symptoms. It is an individual's mental state at the time of the offence that is relevant (57). Although this plea may be put forward for any offence, but in practice it is usually put forward only for murder. Such a plea is rare.

The 1843 M'Naghten rules (relevant to England and Wales) set two criteria by which to judge insanity: firstly that the individual suffered from a mental disorder at the time of offence, and secondly that this lead to the absence of mens rea (a guilty mind). Involuntary manslaughter means manslaughter where there was no malice aforethought.

Diminished Responsibility

This law applies only to a charge of murder. The psychiatric defence of diminished responsibility (raised only by the defence) reduces the murder charge to manslaughter. The offender may plead that at the time of the offence, he or she had diminished responsibility. The offender has to show that at the time of murder, there was abnormality of mind, whether arising from a condition of arrested or retarded development of mind or any inherent causes or induced by disease or injury, that substantially impaired his or her mental responsibility for the act.

Infanticide

As discussed above, infanticide is defined as having occurred when a woman by any wilful act caused the death of her child under the age of 12 months, but at the time of the act or omission the balance of her mind was 'disturbed by reason of her not being fully recovered from the effect of giving birth to the child or the effect of lactation consequent upon the birth of the child'. A conviction for infanticide usually results in a probation order, often with a condition of psychiatric treatment.

Amnesia

Assessment of amnesia is commonly required for offenders, as at least 25 percent of those charged with homicide claim amnesia for the offence. However, the legal significance of amnesia is very restricted. The fact that an individual cannot remember events at the material time will not per se affect his fitness to plead or negate the presumption that he intended the consequences of his actions (58). The clinical importance of finding that an accused has amnesia raises the possibility that his mental state may have been abnormal at the time of the offence.

Amnesia may be present in association with various psychiatric and physical conditions. Amnesia in association with organic brain disease in offenders is rare. It can occur after a head injury, or in association with epilepsy, hypoglycaemia, or other causes of organic transient memory loss (e.g., a toxic state). Dissociative amnesia or a dissociative fugue (in which there is an inability to recall one's past) are occasionally seen in offender. Psychological amnesia in relation to offending is quite controversial. In distinguishing between psychological and organic amnesia, one author has emphasised that a dense and global amnesia in which long periods of patient's life are forgotten is attributable to an organic cause only if it is accompanied by impairment of consciousness or severe disruption of intellectual functions. Inconsistencies suggest a psychological aetiology. In psychological amnesia, there is no corresponding difficulty in retaining material learned after the termination of the period for which amnesia is claimed. Moreover, in psychological amnesia, significant material is gradually forgotten over a period of days or weeks (59).

Automatism

Automatism is a psychiatric defence, and can be defined as 'the state of a person who, though capable of action, is not conscious of what he is doing'. It means unconscious involuntary action, and it is a defence because the mind does not go with what is being done'. The basis of this defence is that because the person is not aware of his or her action, he or she cannot have mens rea. Automatism has been divided into two types: a sane automatism which leads to a full acquittal and an insane automatism leading to a verdict of not guilty by reason of insanity and wide range of disposal (60). Medical or organic automatisms may occur in association with epilepsy, the effects of alcohol or drugs (e.g., Episodic Dyscontrol syndrome), hypoglycaemia, transient global amnesia, and during sleep. In an ictal automatism, the patient should be known to suffer from epilepsy, and previously manifested similar automatisms

In most cases of somnambulism and night terrors there is a family history of these disorders and that onset is in childhood or, at the latest, adolescence. Onset in adult life is suspicious. Sleep automatisms occur in slow-wave sleep normally within two hours of going to sleep. There is disorientation on awakening, with amnesia for the event. There may be trigger factors such as drugs, alcohol, fatigue, or stress. There are no attempts at concealment and the usual pattern is to summon help on awakening. The act should normally be out of character.

Sentencing

In the UK, there are a number of options open to the court for the final disposal of mentally disordered offenders.

Section 35 provides for a remand to hospital so that psychiatric report on the accused's mental state can be prepared.

Section 36 provides for a remand of an accused person to hospital for treatment.

Section 37 (hospital order) is a common disposal once an accused is convicted. The convicted offender is sent to a psychiatric hospital for treatment.

Sometimes Section 41 is added to Section 37 to protect public from serious harm transfer. This patient can only be sent on leave or discharged only with consent of the Home Secretary.

Section 38 is the interim mental disorder to evaluate response to hospital treatment for up to six months (while sentencing is awaited).

Section 47/49 implies transferring a sentenced prisoner from hospital with restrictions on discharge.

While sentencing is awaited, Section 48/49 can be applied to transfer an unsentenced prisoner to hospital.

Court Reports

A report may be requested by a court or by the defence solicitors. Psychiatrist should use the report to help the court reach the most appropriate disposal for the patient. The way in which a report is written and the matters it deals with will depend on the purpose for which it is requested. Its content, style, and structure should vary according to the source of the request for the report, the particular offence with which the defendant is charged, or the issue which the court will decide, and whether it is prepared before or after conviction (61).

The report should be within the remit of the solicitor's instructions. If the solicitor's instructions are not clear, they should be clarified. It should always be borne in mind that some reports may be subjected to intense analysis. It is therefore recommended that the writer should carefully consider all the issues and the scrutiny to which the report may be put.

Ethically, the opinion and recommendations of the psychiatrist should exactly be the same, irrespective of the party requesting the report. As an expert witness, it is not only undesirable but unacceptable, to tailor or modify the report to suit a particular party. The writer of the report must resist the temptation into supporting one or the other side and must give his honest professional opinion. It is not the psychiatrist's job to persuade the court to be lenient. In other words, the report should be objective and impartial.

Regarding confidentiality and disclosure of privileged information, the readers are advised to consult latest guidelines of General Medical Council (GMC), and the Royal College of Psychiatrists, London. Generally speaking, guidelines make it clear that in certain serious situations, the psychiatrist might feel duty bound to disclose information without the subject's consent. Information for the report should be sought from various documents and sources, and these ought to be mentioned in the report.

Essential information includes details about the charge, a social enquiry report from a probation officer (if involved), a list of previous convictions (if any), previous hospital admissions records (if any), and previous social and medical reports.

The detailed history will be taken from the patient and, if possible, from the relative or carer (with the permission of the patient). A comprehensive mental state examination should then be performed. Some important questions to consider are:

- Does he or she have a mental disorder and require specific treatment? Can arrangements be made for such treatment, e.g., hospital, out-patient?
- If the client is dangerous, how can the risks be minimised?

It is worthwhile to mention that technical jargon should be avoided and all technical terms should be explained e.g., paranoid/persecutory delusions (false beliefs), auditory and visual hallucinations (voices and visions).

Paragraph numbers and precise headings should be used for clarity. Different authors have recommended various forms for the court reports. One model is as follows:

In the introduction, the psychiatrist's current status and qualifications are mentioned. The report should state when and where the patient was seen, and at whose request the report is being written, what were the sources of information e.g., if any information was obtained from any relative or other informants. The index offence for which the patient is charged and its date, and the plea if known, i.e. guilty or not guilty, should be highlighted.

Family history should include the history of any medical condition, psychiatric disorder and criminal offences. A detailed personal history from birth till the present time is desirable.

In previous personality, details of personality in terms of social interactions, emotions and habits, e.g., drinking, gambling, drugs should be included. Past medical history is followed by past psychiatric history, which should detail previous diagnoses, admissions and treatments to offending. Past forensic history follows next and then details of index offence.

Defendant's mental state at the time of the offence is of paramount importance.

Current mental state examination ought to be very comprehensive.

The second last part of the report contains the psychiatrist's opinion and recommendations.

Apart from the diagnosis, its implications of the defendant's mental health and prognosis should be mentioned. The final part is, what is called the Statement of truth.

Statement of Truth

I understand that my sole duty in writing this report is to ascertain and state facts within my area of competence and expertise.

I understand that this duty overrides any obligations to the person(s) from whom I have received instructions, or by whom I am paid.

I confirm that I have complied with that duty in writing this report.

I believe that the facts I have stated in this report are true, and the opinions I have expressed are correct to the best of my knowledge.

REFERENCES

1. Gunn, J. and Taylor, P. (1993). *Forensic psychiatry*, clinical, legal and ethical issues. Oxford: Butterworth-Heinemann.
2. Monahan, J. (1997). Clinical and acturial predictions of violence. In D. Faigman, D. Kaye, M. Saks and J. Sanders (Eds.), *Modern scientific evidence*: The law and science of expert testimony (pp. 309). MN: West Publishing.
3. Kaye, C. and Lingiah, T. (2000). *Culture and ethnicity in secure psychiatric practice*: Working with difference. London: Jessica Kingsley.
4. Treasaden, I. (2010). Forensic psychiatry. In B. Puri and I. Treasaden (Eds.), *Psychiatry: An evidence based text* (pp. 1153–1213). London: Hodder Arnold.
5. Farrington, D. P. (1993). The psychosocial milieu of the offender. In J. Gunn, P. Taylor (Eds.), *Forensic Psychiatry, clinical, legal and ethical issues* (pp. 252–285). Oxford: Butterworth- Heinemann.
6. Chiswick, D. (2000). Associations between psychiatric disorder and offending. In M. G. Gelder, J. J. Lopez-Ibor Jr and N. C. Andreasen (Eds.), *The new Oxford textbook of psychiatry*. Oxford: Oxford University Press.
7. Thompson, L. D. G. and Robinson, L. (2010). The relationship between crime and psychiatry. In E. C. Johnstone, D. C. Owens, S. Lawrie, A. M. Mcintosh and M. Sharpe (Eds.), *Companion to psychiatric Studies* (8th Edition, pp. 731–767). Edinburgh: Churchill Livingstone.
8. Taylor, P. J. and Gunn, J. (1999). Homicides by people with mental illness. *British Journal of Psychiatry*, 174, 9–14.
9. Fazel, S. and Danesh, J. (2002). Serious mental disorder in 2300010 prisoners: A systematic review of 62 surveys. *The Lancet*, 359, 545–550.
10. Royal College of Psychiatrists. (2007). *Prison and psychiatry*: Adult prisons in England and Wales (College report CR141). London: Royal College of Psychiatrists
11. Fazel, S., Benning, R. and Denish, J. (2005). Suicides in male prisoners in England and Wales 1978–2003. *The Lancet*, 366, 1301–1302.
12. Link, B. G. and Stueve, A. (1994). Psychotic symptoms and the violent/illegal behaviour of mental patients compared to community controls. In J. Monahan and H. J. Steadman (Eds.), *Violence and mental disorder* (pp. 137–159). Chicago: University of Chicago Press.
13. Coid, J. et al. (2006). Violence and morbidity in the national household population of britain Public health implications. *British Journal of Psychiatry*, 189, 12–19.
14. Thompson, L. D. G. and Robinson, L. (2010). The relationship between crime and psychiatry. In E. C. Johnstone, D. C. Owens, S. Lawrie, A. M. Mcintosh and M. Sharpe (Eds.), *Companion to psychiatric Studies* (8th Edition, pp. 731–767). Edinburgh: Churchill Livingstone.
15. Guze, S. B. (1976). *Criminality and psychiatric disorders*. New York: Oxford University Press.
16. Brennan, P. A., Mednick, S. A. and Hodgins S. (2000). Major mental disorders and criminal violence in a Danish birth cohort. *Archives of General Psychiatry*, 57, 494–500.
17. Harsch, S., Bergk, J. E., Steinert, T., Keller, F. and Jockusch, U. (2006). Prevalence of mental disorders among sexual offenders in forensic psychiatry and prison. *International Journal of Law and Psychiatry*, 29, 443–449.
18. Holland. T and Clare, I. C. (2002). Prevalence of criminal offending by men and women with intellectual disability and the characters of offenders: implications for research and service developments. *Journal of Intellectual Disability Research*, 46, 6–20.
19. Hall, I. (2000). Young offenders with intellectual disability. *Advances in Psychiatric Treatment*, 6, 278–286.

20. Chiswick, D. (2000). Associations between psychiatric disorder and offending. In M. G. Gelder, J. J. Lopez-Ibor Jr and N. C. Andreasen (Eds.), *The new Oxford textbook of psychiatry*. Oxford: Oxford University Press.
21. Brennan, P. A., Mednick, S. A. and Hodgins, S. (2000). Major mental disorders and criminal violence in a Danish birth cohort. *Archives of General Psychiatry*, 57, 494–500.
22. Fazel, S. and Danesh, J. (2002). Serious mental disorder in 2300010 prisoners: A systematic review of 62 surveys. *The Lancet*, 359, 545–550.
23. Faulk, M. (1994). *Basic forensic psychiatry* (2nd Edition). Oxford: Blackwell Science.
24. Faulk, M. (1994). *Basic forensic psychiatry* (2nd Edition). Oxford: Blackwell Science.
25. Buchanan, A. (1999). Risk and dangerousness. *Psychological Medicine*, 29,465–473.
26. Monahan, J. (1981). *The clinical prediction of violent behaviour*. US Department of Health and Human Services, publication. Washington DC: US Government Printing Office.
27. Davison, S. (1997) Risk assessment and management–a busy practitioner's perspective. *International Review of Psychiatry*, 9, 201–206.
28. Douglas, K., Webster, C. D., Eaves, D., et al. (2001). *HCR-20 Violence risk management companion guide*. Vancouver: Simon Fraser University.
29. Quinsey, V. L., Harris, G. T., Rice, M. E. and Cormier, C. A. (1998). *Violent offenders, appraising and manageing risk*. Washington DC: American Psychological Association.
30. Webster, C. D., Douglas, K. S., Eaves, D. and Hart, S. D. (1997). HCR-20, *Assessing risk for violence*: Version 2. Vancouver: Simon Fraser University.
31. Wong, S. and Gordon, A. (2001). The violence risk scale. *The Bulletin of the International Society for the Research on Aggression*, 24(2).
32. Quinsey, V. L., Harris, G. T., Rice, M. E. and Cormier, C. A. (1998). *Violent offenders, appraising and manageing risk*. Washington DC: American Psychological Association.
33. Cheswick, D. Dangerousness. In D. Cheswick and R. Cope (Eds.), *Seminars in practical forensic psychiatry* (pp. 210–242). (1995). London: Royal College of Psychiatrists.
34. Pollock, N. and Webster, C. (1990). The Clinical assessment of dangerousness. In R. Bluglass and P. Bowden (Eds.), *Principles and practice of forensic psychiatry* (pp. 489–497). Edinburgh: Churchill Livingstone.
35. Scott, P. (1977). Assessing dangerousness in criminals. *British Journal of Psychiatry*, 131, 127– 142.
36. Stone, J. L., McDaniel, K. D., Hughes, J. R. and Hermann, B. P. (1986). Episodic dyscontrol disorder and paroxysmal EEG abnormalities: Successful treatment with carbamazepine. *Biological Psychiatry*, 21, 208–212.
37. Worral, E. P., Moody, J. P. and Naylor, G. L. (1975). Lithium in non-organic depressives: Anti aggressive effects and red blood cell lithium values. *British Journal of Psychiatry*, 126, 464–469.
38. Cordess, C. (1995). Crime and mental disorder. In D. Cheswick and R. Cope (Eds.), *Seminars in practical forensic psychiatry* (pp 14–51). London: Royal College of Psychiatrists.
39. Bowden, P. (1990). Homicide. In R. Bluglass and P. Bowden (Eds.), *Principles and practice of forensic psychiatry* (pp. 507–521). Edinburgh: Churchill Livingstone.
40. Shaw, J., Appleby, L., Amos, T., et al. (1999).Mental disorder and clinical care in people convicted of homicide: national clinical survey. *British Medical Journal*, 318, 1240–1244.
41. Wasik, M. (1990). Insanity, diminished responsibility and infanticide: Legal aspects. In R. Bluglass and P. Bowden (Eds.), *Principles and practice of forensic psychiatry* (pp. 255–263). Edinburgh: Churchill Livingstone.
42. Gelder, M., Harrison, P. and Cowen, P. (2006). *Shorter Oxford textbook of psychiatry* (5th Edition). Oxford: Oxford University Press.
43. Gill, D. (2007). *Hughes' outline of modern psychiatry* (5th Edition). Chichester: John Wiley and Sons, Ltd.
44. Gelder, M., Harrison, P. and Cowen, P. (2006). *Shorter Oxford textbook of psychiatry* (5th Edition). Oxford: Oxford University Press.
45. Gelder, M., Harrison, P. and Cowen, P. (2006). *Shorter Oxford textbook of psychiatry* (5th Edition). Oxford: Oxford University Press.
46. Snaith, P. and Bennett, G. (1990). Exhibitionism, indecent exposure, voyerism and frottage In R.Bluglass and P. Bowden (Eds.), *Principles and practice of forensic psychiatry* (pp. 671–676). Edinburgh: Churchill Livingstone.
47. Mullen, P., Pathe, M. and Purcell, R. (2000). *Stalkers and their victims*. Cambridge: Cambridge University Press.
48. Summit, R. and Kryso, J. (1978). Sexual abuse of children: A clinical spectrum. *American Journal of Orthopsychiatry*, 48, 237–25.
49. Finkelhor, D. (1979). *Sexually victimized children*. New York: Free Press.
50. Gill, D. (2007). *Hughes' outline of modern psychiatry* (5th Edition). Chichester: John Wiley and Sons, Ltd.
51. Enayati, J., Grann, M., Lubbe, S. and Fazel, S.(2008). Psychiatric morbidity in arsonists referred for forensic psychiatric assessment in Sweden. *Journal of Forensic Psychiatry and Psychology*, 19(2), 139–147.
52. Thompson, L. D. G. and Robinson, L. (2010). The relationship between crime and psychiatry. In E. C. Johnstone, D. C. Owens, S. Lawrie, A. M. Mcintosh and M. Sharpe (Eds.), *Companion to psychiatric studies* (8th Edition, pp. 731–767). Edinburgh: Churchill Livingstone.
53. Prins, H. and Tennent, G. (1985). Motives for arson (fire raising). *Medicine, Science and the Law*, 25, 275–278.
54. Bluglass, R. (1990). Shoplifting. In R. Bluglass and P. Bowden (Eds.), *Principles and practice of forensic psychiatry* (pp. 787–795). Edinburgh: Churchill Livingstone.
55. Mcelroy, S. L., Pope, H. G., Hudson, J. I., et al. (1991). Kleptomania: A report of 20 cases. *American Journal of Psychiatry*, 148, 652–657.
56. James, D. V., Duffield, G., Blizard, R. and Hamilton, L. W. (2001). Fitness to plead. A prospective study of the inter-relationships between expert opinion, legal criteria, and specific symptomatology. *Psychological Medicine*, 31, 139–150.
57. Thompson, L. (2008). The forensic mental health system in the United Kingdom. In K. Soothill, P. Rogers and M. Dolan (Eds.), *Handbook of forensic mental health* (pp. 19–63). Devon: Willan Publishing.
58. Howard, C. (1990). IV. 7. 9 Amnesia. In R. Bluglass and P. Bowden (Eds.), *Principles and practice of forensic psychiatry* (pp. 291–298). Edinburgh: Churchill Livingstone.
59. Lishman, W. A. (1987). *Organic psychiatry* (2nd Edition). Oxford: Blackwell.
60. Thompson, L. (2008). The forensic mental health system in the United Kingdom. In K. Soothill, P. Rogers and M. Dolan (Eds.), *Handbook of forensic mental health* (pp. 19–63). Devon: Willan Publishing.
61. Bowden, P. (1990). The written report and sentences. In R. Bluglass and P. Bowden (Eds.), *Principles and practice of forensic psychiatry* (pp. 183– 197). Edinburgh: Churchill Livingstone.

CHAPTER 15

Perinatal and Psychiatric Disorders Specific to Women

Some studies have shown that before puberty, both males and females are equally at risk for developing some psychiatric disorders, e.g., mood disorders. After menstruation starts, there is increased tendency for unipolar depression in women as compared with men. Some women are at increased risk for mental health issues during certain times such as premenstrually, postpartum, and perimenopause. While treating women during pregnancy there has to careful consideration of the risks of medication to the unborn child. The risk of untreated psychiatric illness, during pregnancy has to be accounted for as there are high chances of relapse. Psychosocial risk factors and intervening life events are also key factors in increasing women's risk for psychiatric illness.

In this chapter, psychiatric disorders in relation to pregnancy, childbirth and the menstrual cycle will be discussed. Although some authors mention that pregnancy appears to protect against psychiatric disorders, more researchers are of the view that psychiatric disorders occurring during or after pregnancy are quite common. Those women with pre-existing disorder (particularly affective and bipolar disorder) are at risk for exacerbation and recurrence of their illness in the postpartum period, and extra vigilance is needed. Moreover, women with pre-existing bipolar disorder are at a high risk of postpartum relapse, even if treatment with mood stabilisers is maintained (1). This risk is probably also higher for those women with schizoaffective disorder but not with schizophrenia, provided medication is maintained (2).

Drug Treatment During Pregnancy and Breastfeeding

A brief overview is being given here, and readers are advised to consult either the 14th edition of Maudsley Guidelines (3) or Psychotropic Drug Directory 2022 (4) for an elaborate account. Pharmacological treatment is routinely discouraged during pregnancy, especially during the first trimester. The teratogenic potential is maximum between 2–9 weeks after conception. Although in many cases, the risk of relapse will be higher than the risk of fetal damage, if necessary, the lowest effective dose for the shortest period necessary should be used, after individual assessments of benefits and risks. Moreover, poly pharmacy should be avoided (5).

It should be remembered that the pharmacokinetics of drugs may change during pregnancy and the doses may need to be adjusted. Discontinuation effects of some medication have also been reported in the newborn (e.g., Benzodiazepines, antidepressants and opiates) and medication should therefore preferably be reduced or withdrawn gradually over the weeks before the delivery is due (6). A large Swedish study demonstrated no significant difference in the major congenital malformations rate between women taking antipsychotics or not. This finding has been replicated in other studies (7). Low serum folate levels have been shown in women taking second generation antipsychotics, increasing the risk of neural tube defects (8). A meta-analysis found no evidence of major malformations or spontaneous abortion with most tricyclics (TCAs) and Selective Serotonin Reuptake Inhibitors (SSRIs) (9). There is limited data available for venlafaxine and mirtazapine. Some authors believe that the risk of lithium has been overestimated in the past (10). Although lithium is associated with three times the risk of any congenital abnormality, and eight times risk of Ebstein's anomaly (defect of tricuspid valve), the absolute risk of this is approximately 1 in 1000 pregnancies (11). A higher incidence of teratogenicity has been reported in women taking a variety of benzodiazepines (12).

Surveys have shown that the majority of women tend to breastfeed. The use of psychotropic medication during lactation requires a careful risk/benefit assessment. Consideration should be given to all available options, the current data on the medication, the benefits of breastfeeding, the risk of untreated mental illness to the mother and the baby, and also the value the mother or the family places on breastfeeding. Pharmacological treatment during lactation remains controversial (13). Moreover, because of the comparatively limited data, it is difficult to recommend specific medications for lactating women. The SSRIs are preferable to the TCAs as, apart from other side effects, as the latter's autonomic side effects may decrease milk supply and lactational reflexes (14). MAOIs are very rarely used in lactating mothers mainly because of dietary restrictions and the potential for dangerous hypertensive crises (15). Although the data on antianxiety medication is variable, it does support the use of short-acting benzodiazepines without metabolites if such medication is necessary during lactation.

Among mood stabilisers, valproic acid and carbamazepine are regarded as compatible with breastfeeding (16). The use of lithium during lactation has not only been contraindicated by the American Academy of Paediatrics (17), but has also been discouraged by various other authors. There is evidence that careful monitoring of the infant is required, especially the infant's hydration status (18).

Postpartum Psychiatric Disorders

Postpartum psychiatric disorders comprise mood, anxiety and psychotic disorders, which are characterised by the onset of symptoms in the weeks or months following birth. Each disorder is associated with a particular symptom constellation that suggests the clinical diagnosis (19). It has been debated whether depressive and anxiety disorders occurring specific to childbirth are distinct from depressive and anxiety disorders occurring at other times (20). It has been suggested that postnatal depression is of shorter duration as compared to depression occurring at other times. However, there is no doubt that postnatal depression and postnatal psychoses are quite serious disorders and carry risks. The rates of mood and anxiety disorders peak during the childbearing years that is between the ages of 18 and 44 years (21). Moreover, women who have borne children before, have higher rates of mood disorders than nulliparous women (22). One study found that one out of seven depressive episodes was related to a childbearing event (23).

The incidence of psychotic disorders is also more likely to be precipitated in association with childbearing. In fact, there is a significant increase in hospital admissions to psychiatric hospital of women having psychoses within the first three months after delivery, and after this period, the rates decline to those normally expected (24). Due to mothers not being well, this results in disturbed mother-infant relationship and the care and bonding of the newborn is adversely affected. Moreover, the early postpartum period carries a high risk of suicide (25).

Regarding postpartum risk factors, family and personal history of depression are the main risk factors (26), but lack of social support, marital conflicts, medical and obstetric complications, and difficult infant (temperamentally) are other important risk factors (27).

Postnatal (Maternity) Blues

Maternity blues is a self-limiting syndrome that affects about 50–80% of women after delivery. Maternity blues are more common in women who have previously given birth. Symptoms include labile mood (alternations between euphoria and low mood), tearfulness, insomnia, fatigue, tension and irritability.

Symptoms usually begin on the second or third day after delivery, peak on the fifth to seventh day and then start to remit by the second week (28). Sometimes, however, the symptoms continue into the fifth week after childbirth. Some clinicians are of the view that these cases should be considered as mild depressive episodes, rather than maternity blues. Postnatal blues may be a marker for late-onset postpartum depression (29).

Postnatal Depression

Non-psychotic depression is more common than puerperal psychosis and occurs later in the postnatal period, usually at around 6 weeks. Postnatal depression not only has an adverse affect on the infant-mother relationship, but also has implications for early cognitive and emotional development (30).

It is imperative to assess the severity of depressive symptoms. Edinburgh Postnatal Depression Scale is a 10–item scale that can be self-administered (31). Another useful scale is The Beck Depression Scale, which is also self-administered (32). If the risk is assessed to be significant, hospital admission should be arranged. It is advisable to rule out thyroid dysfunction.

Antidepressant medication, and if needed, anti-anxiety medication should be commenced. Although newer antidepressant drugs (SSRIs and SNRIs) are better than older tricyclic medication, these drugs have their own side effect profiles. In case of no satisfactory response to adequate doses of medication, and especially for psychotic depression, ECT should be considered, as there might be a risk of suicide or infanticide (33). Transdermal oestrogen therapy has been suggested as being effective in treating postpartum depression (34). Although large doses of progesterone have also been proposed for premenstrual dysphoric disorder and postnatal depression, its efficacy has not been well-established (35). Supportive psychotherapy and interpersonal psychotherapy are effective treatments.

Postpartum Psychosis

Postpartum psychosis is a very serious illness as there is a high risk of suicide and infanticide. It should be managed on in-patient basis. Many hospitals in developed countries now have mother and baby units. Contact between the mother and baby needs to be closely supervised by the nursing staff.

This condition is more frequent in primiparous women and those who have a history of mental illness. Family history of mental illness also increases the risk. There does not seem to be a difference in hormonal levels in those who develop this disorder and those who do not. Traditionally and currently, postpartum psychosis is considered just like other psychoses. There is no established association between postpartum psychosis and obstetric complications. The onset of postpartum psychoses occurs within the first few days of childbirth. Some authors have mentioned the rate as 1 in 500 births, but one study has shown it is 1 in 1000 births (36). Three types of clinical pictures are observed: delirium, mood disorder and schizophreniform disorder. Bipolar disorder and schizoaffective disorders are more common (37).

Symptoms include agitation, restlessness, pressure of speech, poor appetite, sleep disturbance, confusion, hallucinations (can be in any modality and may include auditory hallucinations asking the mother to kill her infant) and delusions of either persecutory or grandiose nature. Most patients with postpartum psychoses recover either fully or to a significant extent, but some with schizophrenia remain unwell on a long-term basis.

Management includes immediate commencement of mood stabilising medication (lithium or valproic acid) along with an antipsychotic medication. The use of electroconvulsive therapy in postpartum psychosis is found to be an effective treatment (38).

Pseudocyesis, Menopause and Hysterectomy

Pseudocyesis (phantom pregnancy) is a rare condition when a woman believes that she is pregnant, although she is not. This usually occurs in young women and is generally not associated with a psychiatric disorder (Couvade refers to an analogous syndrome in the man, who develops these features). There are symptoms of early pregnancy like amenorrhea and abdominal distension. Although the disorder resolves quickly after examination and investigations, the recurrence rate is quite high.

The definition of menopause is that the menstrual periods do not occur for 12 months. This usually happens between the ages of 45 and 55 but in some women may occur earlier. Menopausal symptoms include hot flushing (in a majority of women), sweating, vaginal dryness, headache, dizziness and low mood. Although hormonal replacement therapy may help prevent certain medical conditions, it carries its own risks. Oestrogen has been used to treat menopausal symptoms, but the evidence is not convincing (39). Many studies have demonstrated an increased prevalence of depressive disorder after hysterectomy (40). This may be because these women are distressed by the loss of their childbearing capacity and disturbed by their sense of femininity.

Premenstrual Syndrome (PMS), Premenstrual Tension (PMT)

PMS has a lifetime prevalence of approximately 2% to 4% in menstruating women (41). These women have various psychological and physical symptoms commencing a few days before the menstrual period and ending shortly after the onset of the menstrual cycle. Symptoms include irritability, anxiety, low mood, decreased interest in usual activities, marked lack of energy, hypersomnia or insomnia, sudden urges for food, breast tenderness, abdominal discomfort and bloating. Among those with predisposition to migraine, headaches may increase. Heightened sexual urges, brief hypomanic episodes, and rarely menstrual and premenstrual psychosis have also been described in literature (42). The presence of a concurrent psychiatric disorder like depressive or anxiety disorder should be excluded before the diagnosis of PMS.

Once the diagnosis of severe PMS is confirmed, SSRI medication is considered the first-line treatment. SSRI may be administered daily or intermittently (from ovulation to menses) to be effective. Other medications used to treat this include progesterone, oral contraceptives, bromocriptine, and diuretics. Progesterone seems to have a beneficial effect on the somatic complaints but not on irritability and depressed mood (43). Similarly, the few oral contraceptive studies have not been encourageing (44). Mineral supplements (especially calcium), beta-blockers, calcium channel blockers, thyroxine, light therapy and sleep deprivation have also been tried.

Non-psychopharmacological treatment include special diets (increasing complex carbohydrates and dietary fibre and reducing sugar and salt intake, etc.), exercise, cognitive therapy and relaxation (45).

Premenstrual Dysphoric Disorder

DSM-5 classifies this disorder under the chapter 'Depressive Disorders'. Essential features include mood lability, irritability, dysphoria and anxiety symptoms. These features occur repeatedly during the premenstrual phase of the cycle and remit around the onset of menses or shortly thereafter (46). Diagnostic criteria specifies that in the majority of menstrual cycles, at least five symptoms must be present in the final week before the onset of menses, start to improve within a few days after the onset of menses and become minimal or absent in the week post-menses. One or more symptoms from the first group (marked affective lability, marked irritability or anger or increased interpersonal conflicts, marked depressed mood, marked anxiety) and one or more symptoms from the second group (decreased interest in usual activities, difficulty in concentration, lethargy, marked change in appetite, hypersomnia or insomnia, a sense of being out of control, and physical symptoms such as breast tenderness, or muscle pain) should amount to a total of at least 5 symptoms. Premenstrual syndrome is less severe than premenstrual dysphoric disorder and there is no minimum requirement of five symptoms. Moreover, there is no stipulation of affective symptoms for premenstrual syndrome (47).

Assessment should exclude other mood or anxiety disorders. Treatment includes guiding the patient about identifying the presence and recognising the symptoms. SSRIs can be effective.

REFERENCES

1. Yonkers, K. A., Wisner, K. L., Stowe, Z., et al. (2004). Management of bipolar disorder during *Companion to psychiatric studies* (8th Edition, pp. 783–799). Edinburgh: Churchill Livingstone.
2. Buist, A., Yonkers, K. and Craig, M. (2008). Bergman, U., Rosa, F. W., Baum, C., Wiholm, B. E. and Faich, G. A. (1992). Effects of exposure in pregnancy and the postpartum period. *American Journal of Psychiatry*.
3. Taylor D, Paton, C. and Kapur S.(2012). *The Maudsley prescribing guidelines in psychiatry*(11th edition).London. Informa Healthcare.
4. Bazire, S. (2022). *Psychotropic drug directory*. Gloucestershire: Lloyd-Reinhold Communications LLP.
5. Steel, R. and Cantwell, R. (2010). Perinatal psychiatry. In E. C. Johnstone, D. C. Owens, S. Lawrie, A. A. M. Mcintosh and M. Sharpe (Eds.), *Companion to psychiatric studies* (8th Edition, pp. 783–799). Edinburgh: Churchill Livingstone.
6. Bazire, S. (2012). *Psychotropic drug directory*. Gloucestershire: Lloyd-Reinhold Communications LLP.
7. Reis, M. and Kallen, B. (2008). Maternal use of antipsychotics in early pregnancy and delivery outcome. *Journal of Clinical Psychopharmacology*, 28, 279–288.
8. Koren, G., Cohn, T., Chitayat, D., Kapur, B., Remington, G., Reid, D. M. and Zipursky, R. B. (2002). Use of atypical antipsychotics during pregnancy and the risk of neural tube defects in infants. *American Journal of Psychiatry*, 159, 136– 137.
9. Austin, M. and Mitchell, P. (1998). Psychotropic medications in pregnant women: Treatment dilemmas. *Medical Journal of Australia*, 169, 428– 432.
10. Schou, M. (1990). Lithium treatment during pregnancy, delivery, and lactation: An update. *Journal of Clinical Psychiatry*, 51, 410–413.
11. Steel, R. and Cantwell, R. (2010). Perinatal psychiatry. In E. C. Johnstone, D. C. Owens, S. Lawrie, A. A. M. Mcintosh and M. Sharpe (Eds.), *Companion to psychiatric studies*(8th edition)pp 783-799. Edinburgh.Churchill Livingstone.
12. Bergman, U.,F.W, Baum, C Wilcolm,B E. and Faich, G.A. (1992) Effects of exposure to benzodiazepine during fetal life. *The Lancet*. 340, 694-696.
13. Stowe, Z.N.,Llewellyn, A. Hostetter, A and Nemeroff, C B (2000). The use of psychiatric medications during breastfeeding. In M Steiner, K. A. Yonkers and E. Erikson (Eds) *Mood disorders in women*(pp.329-351).London. Martin Dunitz.
14. Mortola, J.F.(1989) The use of psychotropic agents in pregnancy and lactation, *Pychiatric Clinics of North America*, 12, 69-87
15. 15. Wisner, K.L. and Perel, J.M.(1988)Psychopharmocologic agents and electroconvulsive therapy during pregnancy and the puerperium. In R.L. Cohen (Ed) *Psychiatric consultation in childbirth settings* : Parents and child-orientated approaches (pp 165-206). New York. Plenium Medical Book Company.
16. Briggs, G. G., Freeman, R. K. and Yaffe, S. J. (1994). *Drugs in pregnancy and lactation*. Baltimore: Williams and Wilkins.
17. American Academy of Paediatrics Committee on Drugs. (1994). The transfer of drugs and other chemicals into human milk. *Paediatrics*, 93, 137–150.
18. Stowe, Z. N., Llewellyn, A., Hostetter, A. and Nemeroff, C. B. (2000). The use of psychiatric medications during breat-feeding. In M. Steiner, K. A. Yonkers and E. Eriksson (Eds.), *Mood disorders in women* (pp. 329–351). London: Martin Dunitz.
19. Sichel, D. (2000). Postpartum psychiatric disorders. In M. Steiner, K. A. Yonkers and E. Eriksson (Eds.), *Mood disorders in women* (pp. 313–328). London: Martin Dunitz.
20. Whiffen, E. (1992). Is postpartum depression distinct diagnosis? *Clinical Psychology Review*, 12, 485–508.
21. Weissman, N. M., Livingston, B. M., Leaf, P. J. Et al. (1991). Affective disorders. In L. N. Robins, D. A. Rigeir (Eds.), *Psychiatric disorders in America*: The epidemiological catchment area study (pp. 53–80). New York: Free Press.
22. Gater, R., Tansellal, M., Korten, A. Et al. (1998). Sex differences in the prevalence and detection of depressive and anxiety disorders in general healthcare settings. *Archives of General Psychiatry*, 55, 405–413.
23. Wisner, K. L., Peindl, K. and Hanusa, B. H. (1993). Relationship of psychiatric illness to childbearing status. A hospital based epidemiological study. *Journal of Affective Disorders*, 28, 39–50.
24. Kendell, R. E., Chalmers, J. C. and Platz, C. (1987). Epidemiology of puerperal psychoses. *British Journal of Psychiatry*, 150, 662–673.
25. Apple, L. (1991). Suicide during pregnancy and in the first postnatal year. *British Journal of Psychiatry*, 302, 137–140.
26. Steiner, M., Tam, W. Y. K. (1999). Postpartum depression in relation to other disorders. In L. J. Miller (Ed.), *Postpartum mood disorders* (pp. 47–63). Washington DC: American Psychiatric Press.
27. O'Hara, M. W. and Swain, A. M. (1996). Rates and risk of postpartum depression: A meta- analysis, *International Review of Psychiatry*, 8, 37–54.
28. Kendell, R. E., mcguire, R. J., Connor, Y. and Cox, J. L. (1981) Mood changes in the first three weeks after childbirth. *Journal of Affective Disorders*, 3, 317–326.
29. O'Hara, M. W., Neunaber, D. J. and Zekoski, E. M. (1984). Prospective study of postpartum depression: Prevalence, course and predictive factors. *Journal of Abnormal Psychology*, 93, 158– 171.
30. Stein, A., Gath, D. H., Bucher, J., et al. (1991). The relationship between postnatal depression and mother child interaction. *British Journal of Psychiatry*, 158, 46–52.
31. Cox, J. L., Holden, J. M. and Sagovsky, R. (1987). Detection of postnatal depression: Development of the 10–item Edinburgh Postnatal Depression Scale. *British Journal of Psychiatry*, 150, 782–786.
32. Beck, A. T. and Steer, R. A. (1987). *Manual for the Revised Beck Depression Inventory*. San Antonio: Psychological Corporation.
33. Nonacs, R., Cohen, L. S. (1998). Postpartum mood disorders: Diagnosis and treatment guidelines. *Journal of Clinical Psychiatry*, 59(2), 34–40.
34. Gregoire, A. J., Kumar, R., Everitt, B., et al. (1996). Transdermal oestrogen therapy for treatment of severe postnatal depression. *The Lancet*, 347, 930–933.
35. Freeman, E., Rickels, K., Sondheimer, S. R. and Polansky, M. (1990). Ineffectiveness of progesterone suppository treatment for premenstrual syndrome. *JAMA*, 264, 349–353.
36. Brockington, I. (1996). *Motherhood and mental health*. Oxford: Oxford University Press.
37. Gelder, M., Harrison, P. and Cowen, P. (2006).*Shorter Oxford textbook of psychiatry* (5th Edition). Oxford: Oxford University Press.
38. Reed, P., Sermin, N., Appleby, L., et al. (1999). A comparison of clinical response to electroconvulsive therapy in puerperal and non- puerperal psychoses. *Journal of Affective Disorders*, 54, 255–260.

39. Pearce, J., Hawton, K. and Blake, F. (1995). Psychological and sexual symptoms associated with menopause and the effects of hormone replacement therapy. *British Journal of Psychiatry*, 167, 163–173.

40. Gath, D., Cooper, P. and Day, A. (1982). Hysterectomy and psychiatric disorder. Levels of psychiatric morbidity before and after hysterectomy. *British Journal of Psychiatry*, 140, 335–342.

41. Ramacharan, S., Love, E., Fick, G., et al. (1992). The epidemiology of premenstrual symptoms in a population based sample of 2650 urban women: Attributable risk and risk factors. *Journal of Clinical Epidemiology*, 45, 377–392.

42. Stein, G. (2007). Perinatal psychiatric disorders. In G. Stein and G. W. Gaskell (Eds.), *Seminars in general adult psychiatry* (pp. 635–667). London: The Royal College of Psychiatrists.

43. Freeman, E. W., Rickels, K., Sondhemer, S. J. and Polansky, M. (1990). Ineffectiveness of progesterone suppository treatment for premenstrual syndrome. *JAMA*, 264, 349–353.

44. Freeman, E., Kroll, R., Rapkin, A., et al. (2001). Evaluation of a unique oral contraceptive in the treatment of premenstrual dysphoric disorder. *Journal of Women's Health and Gender-Based Medicine*, 10, 561–569.

45. Stein, G. (2007). Perinatal psychiatric disorders. In G. Stein and G. W. Gaskell (Eds.), *Seminars in general adult psychiatry* (pp. 635–667). London: The Royal College of Psychiatrists.

46. American Psychiatric Association.(2013). *Diagnostic and statistical manual of mental disorders* (5th Edition). Arlington, VA: American Psychiatric Publishing.

47. American Psychiatric Association (2013). *Diagnostic and statistical manual of mental disorders* (5th Edition). Arlington, VA: American Psychiatric Publishing.

CHAPTER

16 Sleep Disorders

Sleep and wakefulness are fundamental neurobehavioural states and these states are organised within a framework of circadian, or 24-hour, rhythmicity. Disruptions of sleep and circadian rhythms have been related to various medical disorders like cardiovascular disease, metabolic syndrome, and diabetes. The relationship between sleep and mental health is far more important. Acute sleep disruption is associated with impaired vigilance and attention, impaired learning, and dysregulation of positive and negative emotions. Sleep disturbances are nearly universal in patients with psychiatric disorders, and conversely, psychiatric symptoms are common in patients with sleep disorders. Sleep disruptions such as insomnia are risk factors for the subsequent development of mental disorders, including mood and anxiety disorders. The presence of insomnia and other sleep disturbances is also associated with worse treatment response and increased likelihood of recurrence in mood disorders. Sleep is, therefore, particularly relevant to psychiatry.

In depression, patients commonly report difficulty in falling sleep, waking up at night and early morning awakening but some have hypersomnia, especially those in the depressive phase of bipolar affective disorder. In the manic phase, most patients are restless and feel a reduced need for sleep. Anxiety disorders (including PTSD) also cause poor quality of sleep. Insomnia is common in alcohol and substance use disorders.

About a third of the children between the ages of one and three years have sleep problems, and because of their lifestyle and late-night social activities, some adolescents are also at a higher risk of sleep disturbance. Snoring can also cause sleep disturbance to the partner. Because of the increasing rates of obesity among women, snoring is now no longer a male issue. Although there are some changes in sleep patterns in the elderly, sleep can be improved in this group and efforts should be made to find the cause (1). As sleep disorders are common, it is desirable that the sleep pattern is explored as a part of general history taking. As many patients can be vague about their sleep, it is important to ask them specific questions. Questions about caffeine, cigarettes, alcohol and drugs should be asked as well. Two useful screening questions are Leeds Sleep Evaluation Questionnaire (2), and St. Mary's Hospital Sleep Questionnaire (3). In some severe and specific cases, special investigations are necessary. These include actigraphy, polysomnography (overnight sleep recording), Human Leucocyte Antigen (HLA) typing for investigation of narcolepsy, toxicology screening for drug problems, measurement of hypocretin, the multiple sleep latency test and psychometric assessment.

In this chapter, an overview of sleep physiology, pathophysiology of sleep disturbance, and the diagnosis and treatment of sleep disorders shall be given.

Normal Sleep

Sleep can be described along multiple different dimensions such as timing, continuity, and depth, and along with multiple levels of analysis, including self-report, behavioural, and physiological.

Sleep can be defined behaviourally as a reversible state of reduced awareness of and responsiveness to the environment. Physiologically it is characterised by some features which differentiate it from other states of relative inactivity, such as coma (4). Sleep occupies about one-third of human life. The main function of sleep is restorative, as it is evident that persistent sleep disturbance usually leads to physical and psychological problems. Sleep also serves homeostatic function and appears to be crucial for normal thermoregulation and energy conservation. There is a rebound of sleep after a period of sleep deprivation, which suggests that sleep loss triggers homeostatic compensation, and sleep is essential to brain function (5).

Prolonged periods of sleep deprivation sometimes lead to ego disorganisation, hallucinations, and delusions. REM-deprived patients may exhibit irritability and lethargy. People have different sleep requirements, although majority of adults sleep from seven to eight hours per night. However, the amount of sleep needed is the amount that is enough to adequately perform next day's duties. Some persons require fewer than six hours of sleep each night to function adequately. Long sleepers are those who sleep more than nine hours. Short sleepers are generally efficient, ambitious, socially adept, and content. Long sleepers tend to be mildly depressed, anxious, and socially withdrawn. Sleep needs increase with physical work, exercise, illness, pregnancy, general mental stress, and increased mental activity (6).

Sleep is made up of two physiological states: Non-Rapid Eye Movement (NREM) sleep and Rapid Eye Movement (REM) sleep. Both are active states. In NREM sleep (composed of stages 1 to 4), most physiological functions are markedly lower than in wakefulness. REM sleep is a qualitatively different kind of sleep, characterised by a high level of brain activity and physiological activity levels similar to those in wakefulness (7). Shortening of REM latency frequently occurs with such disorders as depressive disorder and narcolepsy.

The disorganisation during arousal from stage three or stage four may result in specific problems, including enuresis, somnambulism, and stage four nightmares or night terrors. The most distinctive feature of REM sleep is dreaming. Persons awakened during REM sleep frequently report that they had been having abstract dreams. Dreaming in NREM sleep is typically lucid and purposeful (8).

Sleep Regulation

There are two interacting processes, the circadian process and the homeostatic or recovery process that control the sleep-wake cycle (9). The circadian process is that which regulates the daily rhythms of the body and the brain. The suprachiasmatic nucleus of the hypothalamus acts as the anatomical site of a circadian pacemaker that regulates melatonin secretion and 24–hour sleep-wake cycle. There is role of serotonin in sleep regulation as prevention of serotonin synthesis, reduces sleep for a considerable time.

Drugs and manipulations that increase the firing of noradrenergic neurons, markedly reduce REM sleep and increase wakefulness. Brain acetylcholine is also involved in sleep, particularly in the production of REM sleep. Compared with healthy persons and non-depressed psychiatric controls, patients who are depressed have marked disruptions of REM sleep patterns. Drugs that reduce REM sleep, such as antidepressants, produce beneficial effects in depression.

Sleep Disorders

The clinical assessment of sleep disorders begins with a precise history. This history should evaluate various dimensions of sleep, including quality, quantity, continuity, variability, and daytime sleepiness. A sleep diary is often helpful to assess sleep patterns, and questionnaires can help to identify specific disorders and quantify their severity. In conducting the patient history, the clinician should maintain a focus on the entire 24-hour day, in order to assess both the characteristics of sleep, and its consequences on waking function. When possible, it is also helpful to obtain a sleep history from a bed partner, who may have observations that the patient is unable to make for himself or herself, e.g., unusual behaviours during sleep.

An accurate history of concurrent medical and psychiatric disorders is mandatory. Sleep problems may be caused, and are often exacerbated by a wide variety of medical and psychiatric disorders. Among the most important are pulmonary disorders (chronic obstructive pulmonary disease, asthma), neurologic conditions (degenerative conditions, chronic pain conditions), and disorders that cause impaired mobility. Among psychiatric disorders, depressive and anxiety disorders are amongst the most common corrrelates of insomnia. A large number of medications, including all psychotropic agents, and non-psychotropic drugs can affect the autonomic nervous system, and can cause insomnia or sleepiness. Furthermore, the timing of administration of such medications may also influence their sleep-wake effects.

Patients with sleep disorders can benefit from a general medical evaluation to investigate contributing factors. For example, patients with suspected sleep apnea should have an examination of their upper airway to determine potential sites and causes of airway obstruction. Targeted blood tests may also be useful. For example, iron deficiency and low serum ferritin values are often observed in patients with restless legs syndrome. Fatigue and sleepiness may be associated with endocrine disorders such as hypothyroidism.

In DSM-5, there have been changes from DSM-IV. The diagnosis of primary insomnia has been renamed insomnia disorder to avoid the distinction between primary and secondary insomnia. DSM-5 distinguishes narcolepsy from other forms of hypersomnolence. The breath-related sleep disorders are divided into obstructive sleep apnea hypopnea, central sleep apnea and sleep-related hypoventilation. The subtypes of circadian rhythm sleep disorders have been expanded to include advanced sleep phase type and irregular sleep-wake type, whereas the jet lag type has been removed. Finally, rapid eye movement sleep behaviour disorder and restless legs syndrome have been described as independent disorders.

Insomnia

Insomnia is a common problem encountered in psychiatric practice, is associated with reduced quality of life (10), and has implications for absence from work. It is more common in females. Insomnia is a perceived disturbance in the quantity or quality of sleep. There may be complaints of difficulty in falling asleep, waking at night repeatedly, early morning awakening or not feeling fresh the next day after an apparently full night's sleep. Transient insomnia is for few days to some weeks, whereas chronic insomnia may last from months to years. A brief period of insomnia is most often associated with stress or anxiety. In persistent insomnia, the problem is most often difficulty falling asleep rather than remaining asleep.

Forms of insomnia include the primary insomnias and circadian rhythm sleep disturbances. It is the most common sleep complaint and may be transient or persistent. Sometimes, a psychotic episode or severe depression begins with acute insomnia.

Jet Lag

The effects of jet lag are usually short-lived and transient, but in frequent travellers, insomnia can become a serious problem having implications for performance and mood disturbances (11). This is the most common circadian rhythm disorder and symptoms include daytime fatigue and sleepiness, night time insomnia, mood changes, and difficulty in concentration.

The effect of jet lag is greater when travelling eastwards. The reason for this is that the internal rhythm is slightly longer than 24 hours, so lengthening the day after westward travel is somewhat easier. Melatonin (0.5 mg–5 mg) taken close to local bedtime for up to 4 days, has shown to be effective.

Shift Working

Shift workers are more prone to insomnia as compared to the general population.

Restless Legs Syndrome

This is a sensorimotor, neurological sleep disorder characterised by a desire to move the legs or arms, usually accompanied by uncomfortable sensations e.g., crawling, tingling, burning or itching. When the individual is resting, the symptoms become worse and so the leg movements are made in an effort to relieve the uncomfortable sensations. Symptoms are worse in the evening or night, and in some cases they occur only in the evening or night. The onset of this syndrome is usually in the second or third decade. The cause is not known but it can occur in pregnancy and those who suffer from iron deficiency anaemia or rheumatoid arthritis.

Benzodiazepines are relatively not effective. If present, anaemia should be treated. L-dopa, carbidopa, bromocriptine, pergolide and ropinirole have been used successfully in some cases.

Treatment of Insomnia

This consists of targeting the specific cause (medical and psychiatric disorders). However, it should be borne in mind that certain drugs prescribed for medical conditions can also cause sleep disturbance (12).

Pharmacological treatment is not recommended as a first-line of treatment. Initially, sleep hygiene should be tried. Some suggestions for sleep hygiene are given below: (13)

1. Sleep and arise at the same time daily.
2. Limit daily in-bed time to the usual amount present before the sleep disturbance.
3. It is better to avoid caffeine, nicotine, alcohol or stimulants, in the evening.
4. Avoid daytime naps (except when the sleep chart shows they induce better night's sleep).
5. Establish physical fitness by means of a graded programme of vigorous exercise early in the day.
6. Avoid evening stimulation; substitute radio or relaxed reading for television.
7. Try very hot, 20–minute, body-temperature- raising bath soaks near bedtime.
8. Eat at regular times daily; avoid large meals near bedtime.
9. Practice evening relaxation routines, such as progressive muscle relaxation or meditation.
10. Maintain comfortable sleeping conditions.

Other strategies should be tried before prescribing drugs. Cognitive restructuring attempts to identify and change distorted cognitions about insomnia. Stimulus control therapy emphasises that one only goes to bed when sleepy, and if not asleep within twenty minutes, to get up and engage in a relaxing activity, before returning to bed (14). Other activities like watching TV and writing letters while in bed should be avoided. Relaxing techniques include imagery and muscle relaxation. It is also helpful to think and actually write some positive steps about the next day's plans and activities, before going to bed (the idea is not to ruminate or worry while in bed).

When treatment with hypnotic medication is indicated, it should be of short duration (no more than 3–4 weeks). Apart from this, four other basic principles have been advised (15). Using the lowest effective dose, using intermittent dosing, discontinuing medication gradually and being aware of the possibility of rebound insomnia after discontinuation. Benzodiazepines, and the 'Z' drugs (zopiclone, zolpidem and zalepon) are effective for insomnia. However, obstructive sleep apnoea can be exacerbated by benzodiazepines. Care should also be taken when the patient is taking alcohol as that will potentiate the effects of these drugs. Indiplon and eszopiclone are comparatively new drugs. Although tricyclic antidepressants (e.g., Amitriptyline) are also used, the efficacy is not established. The results for melatonin are inconclusive for use in insomnia (16), although it is helpful in circadian rhythm disorders. Finally, antihistamines are used for insomnia, although only promethazine has demonstrated efficacy in a controlled trial.

Hypersomnia

This manifests as excessive amounts of sleep, or Excessive Daytime Sleepiness (EDS), or sometimes both. The term somnolence should be restricted for patients who complain of sleepiness, have a clearly demonstrable tendency to fall asleep suddenly, and who cannot remain awake. Complaints of hypersomnia are much less frequent than complaints of insomnia. It can be caused by insufficient night time sleep, frequent parasomnias, chronic physical illnesses, psychiatric disorders (e.g., depressive illness), neurological conditions, drug side effects, obstructive sleep apnoea, narcolepsy, Kleine-Levin syndrome, and circadian rhythm disorder.

Transient and situational hypersomnia is a disruption of the normal sleep-wake pattern; it is marked by excessive difficulty in remaining awake and a tendency to remain in bed for unusually long periods or to return to bed to nap frequently during the day.

Kleine-Levin Syndrome

Kleine-Levin syndrome is a relatively rare condition consisting of recurrent periods of prolonged sleep (from which patients may be aroused) with intervening periods of normal sleep and alert waking. During the hypersomniac episodes, wakeful periods are usually marked by withdrawal from social contacts and return to bed at the first opportunity; patients may also display apathy, irritability, confusion, excessive impairment, incoherent speech, excitation or depression. Lithium is known to be helpful in some cases.

Obstructive Sleep Apnoea Syndrome

It tends to occur in patients who snore, although most snorers do not have sleep apnoea. It usually occurs in middle-aged men, but can occur at any age, including children. These patients have smaller airways than normal sleepers. Obstructive Sleep Apnoea (OSA) is characterised by periods of functional obstruction of the upper airway during sleep. This leads to a state of hypoxia and hypercapnia (elevated carbon dioxide levels) that activates the brain stem, leading to an arousal that increases breathing and rectifies the problem (17).

Medical consequences include cardiac arrhythmias, systemic and pulmonary hypertension, and decreased sexual drive or function. OSA is a risk factor for stroke (18). When sleep apnoea is established or suspected, patients must avoid the use of sedative medication, including alcohol, because it can considerably exacerbate the condition, which may then become life-threatening (19). OSA is diagnosed by specialist sleep disorders clinics and by respiratory physicians with special interest in sleep.

Treatment consists of relieving the cause of the respiratory obstruction and encourageing weight loss. Weight reduction is very effective (20), but nasal continuous positive airway pressure (NCPAP) is the treatment of choice. In this the patient wears a nasal mask at night through which a machine blows air at a prescribed pressure. Other procedures include nasal surgery, tracheostomy, and uvulopalatoplasty. SSRIs and theophylline may be helpful.

Narcolepsy

Narcolepsy is estimated to occur in 0.02 to 0.16 percent of adults and shows some familial incidence. It can occur at any age, but it most frequently begins in adolescence or young adulthood. The disorder either progresses slowly or reaches a plateau that is maintained throughout life.

Narcolepsy is a condition characterised by excessive sleepiness (there may be a continuous feeling of sleepiness, or periodic daytime sudden urges for sleep), cataplexy (sudden loss of skeletal muscle tone in response to emotion), hypnagogic and hypnopompic hallucinations, and fragmented night time sleep. The naps can occur while eating, talking, or driving (making this condition dangerous) and during sex, can last 10 to 20 minutes, after which the patient feels refreshed. All parasomnias are increased in narcolepsy, especially sleep paralysis. Narcolepsy results from a disturbance of centres in the brain that control the sleep-wake cycle, there is especially intrusion of REM sleep into wakefulness. The pathophysiology of narcolepsy involves the neuropeptide hypocretin (21).

The symptoms of narcolepsy can be misdiagnosed sometimes as those of anxiety, depression or personality disorder (22). Cataplexy has also been misdiagnosed as a conversion disorder. Narcolepsy is usually treated by a neurologist with special interest in sleep disorders or by specialist sleep centres. Investigations like polysomnography and Multiple Sleep Latency Test are needed as without the diagnosis of cataplexy, the diagnosis of narcolepsy cannot be made.

Although drug therapy is the treatment of choice, optimising alertness and daytime functioning is important. Modafinil does not produce dependence, reduces the number of sleep attacks and improves psychomotor performance in narcolepsy. Stimulant drugs (like methylphenidate, methamphetamine, and pemoline) to reduce daytime drowsiness may be required. Tricyclics, SSRIs and venlafaxine are also used to reduce cataplexy.

Parasomnias

Parasomnias are unusual or undesirable episodes that appear suddenly during sleep or at the threshold between waking and sleeping, and disturb the patient. They are exacerbated by anxiety and are associated with a high incidence of comorbid anxiety or depressive disorder. Some parasomnias can be considered primary sleep disorders, while others can be manifestations of physical conditions (e.g., epilepsy, asthma, cardiac arrhythmias) or psychiatric disorders (e.g., anxiety disorders especially PTSD). Sometimes there is more than one type of parasomnia reported by the same person. It should be remembered that like daytime, panic attacks can also occur at night. Parasomnias usually occur in stages III and IV of sleep and, therefore, there can be a poor recall of the episode.

Parasomnias arising from non-REM sleep include night terrors, sleep walking, sleep bruxism, sleep talking and head-banging. Nightmares, sleep paralysis, and REM behaviour disorder arise from REM sleep.

Night (Sleep) Terror Disorder

Night terrors are much less common than nightmares, and can be familial. Although predominantly a childhood disorder, it sometimes persists into adulthood. About one to six percent of children have the disorder, which is more common in boys than in girls. Polygraphic recordings of night terrors are somewhat like those of sleepwalking; in fact, the two conditions appear commonly in the same person.

Although in a typical case of night terrors, no signs of a seizure disorder are seen (either clinically or on EEG recordings), when night terrors begin in adolescence and young adulthood, they might turn out to be the first symptom of temporal lobe epilepsy. After few hours of going to sleep, the child (during NREM stages III and IV) sits up in a disoriented and terrified state, may scream, but after few minutes returns to sleep. The child either does not, or remembers very little about the episode. The night terror may develop into a sleepwalking episode, and the child may jump out of bed and start walking or running around. This obviously has high risks involved. The environment should, therefore, be made as safe as possible. As episodes are more dangerous in a strange and new environment such as a hotel. thereby having extra locks for doors, and steps to secure windows are recommended.

Explanation and reassurance to the parents is helpful. It is also advisable that attempts are not made to awaken the patient, as this will cause more confusion. If the episodes are frequent and occur more or less around the same time, waking the patient before that time (anticipatory waking), can be helpful (23).

Family situations should be explored particularly for stressful factors. Individual or family therapy is sometimes indicated and is useful. In some cases when medication is required, imipramine, paroxetine, and diazepam at bedtime improves the condition. However, the medication with the most evidence for efficacy is clonazepam (24). This has a long duration of action and it works by decreasing arousal from sleep.

Sleepwalking Disorder

Sleepwalking, also known as somnambulism, consists of automatic behaviour at night (NREM stage III and IV). The sufferer is unresponsive to the surroundings as well as people. Walking around is the usual behaviour, but sometimes people also urinate, dress, wash, and make tea, etc.

An affected person occasionally wakes up, with several minutes of confusion, but more frequently, the person returns to sleep without any recollection of the sleepwalking event.

Sleepwalking usually begins between ages 4 and 8 and tends to dissipate in adolescence. Lifetime prevalence is about 15–20%, peak prevalence being 12 years of age. Stressful periods are associated with increased sleepwalking in affected persons. Although it can be exacerbated by tiredness and sleep deprivation in childhood, it is not associated with psychiatric illness. The disorder can be dangerous because of the possibility of accidental injuries, and making the environment (especially strange and new) safe is of paramount importance. Educating and reassuring the parents is part of the treatment. Pharmacological treatment is the same as for night terrors.

Sleep Bruxism

Bruxism is tooth grinding at night. It occurs most prominently in stage II sleep. 5 to 10 percent of the population has sufficient bruxism to produce noticeable damage to teeth. Bed partners and roommates are consistently awakened by the sound. The sufferers complain of jaw aches or headaches in the morning. Treatment consists of a dental bite plate and corrective orthodontic procedures. Interventions to reduce stress, make healthy life style changes or strategies to improve coping mechanisms are helpful.

Sleep Starts and Sleep Talking (Somniloquy)

Sleep starts are muscle jerks that usually occur in light sleep, mostly during the first part of night. Although it is not a serious problem, sometimes the movements may become severe. Sleep talking is common in children and adults and occurs in light sleep as well. The talking usually involves a few words that are difficult to distinguish. Episodes of sleep talking sometimes accompany night terrors and sleepwalking. Sleep talking alone requires no treatment.

Head Banging

Head banging is quite common. Children engage in rhythmic to-and-fro head rocking, and less commonly, total body rocking. Sometimes this condition persists into adulthood. This is not strictly a disorder of non-REM sleep, as it occurs mostly at the beginning of the night.

Treatment consists of measures to prevent injury such as protection by extra pillows. Explanation and assurance to the sufferer as well as parents is also recommended.

Nightmares

In this disorder, the person wakes up from REM sleep to full consciousness and can recall the full dream (which often involves personal involvement). It is felt that recalling the dream several times during the day, increases the chances of it happening again the following night (25). The peak age in children is 5 or 6 years. Some persons have frequent nightmares as a lifelong condition; others experience them predominantly at times of stress and illness.

No specific treatment is usually required for nightmare disorder. Any identifiable cause should be looked into. Psychotherapy can be helpful. Guided imagery and exposure that attempts to change the imagery from fearful to pleasant content has been successfully used in nightmares sufferers with PTSD (26). Agents that suppress REM sleep, such as tricyclic drugs, may reduce the frequency of nightmares, and benzodiazepines have also been used.

Sleep Paralysis

This can be isolated or associated with narcolepsy. It is characterised by a sudden inability to execute voluntary movements, either just at the onset of sleep or on awakening during the night or in the morning. The cause is unknown, but the mechanism is an intrusion of the atonia (paralysis of skeletal muscles) which can be frightening, as there can be a crushing feeling of the chest. Episodes are more likely when the sleep pattern is disrupted, particularly by sleep loss or erratic timings. Isolated prevalence increases with anxiety disorders. Improving sleep hygiene and reassurance can be helpful. As sleep paralysis is terminated immediately when there is sensory input from the limbs, the sufferer can indicate to the bed partner by small movements or vocalisations. When the partner touches the arm, the episode ends (27). There is no established pharmacological treatment for sleep paralysis.

REM Behaviour Disorder

This disorder is of psychiatric and medico- legal interest (because of the potential injuries inflicted to the partner). It is characterised by episodes of complex, often violent, behaviour and is thought to represent a patient acting out his or her dreams. There is shouting and violent movements, with no awareness of the surroundings. The dreams are very vivid and violent, and the sufferer remembers them. There are often several episodes in a night. It is more common in older men, but occurs in both genders and in patients of all ages.

There is often a history of a small stroke or other CNS insult. There is also an association with Parkinson's disease, Lewy-body dementia and narcolepsy. Diagnosis is based on establishing a typical history and demonstration of REM sleep abnormalities on polysomnography. The most widely used treatment for REM behaviour disorder is clonazepam (0.5 to 2.0 mg a day). Carbamazepine, 100 mg three times a day, is also effective in controlling the disorder. It is important to remember that tricyclic antidepressants, SSRIs and venlafaxine, make this disorder worse.

Circadian Rhythm Sleep Disorders

Circadian rhythm sleep disorders are disturbances of the normal sleep-wake rhythm and include delayed sleep phase syndrome, advanced sleep phase syndrome, jet lag, and shift work sleep disorder.

Delayed Sleep Phase Syndrome

This simply means that sleep times are delayed relative to the desired or socially acceptable schedule. The sufferer has symptoms of both insomnia and hypersomnia. In this syndrome, the circadian system is operating in a delayed relationship to the day-night cues of the external world. The prevalence in the general population is 0.1 and 0.2%. Diagnosis is based on the patient's history and sleep diary for at least two weeks. Actigraphy assists and polysomnography is usually normal. It is also important to rule out psychotropic medication alcohol

The first major therapy for the delayed sleep- phase syndrome is chronotherapy, in which the patient is instructed to shift his or her hours of sleep and waking progressively later each night, until he or she has moved around the clock to a point at which he or she has a more traditional bedtime. An alternative approach is bright-light therapy in which the patient is exposed to bright artificial light in the early morning (28).

Advanced Sleep Phase Syndrome

This is a rare disorder in which habitual sleep and wake times occur 2–3 hours earlier than desired. There is early morning awakening and sleepiness in the late afternoon or early evening. Sleep history, sleep diaries and actigraphy can assist in the diagnosis. Depression has to be excluded. Treatment with bright light in the evening, so delaying sleep, may also delay awakening. Melatonin does not appear to be helpful, but temazepam and zopiclone have been successfully tried (29).

REFERENCES

1. Shochat, T., Loredo, J. and Anccoli-Israel, S. (2001). Sleep disturbance in the elderly. *Current Treatment Options in Neurology*, 3, 19–36.
2. Parrot, A. C. and Hindmarch, I. (1978). Factor analysis of a sleep evaluation questionnaire. *Psychological Medicine*, 8, 325–329.
3. Ellis, B. W., John, M. W., Lancaster, R., Raptopoulos, P., Angelopoulos, N. and Priest, R. G. (1981). *The St. Mary's Hospital sleep questionnaire*: A study of reliability. Sleep, 4, 93–97.
4. Stores, G. and Ebrahim, I. (2007). Sleep disorders. In G. Stein and G. Wilkinson (Eds.), *College seminars in general adult psychiatry* (pp. 588– 615). London: Royal College of Psychiatrists.
5. Wilson, S. and Nutt, David. (2008). *Sleep disorders*. Oxford: Oxford University Press.
6. Sadock, B. J. and Sadock, V. A. (2007). *Kaplan and Sadock's Synopsis of psychiatry*: Behavioural sciences/ clinical psychiatry (10th Edition). Philadelphia: Lippincott Williams and Wilkins.
7. Stores, G. and Ebrahim, I. (2007). Sleep disorders. In G. Stein and G. Wilkinson (Eds.), *College seminars in general adult psychiatry* (pp. 588– 615). London: Royal College of Psychiatrists.
8. Sadock, B. J. and Sadock, V. A. (2007). *Kaplan and Sadock's Synopsis of psychiatry*: Behavioural sciences/ clinical psychiatry (10th Edition). Philadelphia: Lippincott Williams and Wilkins.
9. Borbely, A. A. (1982). A two-process model of sleep regulation. *Human Neurobiology*, 1, 195– 204.
10. Leger, D., Poursain, B. (2005). An international survey of insomnia: Under recognition and under-treatment of a polysymptomatic condition. *Current Medical Research and Opinion*, 21, 1785–1792.
11. Stores, G. and Ebrahim, I. (2007). Sleep disorders. In G. Stein and G. Wilkinson (Eds.), *College seminars in general adult psychiatry* (pp. 588– 615). London: Royal College of Psychiatrists.
12. Schweitzer, P. K. (2005). Drugs that disturb sleep and wakefulness. In M. H. Kryger, T. Roth and W. C. Dement (Eds.), *Principles and practice of sleep medicine* (4th Edition, pp. 499–518). Philadelphia: Elsevier Saunders.
13. Sadock, B. J. and Sadock, V. A. (2007). *Kaplan and Sadock's Synopsis of psychiatry*: Behavioural sciences/ clinical psychiatry (10th Edition). Philadelphia: Lippincott Williams and Wilkins.
14. Gelder, M., Harrison, P. and Cowen, P. (2006). *Shorter Oxford textbook of psychiatry* (5th Edition). Oxford: Oxford University Press.
15. Kupfer, D. J. and Reynolds, C. F. (1997). Management of insomnia. *New England Journal of Medicine*, 336, 341–346.
16. Buscemi, N., Vandermeer, B., Hooten, N., Pandya, R., Tjosvold, L., Hartling, L., Baker, G., Klassen, T. P. and Vohra, S. (2005). The efficacy and safety of exogenous melatonin for primary sleep disorders. A meta-analysis. *Journal of General Internal Medicine*, 20, 1151–1158.
17. Wilson, S. and Nutt, David. (2008). *Sleep disorders*. Oxford: Oxford University Press.
18. Gelder, M., Harrison, P. and Cowen, P. (2006). *Shorter Oxford textbook of psychiatry* (5th Edition). Oxford: Oxford University Press.

19. Sadock, B. J. and Sadock, V. A. (2007). *Kaplan and Sadock's Synopsis of psychiatry*: Behavioural sciences/ clinical psychiatry (10th Edition). Philadelphia: Lippincott Williams and Wilkins.
20. Peppard, P. E., Young, T., Palta, M., Dempsey, J. and Skatrud, J. (2000). Longitudinal study of moderate weight change and sleep disordered breathing. *JAMA*, 284, 3015–3021.
21. Siegel, J. M. (1999). Narcolepsy: A key role for hypocretins (orexins). *Cell*, 121, 164–172.
22. Kryger, M. H., Walld, R. and Manfreda, J. (2002). Diagnosis received by narcolepsy patients in the year prior to diagnosis by a sleep specialist. *Sleep*, 25, 36–41.
23. Stores, G. and Ebrahim, I. (2007). Sleep disorders. In G. Stein and G. Wilkinson (Eds.), *College seminars in general adult psychiatry* (pp. 588– 615). London: Royal College of Psychiatrists.
24. Schenck, C. and Mohowald, M. (1996). Long-term, nightly benzodiazepine treatment of injurious parasomnias and other disorders of disrupted nocturnal sleep in 170 adults. *American Journal of Medicine*, 100, 333–337.
25. Wilson, S. and Nutt, David. (2008). *Sleep disorders*. Oxford: Oxford University Press.
26. Krakow, B., Hollifield, M., Johnston, L., Koss, M., Schrader, R., Arner, T. D., Tandberg, D., Lauriello, J., Mcbride, L., Cutchen, L., Cheng, D., Emmonsn, S., Germain, A., Melebdrez, D., Sandoval, D. and Prince, H. (2001). Imagery rehearsal therapy for chronic nightmares in sexual assault survivors with post-traumatic stress disorder: a randomised controlled trial. *JAMA*, 286, 537–545.
27. Wilson, S. and Nutt, David. (2008). *Sleep disorders*. Oxford: Oxford University Press.
28. Sadock, B. J. and Sadock, V. A. (2007). *Kaplan and Sadock's Synopsis of psychiatry*: Behavioural sciences/ clinical psychiatry (10th Edition). Philadelphia: Lippincott Williams and Wilkins.
29. Wilson, S. and Nutt, David. (2008). *Sleep disorders*. Oxford: Oxford University Press.

Psychosexual Disorders

CHAPTER 17

The majority of men and women occasionally have experiences that could be labelled as sexual dysfunctions or disorders. The most common are occasional failures to obtain or maintain an erection, or to ejaculate before they wish to do so in men, and in women failure to reach orgasm when they desire to do so. Others include sexual fantasies usually considered deviant. Many male adolescents carry out illegal sexual behaviours, that is, sexual offenses, such as sexual exhibitionism, voyeurism, and making obscene phone calls, most of which are not reported to authorities. The decision of what is normal sexual behaviour is arbitrary, determined by social attitudes. Masturbation and homosexuality, strongly condemned in the past as immoral and unnatural and subsequently became classified as sexual disorders, are now accepted as normal expressions of sexuality.

Given that the human sexual response is simultaneously a physiological, psychological, and, usually, relational phenomenon, the safe assumption in considering the aetiology of sexual dysfunction is that it is multifactorial.

Psychosexual problems are quite common and are very important. They are a major cause of personal distress and marital or relationships breakdown. In order to fully understand and treat sexual problems, one needs to have an adequate knowledge and understanding of sexual anatomy, physiology, and response. Unfortunately, this is beyond the scope of the book and readers are suggested to consult a specialist book like Sex Therapy: A Practical Guide (1).

A brief account of the sexual response described by Masters and Johnson (2) will be given here. In both females and males, a four-stage model has been described although some females do not achieve the third (orgasmic) stage. The first stage is the excitement phase, in which sexual arousal develops in response to sexual stimulation. This may be a physical stimulation or a fantasy. The second stage is the plateau phase and when a certain threshold is reached, it triggers orgasm (third stage). In this stage there is an involuntary release of sexual tension and ejaculation. In females, the pubococcygeus muscles contract rhythmically, the number of contractions vary between 5 and 15. After this, there is a resolution phase in which the body changes that have accompanied sexual arousal, return to normal. Males need a certain period before the cycle starts again, but some females are able to achieve multiple orgasms, without loss of arousal. However, contrary to popular belief, the number of orgasms a woman experiences may have no relationship to her degree of sexual satisfaction. About 10% of women never achieve orgasm (3). Some women report less need for orgasm during every session of sex (4).

Before psychosexual disorders are discussed, sexual orientation will be mentioned briefly. Sexual orientation refers to the person's attraction towards members of the same or opposite sex. According to Kinsey (5), many people cannot be strictly divided into homosexuals and heterosexuals as there can be a continuum, and these people can experience, to varying extent, both homosexual and heterosexual attraction and fantasies. They can engage in sexual activities with both sexes and also adopt lifestyles of both sexes. Another author has emphasised six criteria for sexual orientation: Sexual attraction, sexual fantasies, sexual behaviour, affectional relationship preference, lifestyle, and self-identification (6). In 1973, homosexuality per se was removed from the DSM classification of mental disorders and replaced by the category Sexual Orientation Disturbance. This represented a compromise between the view that preferential homosexuality is invariably a mental disorder and the view that it is merely a normal sexual variant. Homosexuality experience may be actual or imagined, and may or may not be accompanied by emotional involvement.

Psychosexual disorders can be grouped under the following headings:

- Gender-identity disorders in which a person's sense of being male or female is at variance with the anatomical sex
- Sexual dysfunctions, in which sexual performance fails to satisfy the subject or partner
- Sexual deviations in which sexual practice departs from convention in a way that distresses the subject or offends others

Gender Identity Disorders

Gender identity refers to the sense one has of being male or female which corresponds to the person's anatomical sex.

Transsexualism

In this disorder, there is a strong, persistent preference for living as a person of the opposite sex. There is dissatisfaction with one's designated birth sex and a desire to have the body of the other. The ICD-10 diagnostic criteria is that it should not be a symptom of any other mental disorder, and the desire has been persistent for at least two years.

Transsexual persons have a persistent preoccupation acquiring the sex characteristics of the other sex, and they wish to dress and live as a member of the other sex. They engage in activities associated with the other sex. They find their genitals repugnant, and many males insist on surgical intervention (removal of the testes and the penis to create an artificial vagina). Oestrogen is taken to create breasts, and men also have electrolysis to remove their hair.

Women bind their breasts or have a double mastectomy. They have a hysterectomy, removal of ovaries and the creation of artificial phallus. They may also take testosterone to build up muscle mass and deepen their voice. Debate continues regarding the capacity for sexual arousal by the patients after sex reassignment surgery.

Cross-Dressing

Cross-dressing is commonly known as transvestism. It is of two types. In dual-role transvestism, the individual wears clothes of the opposite sex to enjoy the temporary experience of membership of the opposite sex, without any desire for a permanent sex change. Moreover, no sexual excitement accompanies the cross-dressing.

In fetishistic transvestism, cross-dressing is done to obtain sexual excitement. Cross-dressing can coexist with paraphilias, such as sexual sadism, sexual masochism, and paedophilia. A combined approach, using psychotherapy and pharmacotherapy (anxiolytics and antidepressants), is often useful in the treatment of cross-dressing.

Sexual Dysfunctions

Sexual dysfunctions are defined as disturbances in the sexual response cycle or as pain during sexual intercourse. They can be lifelong or acquired, generalised or situational (limited to a specific partner or a certain situation). The great majority of sexual problems are multifactorial (7) and can result from psychological factors, physiological factors, or combined factors. Sexual function can be adversely affected by stress of any kind, by emotional disorders, or by ignorance of sexual function and physiology. Sexual disorders can lead to or result from relational problems and sexual dysfunctions can be associated with mental disorders.

Some organic causes of sexual dysfunctions include neurological disorders (multiple sclerosis, peripheral neuropathy), hormonal (pituitary tumours), vascular (blockage of larger vessels), pharmacological (antipsychotics, antidepressants), and pelvic problems (vaginitis, pelvic injuries) (8). Categories of sexual dysfunction include sexual desire disorders, sexual arousal disorders, orgasm disorders and sexual pain disorders.

Sexual Desire and Sexual Arousal Disorders

The presence of sexual desire depends on several factors: biological drive, adequate self- esteem, previous good experiences with sex, good relationship with the partner, and lack of organic reasons causing sexual dysfunction. In some people there can be either insufficient desire for sexual activity or sexual aversion. Lack of sexual desire can result from stress, anxiety, depression, or it can be an indicator of a relationship problem.

Female sexual arousal disorder is characterised by a recurrent partial or complete failure to attain or maintain the sexual response. A cream containing alprostadil has been developed to treat female sexual arousal disorder. The male erectile disorder is quite common and is characterised by the recurrent and persistent partial or complete failure to attain or maintain an erection to achieve vaginal penetration.

A man may be able to perform adequately in certain circumstances but not in others, in which case erectile disorder is a situational problem. The cause can be organic or psychological or a combination of both factors. Vacuum pumps are mechanical devices that patients, without vascular disease, can use to obtain erections. Penile prosthetic devices are available for men with inadequate erectile responses who are resistant to other treatment methods or who have medically caused deficiencies. When vascular insufficiency is present due to atherosclerosis or other blockages, bypass surgery of penile arteries has been attempted in selected cases with some success. The medications to treat erectile disorder are sildenafil, oral phentolamine, alprostadil, an injectable prostaglandin and a transurethral alprostadil.

Female Orgasmic Disorder (Anorgasmia)

Anorgasmia is defined as the recurrent or persistent inhibition of female orgasm although, as mentioned before, there is a range of orgasmic responses in women. Researchers differ in their opinion about orgasms caused by clitoral stimulation and those caused by vaginal stimulation. Some insist they are physiologically identical. The shaft of the clitoris is the masturbatory site preferred by many women, although others report greater satisfaction by vaginal orgasm. An area on the anterior wall of the vagina has been identified in women as a site of sexual excitation. It is known as the G-spot, but again there is a controversy about its existence.

Psychological factors for this disorder include fears of impregnation, rejection by a sex partner, damage to the vagina, hostility toward men, and feelings of guilt about sexual impulses. Regarding management of this problem, good communication with the partner is essential. Pelvic exercises to strengthen the pubococcygeus muscles are recommended for those women who have been orgasmic before, but are now anorgasmic. The women are suggested to initially masturbate, sometimes using a vibrator. A small suction cup is used that fits over the clitoral region and draws blood into the clitoris. Vibrators used to stimulate the clitoral area have been successful in treating anorgasmic women. Becoming Orgasmic by Heiman and Lopiccolo is a helpful book (9) for this disorder.

Male Orgasmic Disorder and Premature Ejaculation

The incidence of the male orgasmic disorder is much lower than the incidence of premature ejaculation or impotence. Sometimes it is called inhibited orgasm or retarded ejaculation. With this problem a man achieves delayed ejaculation during intercourse with great difficulty, if at all. Male orgasmic disorder is managed initially by extravaginal ejaculation and then by gradual vaginal entry after stimulation to a point near ejaculation.

Premature ejaculation is quite common and effects about 25% of men (10). In premature ejaculation, a man regularly ejaculates before or immediately after entering the vagina. Difficulty in ejaculatory control can be due to anxiety regarding the sex act, especially in young and inexperienced men.

The stop-start technique is commonly used for premature ejaculation (11). The man is taught to delay ejaculation by self-stimulation, and then stopping the stimulation before ejaculatory point is reached. After the sexual urge is diminished, he starts the stimulation again.

Squeeze technique is similar to the stop-start technique. In this the man or the woman stimulates the erect penis until the earliest sensations of approaching ejaculation are felt. At this point, the woman forcefully squeezes the coronal ridge of the glans, the erection is diminished, and ejaculation is inhibited. These exercises are repeated and they gradually raise the threshold of ejaculation (12). The technique is then applied during sexual intercourse.

Clomipramine and other SSRIs are also used for this disorder, the drugs being taken half an hour before the intercourse.

Sexual Pain Disorders

DSM-5 has merged vaginismus and dyspareunia into one diagnostic category of genito-pelvic/ penetration disorder. Dyspareunia is recurrent or persistent genital pain occurring in either men or women before, during, or after intercourse. Vaginismus is an involuntary muscle constriction of the outer third of the vagina that interferes with penile insertion and intercourse. Dyspareunia is more common in women than in men and frequently coincides with vaginismus. Repeated episodes of vaginismus can lead to dyspareunia and vice versa. Dyspareunia should not be diagnosed when an organic basis for the pain is found or when, in a woman, it is caused exclusively by vaginismus or by a lack of lubrication. Chronic pelvic pain is a common complaint in women with a history of rape or childhood sexual abuse. Painful intercourse can result from tension and anxiety about the sex act that causes women to involuntarily contract their vaginal muscles.

In cases of vaginismus, the main emphasis is on gradual retraining of the muscles surrounding the vagina to relax. The advice is to dilate vaginal opening with fingers or with graded dilators. When intercourse is attempted, it is preferable at first, for the woman to be on the top position (as she can then control the depth of penetration). Dilators are also used to treat cases of dyspareunia.

Sexual Deviations (Paraphilias)

Paraphilias (perversions) are largely male conditions. They are sexual acts that are deviations from normal sexual behaviours, are necessary for some persons to experience arousal and orgasm, and usually interfere with the capacity to establish sexual relationships.

The sexual activity of these persons is restricted to specific deviant stimuli. The essential features of paraphilias are recurrent, intense sexual urges, and sexually arousing fantasies generally involving: non-human objects; the suffering or humiliation of one's self or one's partner; or children or other non-consenting persons. Paraphilias may exist as an isolated and discrete anomaly in a stable personality, but many people have personality disorders, substance dependence, anxiety and affective disorders (13).

Exhibitionism

This is the most common of the paraphilias and is almost entirely present in heterosexual males. About two-thirds are married (14). Rarely do women, suffering from psychoses or intellectual disability, display this paraphilia. These women repeatedly expose breasts and very rarely their genitalia. Exhibitionism is the recurrent urge to expose the genitals to a person of the opposite sex, who is either a stranger or an unsuspecting person, without inviting or intending closer contact. Sexual excitement usually, but not invariably, occurs in anticipation of the exposure, and orgasm is brought about by masturbation during or after the event. If the victim shows fright, surprise, or disgust, the exhibitionist's excitement is enhanced.

There are two types of exhibitionists (15). Majority of men (about 80%) expose a flaccid penis. The second type expose an erect penis. They usually have antisocial personality and show no remorse or guilt. This group has poor prognosis.

Fetishism

Fetishism almost always occurs in men, who rely on some non-living object as a stimulus for sexual arousal and satisfaction. The sexual focus is on objects of the opposite sex (e.g., shoes, gloves, leather garments, and stockings). These objects have a central importance in achieving sexual arousal and orgasm (16). For homosexual fetishists, men's shoes are the most important object of sexual arousal (17). Some authors regard fetishistic behaviours along a spectrum that ranges from slight preference to a stage where the fetish object becomes a substitute for the partner entirely (18). Usually, the disorder begins by adolescence, runs a chronic course, and is difficult to treat.

Transvestic fetishism predominantly occurs in men. It is described as fantasies and sexual urges to dress in opposite gender clothing, as a means of arousal and as an adjunct to masturbation or intercourse. It typically begins in childhood or early adolescence.

Frotteurism

Frotteurism is characterised by recurrent, intense, sexual urges, and sexually arousing fantasies, involving touching and rubbing against a non-consensual person.

Usually, a man rubs his penis against the buttocks or other body parts of a fully clothed woman to achieve sexual satisfaction or orgasm. At other times, he may use his hands to rub an unsuspecting victim. The acts usually occur in crowded places, particularly in subways and buses. Those with frotteurism are extremely passive and isolated, and frottage is often their only source of sexual gratification.

Paedophilia

There has been a wide recognition in recent years that child sexual abuse is much more widespread than had been previously recognised. Paedophilia is the most common paraphilia, and now a matter of considerable concern. As a consequence of this paraphilia, children are frequently physically and psychologically damaged, many of them suffering permanent psychological harm and sexual maladjustment. It has been suggested that paedophiles account for about 30 percent of all homosexuals and are older than the other homosexuals. It has also been found that a considerable number of paedophiles are middle-aged and married.

Paedophilia involves recurrent intense sexual urges and sexually arousing fantasies of children. The age of children is generally 13 years or younger. The age of the paedophile is arbitrarily set at 16 years or older. Some paedophiles are attracted exclusively to children of a particular age. The level of contact ranges from touching, masturbating (or mutually masturbating), undressing, genital fondling, penetration with fingers or objects, and oral sex. Vaginal or anal penetration occurs infrequently, except in cases of incest. 95 percent of paedophiles are heterosexual. Some authors have classified paedophilia as primary or secondary (19). The primary paedophile is characterised by a consistent interest in children. It has been suggested that the repetitive fantasies of the paedophile resemble the repetitive phenomenon of obsessive-compulsive disorder.

Moreover, SSRIs have shown some response in a number of people suffering from this disorder (20). Although a majority of paedophiles do not have psychiatric disorder, some have a history of ADHD, major depression, and anxiety disorder (21).

Sexual Masochism

There is no distinct dividing line between sexual masochism and sexual sadism and the two predispositions are often interchangeable and exist in the same individual (22). Sexual masochism is more common among men than among women. The essential feature of this disorder is the urge to gain sexual gratification from the experience of being cruelly treated or humiliated. Although there are elements of sadomasochistic behaviour in ordinary sexual interplay, persons with sexual masochism have a recurrent preoccupation with sexual urges and fantasies involving the act of being humiliated, beaten, bound, or being defiled by being defecated or urinated on. Some people self-mutilate by arranging elaborate apparatus to inflict pain (for instance electrically) or engage in bondage (23). It has been suggested that the number of people who engage in sadomasochistic behaviour is not small (24). About 30 percent of those with sexual masochism also have sadistic fantasies. It had previously been assumed that women who take part in such activities were only prostitutes acting on behalf of their male clients, but later studies have shown that women who are not prostitutes also participate in masochistic activities (25).

Auto-eroticism or hypoxyphilia is a dangerous form of sexual masochism which involves sexual arousal and orgasm by means of oxygen deprivation. This is achieved by means of ligatures, noose, plastic bag, chest compression, or by using amyl nitrate (a vasodilating agent which temporarily decreases oxygen supply to the brain) (26). Death accidentally occurs sometimes. There are possibly 150 to 200 deaths per year in UK as a consequence of this activity (27).

Sexual Sadism

The onset of this disorder is usually before the age of 18 years and most persons with sexual sadism are male. In sexual sadism, there is sexual arousal, habitually and in preference to heterosexual intercourse, by inflicting pain on another person, by bondage or by humiliation (beating or whipping). The recurrent intense desire to give suffering to another provides sexual arousal and excitement.

DSM-5 criteria requires at least six month period of having recurrent and intense sexual arousal from the physical or psychological suffering of another person, as manifested by fantasies, urges, or behaviour (28). It usually comes to attention only in cases of rape, brutality, and lust murder (some sadistic rapists kill their victims after having sex). In some cases, these persons have underlying schizophrenia.

Voyeurism

Voyeurism, also known as scopophilia (the love of seeing), characterised by the recurrent preoccupation with fantasies and acts involving observing persons who are naked or engaged in sexual activity. Observing the sexual activity of others repeatedly is the preferred means of sexual excitement. Masturbation may take place during or after the event. This paraphilia is most common in heterosexual men, whose heterosexual activities are usually inadequate (29).

Telephone and Computer Scatologia

Telephone scatologia is characterised by obscene phone calling. Tension and arousal begin in anticipation of phoning; the recipient of the call listens while the telephoner (usually male) verbally exposes his preoccupations. The conversation is accompanied by masturbation, which is often completed after the contact is interrupted.

Persons also use interactive computer networks, sometimes compulsively, to send obscene messages by electronic mail and to transmit sexually explicit messages and video images (30).

Necrophilia

Necrophilia is an obsession with obtaining sexual gratification from having sex with dead people. Persons with this disorder find corpses in morgues or dig graves. This is a very rare disorder but may be associated with murder (31).

Partialism

Persons with this disorder concentrate their sexual activity on one part of the body to the exclusion of all others. Mouth genital contact such as cunnilingus (oral contact with a woman's external genitals), fellatio (oral contact with the penis), and anilingus (oral contact with the anus) is associated with normal foreplay for some people. But when a person uses these activities as the sole source of sexual gratification and cannot have or refuses to have coitus, a paraphilia exists.

Zoophilia

In this disorder animals are used for sexual activities, including intercourse, masturbation, and oral genital contact. Sex with animals may be a temporary activity because of unavailability of normal sexual contact with partner. When it becomes a persistent and the sole source of sexual gratification, it is a disorder.

Coprophilia, Klismaphilia, Urophilia and Apotemnophilia

Coprophilia is sexual pleasure associated with the desire to defecate on a partner or to be defecated on.

Klismaphilia is the use of enemas as part of sexual stimulation.

Urophilia, a form of urethral eroticism, is interest in sexual pleasure associated with the desire to urinate on a partner or to be urinated on.

Apotemnophilia refers to individuals who become sexually aroused by people who are in some way crippled or have an amputation (32).

Masturbation

Masturbation is a normal activity that is common in all stages of life. It can be defined as a person's achieving sexual pleasure which usually results in orgasm by himself or herself (autoeroticism). Masturbation is abnormal when it is the only type of sexual activity performed in adulthood, and when it is consistently preferred to sex with a partner.

Sex Addiction and Compulsivity

Some persons entire life revolves around sex- seeking behaviour and activities, and they spend an excessive amount of time in such behaviour. Nymphomania signifies a woman's excessive or pathological desire for coitus. These patients usually have one or more sexual disorders. The woman often has an intense fear of losing love and, through her actions, attempts to satisfy her dependence needs rather than gratify her sexual impulses. This disorder is a form of sex addiction.

Prognosis and Treatment of Paraphilias

Early age of onset, a high frequency of acts, no guilt or shame about the act, and substance abuse are poor prognostic features. The course and the prognosis are better when patients have a history of normal intercourse in addition to the paraphilia. Other good prognostic indicators include the presence of only one paraphilia, normal intelligence, the absence of non-sexual antisocial personality traits, and the presence of a successful adult attachment (33). Antipsychotic or antidepressant medication is indicated for the treatment of schizophrenia or depressive disorders if the paraphilia is associated with these disorders. Antiandrogens, such as cyproterone acetate and medroxyprogesterone acetate may reduce the sexual drive. Cognitive-behavioural therapy is effective in stopping and modifying abnormal behaviour. Finally, insight-oriented psychotherapy has also been tried successfully in some people.

REFERENCES

1. Hawton, K. (1985). *Sex therapy. A practical guide.* Oxford: Oxford University Press.
2. Masters, W. H. and Johnson, V. E. (1966). *Human sexual response*. London: Churchill.
3. Masters, W. H., Johnson, V. E. and Kolodny, R.C. (1995). *Human sexuality* (5th Edition). New York: Harper Collins.
4. Hawton, K. (1985). *Sex therapy. A practical guide.*Oxford: Oxford University Press.
5. Kinsey, A. C., Pomeroy, W. B. and Martin, C. E. (1948). *Sexual behaviour in the human male.* Philadelphia: Saunders.
6. Klien, F., Sepekoff, B. and Wolf, T. J. (1985). Sexual orientation: A multiple variable, dynamic process. *Journal of Homosexuality*, 11, 35.
7. Kinsey, A. C., Pomeroy, W. B. and Martin, C. E. (1948). *Sexual behaviour in the human male*. Philadelphia: Saunders.
8. Crowe, M. (1998). Sexual therapy and the couple pages. In H. Freeman, I. Pullen, G. Stein and G. Wilkinson (Eds.), *Seminars in psychosexual disorders* (pp. 59–83). London: Royal College of Psychiatrists.
9. Heiman, J. R. and lopiccolo, J. (1999). *Becoming orgasmic* (2nd Edition). London: Piatkus.
10. Sanders, D. (1987). *The woman report on men*.London: Sphere Books.
11. Semans, J. H. (1956). *Premature ejaculation, a new approach.* Southern Medical Journal, 49, 353–357.
12. Sadock, B. J. and Sadock, V. A. (2007). *Kaplan and Sadock's Synopsis of psychiatry*: Behavioural sciences/ clinical psychiatry (10th Edition). Philadelphia: Lippincott Williams and Wilkins.
13. Brockman, B. and Bluglass, R. (1997). A general psychiatric approach to sexual deviation. In I.Rosen (Ed.), *Sexual deviation* (3rd Edition). Oxford: Oxford University Press.
14. Gayford, J. J. (1981). Indecent exposure: A review of the literature. *Medicine, Science and the Law*, 21, 233–242.
15. Rooth, F. G. (1971). Indecent exposure and exhibitionism. *British Journal of Hospital Medicine*, 5, 521–533.
16. Sims, A. C. P. (1988). *Symptoms in the mind: An introduction to descriptive psychopathology*. London: Balliere Tindall.
17. Weinberg, M. S., Williams, C. J. and Calhan, C. (1994). Homosexual foot fetishism. *Archives of Sexual Behaviour*, 23, 611–626.
18. Gebhard, P. H. (1969). Fetishism and sado- masochism. In J. H. Masermann (Ed.), *Dynamics of deviant sexuality* (pp. 71). New York: Grune and Stratton.
19. Glasser, M. (1990). Paedophilia. In R. Bluglass and P. Bowden (Eds.), *Principles and practice of forensic psychiatry*. Edinburgh: Churchill Livingstone.
20. Bradford, J. W. M. (2001). The neurobiology, neuropharmacology and pharmacological treatment of the paraphilias and compulsive behaviour. *Canadian Journal of Psychiatry*, 46, 26–33.
21. Kafka, M. P. and Prentky, R. A. (1988). Attention deficit hyperactivity disorder in males with paraphilia and paraphilia related disorders: A comorbidity study. *Journal of Clinical Psychiatry*, 59, 388–396.
22. Brockman, B. and Bluglass, R. (1997). A general psychiatric approach to sexual deviation. In I.Rosen (Ed.), *Sexual deviation* (3rd Edition). Oxford: Oxford University Press.
23. Brockman, B. and Bluglass, R. (1997). A general psychiatric approach to sexual deviation. In I.Rosen (Ed.), *Sexual deviation* (3rd Edition). Oxford: Oxford University Press.
24. Storr, A. (1990). Sadomasochism. In R. Bluglass and P. Bowden (Eds.), *Principles and practice of forensic psychiatry*. Edinburgh: Churchill Livingstone.
25. Baumeister, R. F. (1988). Gender difference in masochistic scripts. *Journal of Sex Research*, 25, 478–499.
26. Trigell Pand Kirk, G. (2007). Psychosexual medicine for psychiatrists. In G. Stein and G. Wilkinson (Eds.), *College seminars in general adult psychiatry* (pp. 668–696). London: Royal College of Psychiatrists.
27. Hucker, S. (1990). Sexual asphyxia. In R. Bluglass and P. Bowden (Eds.) *Principles and practice of forensic psychiatry* Edinburgh: Churchill Livingstone.
28. American Psychiatric Association.(2013). *Diagnostic and statistical manual of mental disorders* (5th Edition). Arlington, VA: American Psychiatric
29. Gelder, M., Harrison, P. and Cowen, P. (2006). *Shorter Oxford textbook of psychiatry* (5th Edition). Oxford: Oxford University Press.
30. Sadock, B. J. and Sadock, V. A. (2007). *Kaplan and Sadock's Synopsis of psychiatry*: Behavioural sciences/ clinical psychiatry (10th Edition). Philadelphia: Lippincott Williams and Wilkins.
31. Hucker, S. J. and Stermac, L. (1992). The evaluation and treatment of sexual violence, necrophilia, and asphyxiophilia. *Psychiatric Clinics of North America*, 15,703–719.
32. Goodman, R. E. (1998). The paraphilias: an evolutionary and developmental perspective. In H. Freeman, I. Pullen, G. Stein and G. Wilkinson (Eds.), *Seminars in psychosexual disorders* (pp. 142– 155). London: Royal College of Psychiatrists.
33. Sadock, B. J. and Sadock, V. A. (2007). *Kaplan and Sadock's Synopsis of psychiatry*: Behavioural sciences/ clinical psychiatry (10th Edition). Philadelphia: Lippincott Williams and Wilkins.

Eating Disorders 18

In the current psychiatric nomenclature of the Diagnostic and Statistical Manual of Mental Disorders, Fifth Edition (DSM-5), the feeding and eating disorders category includes three previously defined eating disorder syndromes: Anorexia Nervosa, Bulimia Nervosa, and Binge-Eating Disorder. The three conditions that were modified and moved from the section on Feeding and Eating Disorders of Infancy or Early Childhood in DSM-IV-TR are Pica, Rumination Disorder, and Avoidant/ Restrictive Food Intake Disorder.

It has been debated whether the various eating disorders are fundamentally different. They share the core symptoms e.g., preoccupation with food, disturbed body perception, and inadequate sexual behaviour. Bulimic eating disorders appear to exist on a continuum of clinical severity, from binge-eating disorder (least severe), through non-purging type bulimia nervosa (intermediate severity), to purging-type bulimia nervosa (most severe). The spectrum hypothesis considers all eating disorders as different manifestations of a single disorder or syndrome.

The term disordered eating behaviour is used to indicate those instances in which the nutritional disturbances arise from the person's abnormal eating behaviour patterns, rather than from medical or social factors. For example, fasting for religious or political purposes would not be classified as an eating disorder. Overweight means that weight is higher than normal. Obesity implies there is an excess of body fat that is, but not always, the result of increased food intake and decreased physical activity.

Obesity is one of the major health problems of the developed world and is also becoming more common in developing countries. An increase in the intra-abdominal fat is the primary cause of insulin resistance, which in turn, leads to hypertension, high blood fats, diabetes mellitus, and atherosclerosis. There is, understandably, increased mortality. It is more prevalent in females and in the lower social class. Obesity is not considered a psychiatric disorder because it is not associated with consistent behavioural and psychological problems. However, some people, especially females, may feel depressed as a consequence of obesity. Management strategies for obesity include behavioural therapy for weight control, emphasis on healthy eating, encourageing physical activities, pharmacological as well as surgical treatment, the last one for extreme cases.

Anorexia nervosa and bulimia nervosa are considered eating disorders because they are associated with a defined and consistent group of behavioural and psychological issues. Other eating disorders which do not fulfil the diagnostic criteria for anorexia nervosa or bulimia nervosa are classified under the groups, called atypical eating disorders or eating disorders not otherwise specified. Binge-eating disorder which indicates bulimia without compensatory behaviours to prevent weight gain, is more common than anorexia nervosa and bulimia nervosa, and is included as eating disorder not otherwise specified. Binge-eating disorder is associated with obesity and has a better outcome than bulimia nervosa. Patients suffering from atypical eating disorders or eating disorders not specified, may go on to develop anorexia nervosa or bulimia nervosa, but it is very rare that anorexia nervosa patients develop bulimia nervosa and vice versa.

ICD-10 Classification of Eating Disorders

- Anorexia nervosa
- Atypical anorexia nervosa
- Bulimia nervosa
- Atypical bulimia nervosa
- Overeating associated with other psychological disturbances
- Vomiting associated with other psychiatric disorders

Anorexia Nervosa

Anorexia nervosa is a condition characterised by self-induced weight loss, preoccupation with body weight and food, peculiar patterns of handling food, intense fear of gaining weight, disturbance of body image and amenorrhea. It is usually seen in adolescent girls and young women. It occurs less commonly in prepubertal children, middle-aged women or men. Patients perceive themselves as being fat even though they are emaciated. They are quite convinced about their body being overweight and are either preoccupied with the methods to reduce their weight or to prevent having a further gain. The obsessions concerning food and weight are egosyntonic in these patients. The core psychopathology is usually an overvalued idea rather than a delusion.

These patients are continually engaged to either maintain or increase their weight loss. Patients avoid high energy foods, drastically reduce their daily intake, abuse laxatives and diuretics, and indulge in strenuous exercise. Since they typically dread gaining weight, they very frequently watch mirrors to reassure themselves that they are not gaining weight. Their denial of the gravity of medical implications of their malnourished state allows them to believe that slimness can solely define their self-worth.

The idea that the self-worth may be increased by being slim is usually (but not always) the initial motivation for caution in eating which then leads to anorexia nervosa. Many people who are trying to be slender usually give up the efforts to lose further weight in response to their bodies' regulatory responses. Somehow, for some reasons, the future anorectic patients persist in their efforts at losing further weight and become caught up in the vicious cycle. Unfortunately, the more these patients try to control their eating and weight, the more this seems to be out of control, which maintains their abnormal behaviour.

Some patients suffering from anorexia nervosa also suffer from depressive disorder, and others may have symptoms like irritability, social withdrawal, obsessional ruminations, and disturbed concentration. Very often, patients with anorexia nervosa develop an obsession with cleanliness and become excessively involved in housecleaning activities. Obsessive-compulsive disorder is considerably higher in first degree relatives of anorexia nervosa. There is a high comorbidity with depressive disorder which is present in almost 70% of cases of anorexia nervosa. A calculation of the individual's Body-Mass Index (BMI) is the best way to measure the extent to which an individual is underweight or overweight. The BMI can be calculated by dividing the individual's weight by the square of his or her height.

The diagnostic criteria of ICD-10 and DSM- 5 are very similar. DSM-5, however, divides anorexia nervosa into two subtypes. The classical form is called restricting type while the other category is called binge-eating/purging type. Patients suffering from the latter type regularly indulge in binging and purging behaviour. DSM-5 has eliminated the requirement of amenorrhea for anorexia nervosa. For bulimia nervosa, there is now a reduction in the required minimum average frequency of binge-eating and inappropriate compensatory behaviour frequency from twice to once weekly.

ICD-10 Diagnostic Criteria for Anorexia Nervosa

All of the following are required:

a. Weight is maintained at least 15% below that expected (either lost or never achieved), or Quetelet's body-mass index is 17. 5 or less.
b. Weight loss is self-induced by avoidance of food causing fatness and by one or more method of weight loss: Self-induced vomiting; self-induced purging; excessive exercise; use of appetite suppressants and/or diuretics.
c. Self-perception of being too fat. There is psychopathology involving an over-valued idea about body-image distortion, and dread of fatness dominates the patient's life.
d. A widespread endocrine disorder involving the hypothalamic-pituitary-gonadal axis exists. There is amenorrhoea in women and loss of sexual interest in men.
e. In case the onset is prepubertal, the sequence of pubertal events is delayed or even arrested.

Restricting Type

During the current episode of anorexia nervosa, the person has not regularly engaged in binge-eating or purging behaviour (i.e. self-induced vomiting or the misuse of laxatives, diuretics or enemas).

Binge-Eating/Purging Type

During the current episode of anorexia nervosa, the person has regularly engaged in binge-eating or purging behaviour.

Differential Diagnosis of Anorexia Nervosa

Somatic causes of weight loss in patients e.g., Chronic debilitating diseases, brain tumours, Crohn's disease, malabsorption syndrome, diabetes mellitus, hyperthyroidism, Addison's disease, Human Immunodeficiency Virus (HIV)/Acquired Immunodeficiency Syndrome (AIDS), and chronic infectious disease, need to be distinguished. However, it is not advisable to encourage extensive and invasive medical investigations if the patient's symptoms can be explained adequately by the diagnosis of anorexia nervosa or any other eating disorder. The physical signs that help to confirm the diagnosis of an eating disorder are Russell's sign (calluses on the knuckles or back of the hand due to repeated self-induced vomiting over long periods of time), erosion of teeth, parotid and submandibular gland hypertrophy, hypercarotenemia and lanugo hair.

Depressive, anxiety, and obsessional symptoms are quite common, and there may be features of personality disorder. Patients suffering from clinical depression may lose weight with the loss of appetite or motivation to eat. However, people with anorexia nervosa do not lose appetite; rather they choose not to eat in spite of hunger and desire for food. Similarly, unlike anorexia nervosa, they do not exhibit excessive concern about their body shape or the caloric content of food. Moreover, unlike those who are depressed, people with anorexia nervosa are pleased about their weight loss. Anxiety about eating with others may be a symptom of social phobia.

Atypical Anorexia Nervosa

This term is used for those cases of eating disorders in which one or more key features of anorexia nervosa, such as amenorrhoea or significant weight loss, are absent but who otherwise present a fairly typical clinical picture. In addition, those patients who have all the main symptoms but only to a mild degree are also described by this term. However, this term should not be used for eating disorders that resemble anorexia nervosa but are due to known physical illness.

Epidemiology of Anorexia Nervosa

Anorexia nervosa has low prevalence, usually has a long course and is associated with serious medical and psychiatric morbidity as well as high mortality. A third of patients fail to recover and many among this group die prematurely (1). Another 9–14 year follow-up showed that over 20% of patients were unable to support themselves independently (2). Incidence of new cases is 7 per 100,000 (3). Females are ten times more likely to have this disorder. The lifetime risk for females is between 0.2% and 0.5%. The possible reasons for this female preponderance includes the effects of oestrogen and zinc on neurotransmitters, the fact that weight gain and excessive fatty tissue associated with puberty are more prominent in girls, and the higher importance females attach to their weight and the shape of their body. There is no substantial evidence that this disorder is increasing among males.

However, the age of onset is widening as now more prepubertal children and older people are increasingly being affected. Patients with anorexia disorder are 30 times more likely to die as a result of suicide as compared to the general population. Unlike the commonly held view, anorexia nervosa is not restricted to the upper and middle class but is distributed evenly between different social classes in the developed countries. Although it is also present in developing countries, the incidence is quite low.

Aetiology

In seventy percent of the cases the onset of anorexia nervosa follows a life event (4). The precise cause and pathogenesis for anorexia nervosa (and bulimia nervosa) is unknown. The aetiology is usually seen as multi-factorial or multidimensional, taking into account genetic factors, social factors, psychological causes and family causes. It is thought that perfectionism, asceticism, obsessionality and maturity fears may be vulnerability factors.

Regarding biological factors, one hypothesis is that there may be abnormal regulation of body composition and appetite. Evidence to support this model is the tendency for leanness to run in families. Another biological model states that temperamental traits, such as harm avoidance and persistence, may be either moderating or mediating factors (5).

Many persons develop amenorrhoea before weight loss has occurred, and return to a normal menstrual cycle often lags behind the return to normal body weight. This fact has given support to the view there is a primary hypothalamic dysfunction in patients with anorexia nervosa. The resumption of menses in anorexia nervosa is associated with marked psychological improvement after weight gain.

It has been postulated, that anorexia nervosa constitutes a phobic avoidance response to food, resulting from the sexual and social tension generated by the physical changes associated with puberty. Slimness as a feature of attractiveness is advocated in some cultures (especially Western). Some people diet for the purpose of being more attractive while others for being more professionally competent. For example ballet dancers, jockeys and gymnasts, have a higher risk for developing an eating disorder. It has also been postulated that some women diet vigorously in response to the stress caused by professional and social demands. According to some authors, dieting behaviour is the instigating and common stimulus that leads to the development of serious eating disorders. Psychological and physiological reinforcement of the maladaptive eating behaviour constitutes a sustaining cycle of core dysfunctions in eating disorder behaviour. Unlike the commonly held view, there is little evidence to support gross disturbance in family functioning (6). Although anorexia develops in all social classes, there is a tendency for women with anorexia nervosa to join in the efforts to attain a higher ranking (7).

Medical Complications of Anorexia Nervosa

Anorexia nervosa causes a wide variety of physical problems, many of which are quite significant.

- Neurological: Seizures, peripheral neuritis, increase in ventricular size in brain, decrease in brain substance
- Cardiovascular: Bradycardia, hypotension, poor circulation, arrhythmias, faints, prolonged Q-T interval, cold, blue peripheries, cardiomyopathy, mitral valve prolapse, peripheral oedema and heart failure
- Metabolic: Hypoglycaemia, hypercholesterolaemia
- Endocrine: Amenorrhoea and reduced fertility, increased growth hormone, decreased oestrogens and testosterone
- Haematological: Leucopenia, anaemia
- Gastrointestinal: Parotid enlargement, de-ntal caries, delayed gastric emptying, acute gastric dilatations, peptic ulcers, superior mesenteric artery syndrome, constipation, acute pancreatitis and hepatitis
- Renal: Acute/chronic renal failure, renal stones
- Musculoskeletal and skin: Osteoporosis, stunted growth, pathological fractures, muscle cramps, lanugo hair, purpura and conjunctival haemorrhage, brittle hair and nails
- Other: Hypothermia, bacterial infections, increased miscarriages, vulnerability to infections

Course and Prognosis

The average duration of the disorder is 6 years (8). The shorter the history, the better will be the prognosis. One-fifth of patients make full recovery. In severe cases with long history (30 years), there can be 15–20% mortality. Approximately one half of the deaths result from medical complications and the rest result from suicide. About 25% remain chronically ill, either maintaining a low body weight or developing bulimia with wide fluctuations in weight.

Those patients who recover from anorexia nervosa, usually return to normal life. Patients can achieve pregnancy and normal childbirth. There is no permanent damage to the heart or kidneys However, permanent damage such as loss or erosion of teeth, Karsakoff 's syndrome and osteopenia may occur. Constipation, bloating, and abdominal pains can sometimes last for decades. Osteoporosis may lead to chronic pain and disability.

Poor Prognostic Factors are:

- Later age of onset
- Long duration of illness
- Presence of vomiting in malnourished patient
- History of personality problems
- Disturbed family relationships

Favourable Prognostic Factors are:

- Absence of severe emaciation (i.e. body mass index >17)
- Absence of serious medical complications
- High motivation to change
- Supportive family and friends

Assessment

Even if the diagnosis is obvious, it is essential to do a usual and comprehensive mental state examination. Similarly, the routine psychiatric history should include special attention to details regarding weight, and eating patterns. Lifetime weight history (including highest ever and premorbid stable weight), history of restricted eating, use of abnormal weight control methods (vomiting, laxatives and diuretics, etc.), presence of binging, ideas of loss of control of weight and eating, disturbance of body image, and use of exercise, are mandatory details (9). As it is common for people to deny their dieting behaviours and to downplay the severity of their symptoms, clinicians should maintain a high level of suspicion for this disorder.

Assessment of physical state is similarly very important, as there is a significant mortality from physical complications. ECG, full blood count, urea and electrolytes, glucose, calcium and phosphate levels, thyroid function tests, bone density, and liver function tests are some of the essential investigations. It is important to rule out organic causes of weight loss e.g., Inflammatory bowel disease, malignancy, diabetes or hypothyroidism.

Management

Although there is not much problem diagnosing anorexia nervosa, its management poses challenges. Some patients are ambivalent about treatment while others exhibit significant resistance. The disorder causes disability in physical, psychological and social domains.

Patients in the early phase of the disorder are quite reluctant to admit that there is something wrong and that they need treatment. They may, however, be concerned about their poor concentration that affects their day-to-day activities e.g., studies, or they might be concerned that their hair is falling out. In fact, it helps to concentrate on the physical complaints, since patients find it much easier to talk about their physical concerns. Since treatment of physical problems is generally accepted easily and is appreciated, it helps in developing rapport and therapeutic alliance. As these patients can be quite resistant to treatment, it is, therefore, very important to engage these patients in a constructive dialogue. The need for a confident and trusting working relationship cannot be overstated.

At presentation, many patients are ambivalent about treatment, and few wish to gain weight in spite of their life-threatening emaciation. Motivational interview techniques can be very helpful. Reflective listening and empathic understanding are used to enhance motivation. The correction of mistaken assumptions and clarification of negative issues, such as the profound psychological, social and medical consequences of starvation, are key components of treatment.

As family plays an important role, it is also very desirable to have a good relationship with the family members who, also need to be given essential information and education. There are often powerful feelings of guilt and anger that family members hold towards the patient. Families need to be advised against constant nagging about eating or getting over-involved with the patient. There is a need to minimise the time of untreated symptoms early in the illness. On the other hand, those patients who have a persistent and chronic course need help with the factors which are contributing to the maintenance of the symptoms. Recovery from anorexia nervosa becomes difficult the longer duration the illness has persisted (10).

One of the main aims of management is restoration of weight that is normal and sustainable. Patients are encouraged to develop a regular pattern of eating. The weight target is usually the average one (BMI 18–25). The second important task is to attempt to disentangle the ideas about eating and weight from issues such as self-esteem. The medical manifestations of anorexia nervosa that impair physical function or are threats to life must be treated promptly.

Medication

There is little evidence that drug treatments are helpful in modifying and improving weight or the basic psychopathology of anorexia nervosa. However, there may be some role of drugs in the treatment of some symptoms (e.g., bloating). Moreover, medication may be needed to treat comorbid disorders e.g., Antidepressant therapy for depressive disorder. There is some evidence that fluoxetine may prevent relapse after in-patient treatment.

Dietary Plan

For in-depth dietary advice the expertise of a dietician is sometimes needed but is not essential as most patients only lack the common sense about diet. The idea is to encourage the patient to have a gradually increased food intake at a pace that is manageable for the patient. It is helpful to give regular vitamin supplements to those patients who are quite malnourished.

Treating Medical Complications

All the medical manifestations of anorexia nervosa which have consequently developed have to be adequately treated. For example, it is urgently desirable to restore normal electrolytes, and treat severe anaemia and hypothermia. Osteoporosis is another serious and common complication of chronic anorexia. Similarly, hypokalaemia, associated with vomiting and purgative use can be extreme.

In-Patient Treatment

A third of patients do not make satisfactory improvement on an out-patient basis and require admission. This group usually has a comparatively poor prognosis. In some cases, compulsory admission is indicated and food is considered treatment under the Mental Health Act.

Admission is required when the physical status of the patient deteriorates to the extent of posing danger to life, there is a risk of suicide, for the treatment of a comorbid disorder, intolerable family situation or failure of out-patient treatment. A BMI of less than 13.5 is considered dangerously low.

One of the main goals of treatment is to promptly assist weight gain, and restore nutritional status. A skilled multi-disciplinary team can establish collaborative working relationships with patients. A target weight should be negotiated and agreed upon with the patient. The aimed calorie intake would be 3000 calories a day as a weight gain of 1–2 kg per week is a reasonable target for in-patients (a lower rate of weight gain is generally acceptable for out-patients). As fats, carbohydrates and proteins are all necessary components of a healthy diet, a mixed diet is, therefore, encouraged. The attitude of the clinician(s) needs to be reassuring, sympathetic, and encourageing. Dedicated and skilled nursing staff are invaluable in helping these patients. There is no evidence to suggest that strict regimes are any more effective than those that are more lenient (11). Harsh behavioural regimes are not effective in terms of long-term compliance and acceptability by the patient.

Psychotherapeutic Interventions

Thinness is held as the principal construct on which patients base their self-esteem and self- worth. Cognitive Behaviour Therapy (CBT) is aimed at rectifying faulty beliefs about food and weight and is also helpful in changing the characteristic ascetic, self-punitive, and self-denying beliefs from which the abnormal behaviour derives. In CBT, there is explicit emphasis on beliefs, assumptions, and schematic processing, which are accountable for maladaptive emotions and behaviours.

Family therapy in anorexia nervosa is based on the premise that a change in the family system will result in a reduction in abnormal eating behaviour. Family therapy produces a good long-term outcome in young patients with a short duration of illness. Many studies have demonstrated the effectiveness of family therapy applied early in the course of the illness (12). Cognitive analytical therapy, supportive psychotherapy, interpersonal therapy and psychodynamic therapy have also been tried with sporadic success.

Bulimia Nervosa

This disorder is related to anorexia nervosa by virtue of sharing the same psychopathology (a morbid dread of fatness and distorted body image). There is often, but not always, a history of an earlier episode of anorexia nervosa, the interval between the two disorders ranging from a few months to several years. Bulimia nervosa usually begins from a period of a few weeks to a year or even longer after dieting. It is a syndrome characterised by repeated bouts of overeating and excessive preoccupation with the control of body weight. Patients adopt extreme measures to mitigate the 'fattening 'effects of the ingested food. Although binge-eating behaviour is an essential criteria, there is little consensus on what constitutes a binge and what is acceptable as the minimum binge frequency for bulimia nervosa.

According to some authors, binge-eating is defined as eating more than most people would in similar circumstances in a similar period of time. The average length of a binging episode is about one hour. The sense of losing control is a significant subjective aspect that occurs in binge-eating. The food consumed during a binge episode usually has a high dense calorie content. Some patients have abrasions and scars on the backs of their hands from sticking their fingers down their throat to induce vomiting. Many patients with bulimia nervosa have been at the upper end of a normal weight range or slightly overweight. After developing the disorder, they usually choose a weight at the lower end of a normal weight. About ten percent of patients have been markedly over weight. Although patients with bulimia nervosa may be concerned about their weight, they are less distressed as compared to those suffering from anorexia nervosa and are consequently less driven in their efforts to lose weight. One reasonable explanation for this is that the actual binge-eating episode provides them a sense of relief from anxiety and can thus become a rewarding behaviour. The recurrent use of inappropriate compensatory behaviours to avoid weight gain (purging) include self-induced vomiting, laxative or very restrictive dieting.

Bulimia nervosa is further classified into letter purging and non-purging type. Patients in the latter group use strict dieting, fasting or vigorous exercise but do not regularly engage in purging. These patients tend to be obese. People with bulimia nervosa are often impulsive and in contrast to anorexia nervosa, indulge in taking over doses or cutting their wrists. Unlike anorexia nervosa, bulimia nervosa has a better prognosis and a shorter course. Bulimia nervosa has a prevalence rate of about 1 percent in adolescent and young adult women. The bias towards females is not as strong as anorexia nervosa. It is associated with personality disorders and substance abuse. There is a significant prevalence with mood disorders and substance abuse is not unusual.

Bulimia nervosa patients who engage in self- induced vomiting and abuse purgative or diuretic medications are prone to develop the same medical complications as anorexia nervosa patients involved in this behaviour. About half of the patients with bulimia nervosa make a full recovery (with cognitive-behaviour therapy). After a 10 year follow-up, about 10% of patients still meet the criteria. Aetiology includes general risk factors of psychiatry disorder and the risk factors for dieting. There can be a family history of depression, adverse childhood experiences, personality traits like perfectionism and low self-esteem, and inherited abnormality in the regulation of weight and eating.

ICD-10 Diagnostic Criteria

For a definite diagnosis, all of the following are required:

- Persistent preoccupation with eating, and an irresistible craving for food; the patient succumbs to episodes of overeating in which large amounts of food are consumed in relatively short periods of time.
- Attempts to counteract the 'fattening' effects of food by self-induced vomiting; purgative abuse, alternating periods of starvation; use of drugs such as appetite suppressants, thyroid preparations or diuretics.
- Self-perception of being too fat. The patients set themselves a sharply defined weight threshold, well below the premorbid weight that constitutes the optimum or healthy weight.

Differential diagnosis of bulimia nervosa includes, upper gastrointestinal disorders leading to repeated vomiting (but where characteristic psychopathology is absent), a more general abnormality of personality (the eating disorder may co-exist with alcohol dependence and small offences as shoplifting), and depressive disorder (bulimic patients often experience depressive disorders). Rarely, central nervous system tumour may be associated with bulimic behaviours. Overeating episodes also occur in the Kluver-Bucy syndrome, which consists of visual agnosia, compulsive licking and biting, inability to ignore any stimulus, and hypersexuality. Kleine-Levin syndrome is another rare syndrome associated with hyperphagia. It is characterised by periodic hypersomnia lasting for several weeks.

Atypical Bulimia Nervosa

This term is used for those individuals in whom one or more key diagnostic features of bulimia nervosa is absent, but who otherwise present a fairly typical clinical picture. Most commonly it applies to people with normal or even excessive weight but with typical periods of overeating followed by vomiting or purging.

Management

Management of bulimia nervosa is comparatively easier than anorexia nervosa. There is research-based evidence for the effectiveness of cognitive behaviour therapy, interpersonal therapy, nutritional counselling and the use of antidepressant drugs, especially SSRIs.

Admission is rarely required and most patients are treated on an out-patient basis. There is usually no need for weight restoration.

Overeating Associated with Other Psychological Disturbances

According to ICD-10 classification, when distressing events lead to overeating and obesity, the condition is coded under this heading. Bereavements, accidents, surgical operations, and emotionally distressing events may be followed by 'reactive obesity'. Individuals who are predisposed to weight gain are particularly vulnerable.

Vomiting Associated with Other Psychological Disturbances

Apart from the self-induced vomiting of bulimia nervosa, repeated vomiting may occur in dissociative disorders, hypochondriacal disorders and pregnancy.

REFERENCES

1. Treasure, J. (1999). Chapter 7. In M. Lader and D. Naber (Eds.), *Difficult clinical problems in psychiatry*. London: Martin Dunitz.
2. Hjern, A., Lindberg, L. and Lindblad, F. (2006). Outcome and prognostic factors for an adolescent female in-patients with anorexia nervosa: 9–14 year follow-up. *British Journal of Psychiatry*, 189, 428–432.
3. Turnbull, S., Ward, A., Treasure, J., et al. (1996). The demand for eating disorder care: a study using the general practice research data base. *British Journal of Psychiatry*, 169, 705–712.
4. Schmidt, U. H., Tiller, J. M., Andrews, B., et al. (1997). Is there a specific trauma precipitating the onset of anorexia nervosa? *Psychological Medicine*, 27, 523–530.
5. Treasure, J. and Holland, A. (1995). Genetic factors in eating disorders. In G. Szmukler, C. Dare and J. Treasure (Eds.), *Handbook of eating disorders:* theory, treatment and research. Chichester: Wiley.
6. Schmidt, U. H., Tiller, J. M. and Treasure, J. (1993). Setting the scene for eating disorders: childhood care, classification and course of illness. *Psychological Medicine*, 23, 663–672.
7. Gillberg, C. and Rastam, M. (1998). The aetiology of anorexia nervosa. In W. H. Hoek, J. Treasure and M. Katzman (Eds.), *The integration of neurobiology in the treatment of eating disorders*. Chichester: Wiley.
8. Herzog, W., Schellberg, D. and Deter, H. C. (1997). First recovery in anorexia nervosa patients in the long-term course: a discrete time survival analysis. *Journal of Consulting and Clinical Psychology*, 65, 169–177.
9. Palmer, R. L. (1996). The Management of anorexia nervosa. *Advances in psychiatric treatment*. London: The Royal College of Psychiatrists.
10. Von Holle, A., Pinheiro, A. P., Thornton, L. M., Klump, K. L., Berrettini, W. H., Brandt, H., et al. (2008). Temporal patterns of recovery across eating disorder subtypes. Australian and New Zealand *Journal of Psychiatry*, 42, 108–117.
11. Touyz, S. W., Beaumont, P. J. V., Glaun, D., et al. (1984). A comparison of lenient and strict operant conditioning programmes in refeeding patients with anorexia nervosa. *British Journal of Psychiatry*,144, 517–520.
12. Morgan, G. (2011). Early intervention in anorexia nervosa. *The British Journal of Psychiatry*, 199, 432.

Psychological Methods of Treatment

19

Psychotherapy is broadly defined as being composed of three distinct components: a healing agent, a sufferer, and a healing or therapeutic relationship. Psychotherapy is the systematic use of a human relationship for therapeutic purposes of alleviating emotional distress by effecting enduring changes in a patient's thinking, feelings, and behaviour. The mutual engagement of the patient and the psychotherapist, both cognitively and emotionally, is the foundation for effective psychotherapeutic work.

Psychological methods of treatment and psychotherapy are more or less synonymous. Sometimes psychological help is given informally by other people in the form of advice or guidance. Psychotherapy differs from this sort of support in the sense that psychotherapists have specialist training and focus their practice according to various theoretical constructs (1).

Clients seek psychotherapy for various reasons including understanding of self, symptom relief, improved well-being, improvement in relationship(s), and to gain autonomy. Therapists attempt to relieve the distress or malfunctioning through psychological means. The main goals of psychotherapy are to help in gaining insight, and to bring about modifications of troublesome feelings and attitudes.

The primary aim of all therapies is to enhance insight into the conflicting or problematic areas of life. Clients' habitual ways of thinking, feeling and behaving are clarified, highlighted and challenged by the therapist. They are helped to correct the maladaptive attitudes, emotions and behaviours which adversely affect their day-to-day functioning or cause interpersonal difficulties. The therapist attempts to consolidate their abilities which have either not been adequately developed or are temporarily not accessible to them because of stressful events. Instead of the self-defeating and inadequate coping mechanisms, more effective strategies are explored, encouraged and reinforced by repetition.

Although all therapies attempt to influence the client in three ways—cognitively, emotionally and behaviourally, some would lay emphasis on one area more than the other two. Understanding of the unconscious process is a core feature of psychodynamic psychotherapy, and the emphasis that this form of therapy places on the relational aspects of transference (explained later), is a key technical difference from cognitive-behavioural therapy (2). There are a number of common factors in all types of psychotherapies (3).

1. Non-judgemental and empathic attitude of the therapist
2. A trusting and confiding relationship
3. Structure and boundaries which formalise the setting
4. Instillation of hope
5. A theoretical rationale for treatment
6. A recognizable treatment process

Therapeutic Relationship

A robust review of literature has demonstrated that the largest variation in therapy outcome is accounted for by pre-existing client factors, such as expectations for change and severity of the disorder, and the therapeutic relationship is the second largest proportion of change (4). This applies to all types of psychotherapies. Various other studies have also attributed the improvement by psychotherapy to the therapeutic relationship (5) and emphasise that the relationship between the therapist and the client is a very significant factor in bringing about the positive changes.

The personal influence of the therapist is crucial for the success of all types of psychotherapies, and as implied already, establishing the therapeutic alliance is one of the vital components. It has been demonstrated that the personality of the therapist contributes to the success or failure of psychotherapy. For therapists to be effective, they should themselves have the capacity for psychological insightfulness that includes the ability to self-criticise. In the past it was felt that in order to practice psychodynamic psychotherapy, therapists should first undergo a personal analysis. Although this is at times helpful, it is no longer considered necessary or practical. The main reason is that a personal analysis of the therapist does not guarantee or ensure that counter transference problems, or acting out by the therapist will not occur (6).

Psychotherapeutic skill depends to a great extent on the ability of the therapist to be genuinely interested in the symptoms of the client, while at the same time remaining detached enough to observe the psychotherapeutic process as it proceeds (7). Clients usually regard their therapist as a powerful healing authority, which itself contributes significantly to alleviating anxiety, and instilling hope and positive thinking. But the most important effect of therapy is educational. By gaining insight into their issues (especially in psychodynamic therapy) and learning how past experiences and unconscious conflicts shape the unwanted behaviours, learn new and better ways to cope with their current and future issues. However, not all people are suited for therapy, and certainly not everybody benefits from it. In fact, the book, Psychotherapy for Better or Worse (8) is based on the premise that psychotherapy can be detrimental when used improperly. It also needs to be remembered that psychotherapy may serve the needs of the therapist rather than the client. For example, some therapists may have an excessive sense of importance and may use the sessions for their own glorification. Moreover, therapists may even act out their own unconscious sadistic or competitive impulses by continually criticising the clients or even passing moral judgements. In some unfortunate cases, social or even sexual relationships between a therapist and the client may subsequently develop.

Assessment

Assessment is one important part of psychotherapy. It is essentially needed to select those people who are likely to benefit from psychotherapy, and to exclude those who are not likely to gain much from it. It also helps in predicting the probable outcome and the likely duration of the psychotherapeutic process.

What is psychotherapy assessment for? This framework can be summarised as two main decisions: first, the appropriateness of any psychological treatment approach; and the second, the choice of which particular psychological treatment method. These decisions involve knowledge gained from research (evidence-based practice) and views based on systematic clinical experience (practice-based evidence) (9).

Psychological mindedness is not only desirable but almost mandatory. It refers to an individual's capacity for reflection and introspection. It also includes an ability to appreciate the links between current problems with the past experiences. It has been demonstrated that psychologically minded people generally have some insight into their problems even before they commence therapy.

While assessing the suitability, it is not only imperative to ascertain the 'psychological mindedness' but also the ego strength of the client. The capacity to tolerate frustration, the ability to postpone immediate gratification, the willingness to examine the unpleasant aspects of oneself, the coping mechanisms being used, and interpersonal relations are all very important aspects for the suitability of psychotherapy. Those clients who have florid psychotic symptoms, are actively abusing illicit substances or pose high risks to themselves and others, are not suitable for psychotherapy. A psychiatric diagnosis is usually felt to be necessary, but is not sufficient in evaluating a client for psychotherapy (10).

Types of Psychotherapies

There are various types of psychotherapies for various psychiatric disorders and other problems (marital conflicts, low self-esteem, etc.) Some therapies have more evidence than the others regarding effectiveness and are practised more commonly. However, this is only a partial explanation, and the popularity of a particular type of therapy may also be dependent on the resources and availability of the relevant psychotherapist.

Some of the therapies are: Counselling, psychodynamic psychotherapy, client or person- centred therapy, existential therapy, personal construct therapy, gestalt therapy, transactional analysis Cognitive Behavioural Therapy (CBT), rational emotive therapy, family therapy, group therapy, interpersonal therapy, cognitive analytic therapy and dialectical behavioural therapy. Some psychotherapies will be discussed briefly, as it is beyond the scope of this book to provide an exhaustive account of all the therapies.

Counselling

Counselling is a broad term and applies to a kind of helpful psychological activity for mental health issues. It is also practised for non-psychiatric problems. National Institute of Clinical Excellence (NICE) defines it as a discrete, usually time-limited, psychological intervention where an intervention may have a facilitating approach often with a strong focus on the therapeutic relationship, but may be structured and at times directive (11).

It is a typically brief intervention that helps people cope with difficult circumstances by restoring their capacity to resolve problems. Counselling rarely comprises more than five sessions. In contrast to psychotherapy, which is person-oriented, counselling is problem-oriented (12). Counselling is suitable for problems that are usually not very severe, and for people having difficulties with recent onset and a clear triggering event. Techniques of counselling include active listening, and probing in an empathetic way without being judgmental. There is unburdening and sharing of problems, and ventilation of feelings.

Cognitive Therapy

Cognitive therapy is commonly and successfully used for depressive and anxiety disorders. It is very structured and usually lasts from 12 to 16 weeks. It is based on the theory that people react differently to stress and life, through a combination of cognitive, affective, motivational and behavioural responses (13). There are many proponents of cognitive theory but the most widely researched is Beck's approach (14).

According to Beck, it is not the specific stress or event that is responsible for an individual's feelings and behaviour, but the way that individual perceives that stress or event. Elaborating on the psychopathology of depression, Beck has identified three components: (1) Negative cognitive set (cognitive triad); (2) negative beliefs, silent assumptions, and automatic thoughts; and (3) cognitive errors or distortions (15). Most depressed people have negative and automatic thoughts about themselves, their world and their future. These negative thoughts are reinforced through faulty information processing, setting a vicious cycle in which a low mood enhances the intensity of negative thinking. This subsequently has an adverse result and increases the emotional, cognitive and behavioural disturbances (16). Cognitive therapy is very effective in the treatment of depression and is specifically designed to modify patterns of habitual negative thinking. It aims to improve the depressed mood by making the client aware of the habit of negative thinking, interpreting all events in their worst possible light and erroneously making generalised pessimistic conclusions from an isolated incident.

The therapist uses various techniques to alleviate the negative thought patterns and beliefs. These techniques are designed to help the patient recognise, challenge, and modify irrational or dysfunctional beliefs, ideas, perceptions, and self-statements that are assumed to cause pathological emotional reactions to negative or stressful events. The general term for modifying such beliefs is called 'cognitive restructuring'. Cognitive therapy also uses skills training, relaxation, assertive training, social skills training, role-playing, behavioural rehearsal, and exposure therapy. Clients are expected to do homework between sessions e.g., self-monitoring. Cognitive therapy is frequently combined with behavioural therapy (CBT). Apart from depressive and anxiety disorders, therapists claim that it is also effective for psychotic symptoms in some patients.

Behaviour Therapy

The central tenet of behaviour therapy is that psychological distress results from learned behaviour and this behaviour can be unlearned (17). In behaviour therapy, there is a systematic application of principles of learning. The aim of behaviour therapy is to modify maladaptive behaviour caused by faulty learning and substitute it with adaptive behaviour. The patient is helped to acquire this adaptive behaviour by means of various techniques based on learning principles. There is no effort to explore the client's childhood issues, etc. Behaviour therapy has shown to be effective (and treatment of choice) for phobic disorders including agoraphobia, obsessive-compulsive disorder and sexual dysfunction. It is also effective for tics, obesity, bulimia, anorexia nervosa, anger management and marital problems (18).

A behavioural analysis is undertaken and ABC model (Antecedents, Behaviours and Consequences) is applied (19). Some of the techniques used by behaviour therapists are as follows: In systematic desensitisation, the individual is trained to relax and then gradually expose him to anxiety-provoking situations in the imagination or reality. The patient is first trained to relax using the principle of progressive relaxation. In flooding/implosive therapy, huge anxiety is elicited. The patient is instructed to imagine the most stressful situation for long periods of time. Anxiety of the patient, after reaching a peak level, will show spontaneous reduction. Aversion therapy involves the elimination of undesirable behaviour by means of punishment. The aim is to stop maladaptive behaviour for a period of time during which an opportunity is given to learning more adaptive behaviour.

Modelling involves learning by imitation and has proved successful in the treatment of phobias and in teaching social skills.

In assertive training, the therapist guides the client in role-playing during the therapy session, showing him how to adopt a more assertive role. The therapist also guides him to practise his newly learnt responses in real-life situations.

Token economy has proved very successful in modification of severely maladaptive behaviour such as that shown by psychotic and mentally retarded individuals. In this method, appropriate behaviour is rewarded by tokens which can later be exchanged for desired objects or privileges.

Response shaping is used for establishing responses which are not initially in the individual's behaviour repertoire. Responses that approximate or resemble the desired behaviour are rewarded. Through successive approximations, the desired behaviour is learned.

Person-Centred Therapy

This was previously known as client-centred therapy. In this therapy, non-directive techniques are used and diagnostic labelling of persons is not justified. The fundamental and pervasive concept in this form of therapy is trust (20). Another important concept in this therapy is self-actualization, which implies that individuals seek and are capable of healthy development which leads to a full expression of themselves (21). The therapist tries to understand the client's world in whatever way the client wishes to share it. The client is encouraged to talk openly about his feelings and attitudes. The therapist reflects and clarifies the feelings of the client. The therapist must possess three qualities: genuineness, unconditional positive regard for the client and empathy. It is assumed that through 'talking it out' in a warm and permissive atmosphere, the client will come to see certain relationships between his feelings and behaviour and thus a way will be paved for his greater emotional adjustment and integration of personality.

Existential Therapy

Existential psychotherapy perceives the client as an existing, immediate person, and not as a composite of drives, archetypes, or conditioning (22). In this therapy (based on existential schools of philosophy), the focus is on uniqueness of the individual and the freedom of choice. Efforts are directed to explore important life themes like despair, isolation, death and the meaning or meaninglessness of life. Rather than prescribing techniques and methods, this therapy is an attitudinal approach to the issues of living (23).

The aim is to guide the individual to realise their potential and to accept responsibility for their actions. The central task of the existential psychotherapist is to understand the client as a being in the world. Existentially orientated therapists help the patient to discover new potentialities for personal satisfaction and growth (24). Psychopathology is considered in many cases to be caused by feelings of alienation, depersonalisation and loneliness, and by lack of a meaningful and fulfiling existence.

Gestalt Therapy

This approach is based on the premise that people must find their own way in life and accept personal responsibility if they hope to achieve maturity (25). The term gestalt means whole. Gestalt therapy focuses on the 'wholeness' of the individual and on the integration of thought, feeling and action. Aim of the therapy is to help the individual become aware of himself as a whole in the present, to work through unresolved conflicts and to take responsibility for his thoughts, feelings and actions. The therapist emphasises on the individual's experiences in the present moment and personal responsibility.

Rational Emotive Therapy

The basic goals of this therapy are to help people to live happier lives by minimising emotional turmoils, decreasing self-defeating self- behaviours, and becoming self-actualised (26). Other goals are to assist clients to think clearly and rationally, feel more appropriately, and to act more efficiently and effectively (27). This therapy works on the ABC framework, which states that individuals respond to an activating event (A), with emotional and behavioural consequences (C), but these consequences result not from (A) but from the individual belief system (B) (28).

The basic assumption underlying this therapy is that maladaptive emotional reactions are caused by irrational beliefs, self-damageing habituations, wishful thinking and intolerance (29). The task of the therapist is to unmask the client's self-defeating ideas, help him or her understand the role in causing problems. Thus the focus of the therapy is on cognitive change.

Family Therapy

Family therapy is a psychotherapeutic intervention that aims to alter interactions between family members and attempts at the same time to improve the functioning of an individual family member (30). The relationships within the family are improved by helping the members clarify and express their feelings towards one another, show mutual understanding and work cooperatively for the resolution of problems. The focus is on facilitating and improving communication patterns within the family by challenging unhelpful interaction patterns and dysfunctional communications.

The therapy can either be done with the whole family or with an individual. Family therapists who are insight-oriented lay emphasis on the resolution of conflicts within the family while the proponents of behaviour therapy try to modify the specific conditions that appear to be reinforcing maladaptive behaviour. Different models of family therapy include systems, structural, strategic and narrative approach. The structural approach is concerned with how family members relate to each other during the therapy hour and at home. A strategic approach aims to bring change in the symptoms. In the narrative approach, families are encouraged to change stories to positive themes and outcomes. In the systems approach, the therapist analyses the family's typical patterns of relating by treating the family as a group (31). A very useful overview has been provided by some authors (32).

Group Therapy

Many emotional problems arise due to difficulties in interpersonal relationships. These can sometimes be best treated in a group setting, involving a number of individuals. In group therapy individuals can work out their problems in the presence of others, realise their faulty ways of interacting and learn more effective methods of relating to other people.

In the supportive atmosphere of the group, the individuals learn that they are not alone with those problems. Participants can also learn by watching how others behave and react to social situations. The long-term goal is personality change.

Therapeutic factors in group therapy highlighted by Yalom include universality, altruism, instillation of hope, imparting information, corrective recapitulation, group cohesion, socialisation, imitation, existential factors, catharsis, interpersonal learning and self-understanding (33). An updated and extensive review has been done about these therapeutic factors (34).

Cognitive Analytic Therapy

This therapy is an integration of cognitive therapy and psychoanalytic (object-relations) theory. It is a structured and time-limited psychotherapy for personality disorder patients. Clients receive 24 weekly sessions and follow-up by 4 sessions which are spread over six months (35). The borderline personality disorder usually becomes apparent in early adult life. About 60% of cases have suffered severe abuse or deprivation in childhood, and the majority of patients have very disruptive or restricted lives because of lability of mood, inability to hold long-term relationships, repeated self-harm. Nearly 10% of once hospitalised patients die by suicide (36). Cognitive analytic therapy is based on an understanding that human personality is formed by internalising reciprocal role relationships experienced with others during childhood, and then maintained by the current experience of such reciprocal roles in relation to self and others (37).

Various concepts and procedures will be briefly described. Snag is a procedure when the person presumes that they will be blocked or punished for their action. The person will often not be aware of the part played by guilt in this procedure. In traps the person proceeds on the basis of a negative assumption and the resulting behaviour ends up seeming to confirm that negative assumption. Dilemma is another term used in cognitive analytic therapy. A person in a dilemma believes that his or her choice of action is restricted to either of two opposite activities, neither of which is satisfactory. The term role is derived from psychoanalytic object relations theory with the term role replacing the concept of identification with an internal object. It is felt that roles are gradually built into the individual's mind (in psychoanalytic terminology called internalisation), or developed into schema (in cognitive therapy terms) from early childhood in relationships with the parents. The term reciprocal role is used to describe this inter-relationship (38). The patient and therapist together draw up a list of target problems and target problems procedures which are written down in a reformulation letter, and drawn out in a sequential diagrammatic reformulation.

Interpersonal Therapy

Interpersonal Psychotherapy (IPT) is a structured and time-limited (12–16 sessions) therapy which was initially developed for patients with major depressive disorder but later adapted and used for other disorders (substance abuse, eating disorders, anxiety disorders and borderline personality disorder) as well. IPT assumes that the origin and perpetuation of some psychological symptoms occur in a social and interpersonal context. The overall goal is to alleviate the symptoms by addressing the patient's social environment and improving the quality of current interpersonal relations and social functioning in persons with major depressive disorder.

Dialectical Behavioural Therapy

This therapy is becoming increasingly popular for Borderline Personality Disorder patients. People suffering from this personality disorder borderline personality disorder are notoriously difficult to treat. They repeatedly harm themselves, and have dysregulation in the sphere of emotions, relationships, cognition and the sense of self. A pattern of self-mutilation tends to develop as a means of coping with the intense and painful feelings. Dialectical behaviour therapy is an intensive therapy which lasts up to a year. It uses cognitive as well as behavioural techniques. It is based on bio- social theory of borderline personality disorder. Linehan hypothesises that the disorder is a consequence of an emotionally vulnerable individual growing up within a particular set of environmental circumstances which he refers to as 'Invalidating Environment' (39).

Supportive Psychotherapy

The term supportive therapy is used in various ways. Sometimes it is used to refer to a form of psychological treatment given to patients with chronic and disabling psychiatric conditions for whom fundamental change is not a realistic goal (40). One definition stresses on supporting and strengthening the potential for better and more mature ego functioning in both adaptational and developmental tasks (41).

Provision of support to the patient is the main aspect of treatment, and the therapist sustains the patient who is unable to manage his life independently. The task of the therapist is to provide reassurance, encouragement and guidance to the patient but without fostering undue dependency. An attempt is made to help the patient function as efficiently as possible within his limitations. It helps in enhancing the patient's self-esteem and strengthening healthy defences. It also helps in reducing inappropriate behaviour and maximising family and social support. Unlike other psychotherapies, which are based upon theory or concept, supportive psychotherapy is not dependent upon any such concept or theory.

Sex and Marital Therapy

The aim of this therapy is to clarify and improve the relationship between the couple. The therapist plays an active role as a facilitator in helping the couple become aware of the nature of their marital difficulties and learn more satisfying ways of relating to each other. Most marital problems arise due to inadequate communication between couples and due to faulty role expectations. The goal of the therapy is to improve communication patterns, make more use of non-verbal communication, and increase the couple's sensitivity to each other's feelings and needs.

Sex therapy is used for the treatment of psychosexual dysfunction. The broad goals of sex therapy are, (1) to help the individual accept and feel comfortable with his or her own sexuality, (2) to help the individual initiate and maintain sexual relationship, and (3) to help the couple improve the quality of their sexual relationship.

Sex therapy usually begins with educating the patients about sexual anatomy and the physiological processes of intercourse. Anxiety or fears of performance may be reduced by using various desensitisation techniques. In some sexual problems, medical procedures may have to be employed. There is a comprehensive review of sex therapy available (42). It covers all aspects of sexual behaviours, problems, and treatment.

Psychodynamic Psychotherapy

In this type of psychotherapy, the psychoanalytic psychotherapist makes contact with and comprehends, as thoroughly as possible, the patient's subjective inner world so as to engage in an analytical (i.e., interpretive) conversation about it. Psychoanalytic psychotherapy may be further defined in terms of three operations: accepting, understanding, and explaining.

Psychodynamic psychotherapy is based on psychoanalytic theory. According to this theory, thoughts, feelings and behaviour are expressions of conscious factors, as well as of unconscious processes or impulses. Subsequently, unpleasant symptoms may develop because of these expressions. However, these symptoms may provide relief (primary gain) from anxiety which is due to the unacceptable impulses or urges (43). Impulses, desires and experiences which are unacceptable to the individual (at the conscious level) are repressed into the unconscious from which they cannot be retrieved voluntarily. However, these unconscious conflicts, lead to disturbance and maladaptive behaviour. Therapy brings to awareness these unresolved conflicts. It is assumed that when the patient becomes aware of the motives underlying his or her maladaptive behaviour and thought processes, the path is cleared for the restructuring of the personality leading to healthy and effective means of coping.

In psychodynamic psychotherapy, unders- tanding the past is of paramount importance as our childhood years are considered to be the most formative period of our lives (44). The primary focus is on the distress that arises from earlier and unresolved internal conflicts. The therapist seeks to unearth and unravel the possible sources of current anxieties, difficulties and malfunctioning. However, cognitive challenges are also posed to clients in psychodynamic psychotherapy, for example when dichotomised or catastrophising assumptions underlie the transference (45).

Psychodynamic psychotherapy is used across the spectrum of affective, anxiety, and personality disorders. It can only be used with individuals who are motivated, educated and able to verbalise adequately. It is not applicable to psychotic individuals or people of low intelligence. Psychodynamic psychotherapy can be carried out both as a short-term and as a long-term treatment.

It remains controversial in spite of being frequently used in clinical practice. There is conspicuous criticism about the therapist's strong assumption that he or she can know the mind of the client better than the client, the conjectures made about the human mind, and the notion that dynamic unconscious is a license for abuse (46).

Some of the key terms and techniques in psychodynamic psychotherapy are: Free association (clients are encouraged to speak of whatever comes to mind), interpretations, non-verbal comments, intrusive comments, the corrective emotional experience (when clients are re-exposed, under favourable circumstances, to emotional situations which they could not handle in the past), resistance, transference, countertransference, deconditioning, recapitulations and confrontations.

Interpretation is the hallmark of psychodynamic psychotherapy. It is an informative statement based on decoding the client's communication, and brings unconscious material into consciousness. It is of two types; content interpretation, which is the statement based on the substance of the message; and meta interpretation, which refers to the form in which a message is presented.

Although the insight gained by the client with the help of interpretations, does not itself produce change, it does facilitates change, and widens the choices and options for the client.

Transference is the process whereby an individual transfers thoughts, ideas, affects, which are held about early figures in their life, most notably parents, to bear on their current relationships, and experience them similarly. This term is sometimes used inappropriately. Analysis of transference and resolving it is a very important part of psychodynamic therapy. It helps the patient recognise and manage the unconscious feelings and expectations that he or she brings to the new relationships (including the therapist). The patient has to be able to move from a less reflective to a more reflective state of mind, where he or she can bring thought to bear on his or her feelings rather than enacting his or her expectations (47).

Countertransference has been defined in different ways: the emotional reactions of the therapist to the client's transference; all the feelings which the therapist experiences towards the client; or it refers only to those phenomena which are transferences of the therapist to the client. These days, the third definition is generally accepted (48).

For psychodynamic therapy, a psychodynamic formulation based on the assessment provides guidelines for the therapeutic plan. The formulation is an attempt to find a core or central theme which underlies the client's conflicts and anxieties. It coherently weaves together the presenting problems, past difficulties, and the reactions of the client during the interview (49) into what Malan called 'the triangle of insight' (50). A psychodynamic formulation has a number of clinical uses. It assists the therapist to see what a person is doing, thinking and feeling, and to explain why. It helps in anticipating how that person may behave in the future and how they may respond to adverse events and to different treatments. Formulation can also guide the treating psychotherapist by providing a map of treatment (51).

Defence Mechanisms

Some of the defence mechanisms were described by Freud but later his daughter Anna added to the list and Melanie Klein also contributed some of them. Defence mechanisms are psychological strategies by which a person reduces or avoids negative states such as conflict, frustration, anxiety and stress. Most people are motivated to reduce these unpleasant states. Freud regarded these mechanisms as unconscious psychological processes that people develop to alleviate anxiety. All defence mechanisms are based on the distortion of reality to some extent. They are not necessarily harmful but some people often display them in exaggerated form. Defence mechanisms are very useful in understanding many aspects of the day-to-day behaviour of ourselves and other people.

Valiant has divided them into three main groups: immature (e.g., splitting, projection), neurotic (e.g., repression, intellectualisation), and mature (e.g., sublimation, humour) (52).

Repression

This is the most basic defence mechanism and prevents unacceptable desires, motivations or emotions from becoming conscious. It is a process by which a person (unconsciously) prevents painful or dangerous thoughts from entering consciousness.

Rationalisation

It is one of the commonest defence mechanism used in everyday life. A person is able to provide a false but acceptable explanation for behaviour. People also resort to rationalisation to explain away their frustrations.

Sublimation

It is seen as a healthy defence mechanism. Sometimes a motive that causes anxiety may be transformed unconsciously into a different but related motive that is more acceptable to society and to oneself.

Identification

In this defence mechanism, a person increases his feelings of worth by affiliating himself with a person or institution of illustrious standing. This taking on the personal characteristics of another person can serve the purpose of reducing the anxiety.

Reaction Formation

This refers to the unconscious adoption of behaviour opposite to that which would reflect true feelings and intentions.

Suppression

The person avoids stressful thoughts by not thinking about them. This differs from repression in that with suppression the stress provoking thought is there but ignored and blocked by other thoughts, rather than being completely unavailable as is the case with repression. Unlike most other defences, in some cases, persons will consciously initiate suppression.

Regression

Sometimes, when faced with conflict, stress and particularly frustration, a person may return to an earlier stage of life in which the person was secure, and so avoid the present conflict or stress.

Compensation

When a person believes that he or she is inferior in some way the person may attempt to overcome the feelings of inferiority and related anxiety by devoting additional effort to the area of inferiority.

Denial

Sometimes a person behaves as though unaware of something which he may be reasonably expected to know. The person protects himself from unpleasant reality by refusing to perceive or face it. Denial differs from repression in that the person selectively attends and reinterprets, rather than obliterates, the experience forms consciousness.

Displacement

This defence mechanism occurs when emotions are diverted onto someone else because the emotions cannot be expressed to the person concerned or because accepting faults in ourselves will cause anxiety. It is the unconscious process of transferring emotion from a situation or objects with which it is associated, to another which will give a rise to less distress. Through displacement, a person discharges pent-up feelings, of hostility, on objects less threatening than those arousing the feelings.

Isolation

This occurs when a person cuts off emotional charge from hurtful situations or separates incompatible attitudes by logic-tight compartments.

Intellectualisation

In this defence mechanism, the person thinks and speaks in an excessive intellectual manner without feelings.

Undoing

Here a person acts in an inappropriate way which may elicit anxiety, then behaves in the opposite way so as to reverse or balance the original behaviour and thus eliminate the anxiety that the first behaviour engendered.

Acting Out

This is engageing in antisocial or excessive behaviour without regard to negative consequences as a way of dealing with emotional stress.

Splitting

In this the person views himself or others as all good or bad without integrating positive or negative qualities of the person into the evaluation.

Fantasy

This is a mechanism through which a person gratifies his desires by imagining. This is a very common phenomenon.

Projection

By projecting, people project onto other people motives or thoughts of their own that cause them anxiety. Projection is one of the most powerful and dangerous defence mechanisms.

Projective Identification

In this defence mechanism, there is dissociation of unacceptable parts of the personality and projection onto another.

Evidence for Psychotherapies

In spite of the demonstrated general superiority of psychotherapy over no treatment, formidable problems for evaluation remain (53). Although some of the inherent problems in conducting psychotherapy research, especially Randomised Control Trials (RCTs) for psychotherapy cannot be denied, there is impressive empirical evidence for its efficacy. Several controlled studies indicate that psychotherapy either alone or combined with psychotropic medications, when judiciously administered for specific disorders, is a potent and effective treatment modality (54).

Twenty-three RCTs of long-term psychodynamic psychotherapy, for specific psychiatric disorders, provide evidence that psychodynamic psychotherapy is superior to control conditions (treatment as usual or those on waiting lists), and on the whole, as effective as already established treatments (e.g., cognitive behavioural therapy) (55). Fifteen RCTs support the efficacy of short-term psychodynamic psychotherapy for borderline personality disorder, bulimia and anorexia nervosa, somatoform disorders, PTSD, alcohol dependence, opiate dependence and depressive disorders (56).

To conclude, psychotherapy is an effective and efficient way for treating patients with a variety of mental disorders (57). There are many studies advocating the role of various psychotherapies. However, the important question 'what works for whom', posed many decades ago, continues to be debated (58).

Psychotherapies for Specific Psychiatric Disorders

The following is an evidence-based list of psychotherapies (59):

- For major depressive disorder, cognitive-behavioural approaches, interpersonal therapy and short-term structured psychodynamic psychotherapy
- For bipolar disorder, psychoeducation and cognitive-behavioural therapy aimed at relapse prevention
- For specific phobia and social phobia, exposure therapy and cognitive therapy in combination with exposure
- For generalised anxiety disorder, cognitive behavioural therapy and applied relaxation
- For panic disorder with or without agoraphobia, exposure therapy, and cognitive-behavioural therapy
- For obsessive-compulsive disorders, exposure and response prevention, and cognitive restructuring and rational-emotive therapy, in combination with exposure
- For post-traumatic stress disorder, cognitive-behavioural approaches, eye movement desensitisation and reprocessing, and structured psychodynamic psychotherapy
- For anorexia nervosa, inpatient contingency management (in relation to short-term weight gain), family therapy (particularly when offered to younger patients), cognitive-behavioural approaches and cognitive analytic therapy
- For bulimia nervosa, cognitive-behavioural therapy, including dietary management, and interpersonal therapy
- For binge-eating disorder, cognitive-behavioural therapy
- For schizophrenia, family interventions programmes, cognitive therapy for delusions, psychoeducation in combination with psychological intervention
- For borderline personality disorders, dialectical behaviour therapy
- For avoidant personality disorders, social skills training
- For alcohol abuse, brief educational interventions, including motivational interviewing, social skills training, relapse prevention, coping skills training, contingency management, marital therapy
- For sexual dysfunctions, behavioural and cognitive-behavioural treatment approaches aimed at reducing sexual anxiety and improving communication for erectile dysfunction. Exposure-based behavioural techniques for vaginismus, and specific behavioural techniques for premature ejaculation.

REFERENCES

1. Frank, D. F. What is psychotherapy? (1996). In S. Bloch (Ed.), *An introduction to the psychotherapies* (pp. 1–20). Oxford: Oxford Medical Publications.
2. Cutler, J. L., Goldyne, A., Markpwitz, J. C., Devlin, M. J. and Glick, R. A. (2004). Comparing cognitive behaviour therapy, interpersonal therapy and psychodynamic psychotherapy. *American Journal of Psychiatry*, 161, 1567–1573.
3. Frank, J. D. (1982). Therapeutic components shared by all psychotherapies. In J. H. Harvey, M. M. Parks (Eds.), *The master lecture series* (Vol 1): Psychotherapy research and behaviour change (pp. 9–37). Washington DC: American Psychological Association.
4. Bergin, A. E. and Lambert, M. J. (1978). The evaluation of therapeutic outcomes. In S. L. Garfield and A. E. Bergin (Eds.), *Handbook of psychotherapy and behaviour change* (2nd Edition). New York: Wiley.
5. Horvath, A. O. and Bedi, R. P. (2002). The alliance. In J. C. Norcross (Ed.), *Psychotherapy relationships that work.* New York: Oxford University Press.
6. Hollender, M. H. and Ford, C. V. (1990). *Dynamic psychotherapy*. Washington: American Psychiatric Press.
7. Holmes, J. (1991). The psychotherapies and their application to psychiatry. In J. Holmes (Ed.), *Textbook of psychotherapy in psychiatric practice* (pp. 3–29). Edinburgh: Churchill Livingstone.
8. Strupp, H. H., Hadley, S. W. and Gomes- Schwartz, B. (1977). *Psychotherapy for better or worse*: The problem of negative effects. New York: Aronson.
9. Margison, F. and Brown, P. (2007). Assessment in psychotherapy. In J. Naismith and S. Grant (Eds.), *Seminars in the psychotherapies* (pp. 1–27). London: Royal College of psychiatrists.
10. Hollender, M. H. and Ford, C. V. (1990). *Dynamic psychotherapy*. Washington: American Psychiatric Press.
11. NICE. (2007). Clinical guidelines 23 (amended) depression: *Management of depression in primary and secondary care.* London: National Institute for Clinical Excellence.
12. Corsini R. J. (2000). Introduction. In F. E. Peacock (Ed.), *Current psychotherapies* (6th Edition, pp. 1–15). Illinois: Peacock Publishers.
13. Beck, A. T. and Weishaar, M. E. (2000). Cognitive therapy. In R. J. Corsini (Ed.), *Current psychotherapies* (6th Edition, pp. 241–272). Illinois: Peacock Publishers.
14. Beck, A. T. (1983). Cognitive therapy of depression: New perspectives. In P. Clayton and J. Barrett (Eds.), *Treatment of depression: Old controversies and new approaches* (pp. 265–284). New York: Raven Press.
15. Beck, A. T. (1976). *Cognitive therapy and the emotional disorders*. New York: International University Press.
16. Scott, J. (1998). Psychological treatments for depression. In D. Tantam (Ed.), *Clinical topics in psychotherapy* (pp. 18–25). London: Gaskell.
17. Stern, R. S. and Drummond, L. M. (1991). *The practice of behavioural and cognitive psychotherapy*. Cambridge: Cambridge University Press.
18. Drummond, L. (1996). Behavioural psychotherapy. In S. Baloch (Ed.), *An introduction to psychotherapies* (3rd Edition, pp. 137–166). Oxford: Oxford Medical Publications.
19. O'Leary, K. D. and Wilson, G. T. (1975). *Behaviour therapy: Application and outcome*. New Jersey: Prentice Hall.

20. Sharf, R. S. (2000). *Theories of psychotherapy and counselling*. Concept and cases (2nd Edition). New York: Wadsworth.
21. Sharf, R. S. (2000). *Theories of psychotherapy and counselling*. Concept and cases (2nd Edition). New York: Wadsworth.
22. May, R. (2000). Existential psychotherapy. In R. J. Corsini (Ed.), *Current psychotherapies* (6th Edition, pp. 273–302). Illinois: Peacock Publishers.
23. Sharf, R. S. (2000). *Theories of psychotherapy and counselling*. Concept and cases (2nd Edition). New York: Wadsworth.
24. Frank, D. J. (1996). What is psychotherapy? In S. Bloch (Ed.), *An introduction to the psychotherapies* (3rd Edition, pp. 1–20). Oxford: Oxford University Press.
25. Corey, G. (1996). *Theory and practice of counselling and psychotherapy* (5th Edition). California: Brooks/Cole Publishing Company.
26. Ellis, A. and Bernard, M. E. (1985). What is rational emotive therapy (RET). In A. Ellis and M. E. Bernard (Eds.), *Clinical applications of rational emotive therapy* (pp. 1–30). Plenum: New York.
27. Sharf, R. S. (2000). *Theories of psychotherapy and counselling*. Concept and cases (2nd Edition). New York: Wadsworth.
28. Sharf, R. S. (2000). *Theories of psychotherapy and counselling*. Concept and cases (2nd Edition). New York: Wadsworth.
29. Ellis, A. (2000). Rational Emotive Behaviour Therapy. In R. J. Corsini (Ed.), *Current psychotherapies* (6th Edition, pp. 168–204). Illinois: Peacock Publishers.
30. Bentovim, A. and Kinston, W. (1991). Focal family therapy: Joining systems with psychodynamic understanding. In A. S. Gurman and D. P. Kniskern (Eds), *Handbook of family therapy Vol 2.* New York: Brunner/Mazel.
31. Bentovim, A. (1996). Family therapy. In S. Bloch (Ed.), *An introduction to the psychotherapies* (3rd Edition, pp. 238–260). Oxford: Oxford University Press.
32. Bentovim, A. and Kinston, W. (1991).Focal family therapy: Joining systems with psychodynamic understanding. In A. S. Gurman and D. P. Kniskern (Eds), *Handbook of family therapy Vol 2.* New York: Brunner/Mazel.
33. Yalom, I. D. (1985). *The theory and practice of group therapy* (3rd Edition). New York: Basic Books.
34. Crouch, E., Bloch, S. and Wanlass, J. (1994).Therapeutic factors: Interpersonal and intrapersonal mechanisms. In A. Fuhriman and G. Burlingame (Eds.), *Handbook of group psychotherapy*. New York: Wiley.
35. Ryle, A. (1997). *Cognitive analytic therapy and borderline personality disorder*: The model and the method. Chichester: Wiley.
36. Ryle, A. and Golynkina, K. (2000). Effectiveness of time-limited cognitive analytic therapy of borderline personality: Factors associated with outcome. *British Journal of Psychology*, 73, 197– 210.
37. Sheardi, T., Evans, J., Cash, D., Hicks, J., King, A., et al. (2000). A CAT- derived one to three session intervention for repeated deliberate self- harm: A description of the model and initial experience of trainee psychiatrists in using it. *British Journal of Medical Psychology*, 73, 179–197.
38. Murphy, T. and Llewelyn, S. (2007). Cognitive analytic therapy. In J. Naismith and S. Grant (Eds.), *Seminars in the psychotherapies* (pp. 118– 139). London: Royal College of psychiatrists.
39. Linehan, M. M. (1993). *Cognitive behavioural treatment of borderline personality disorder*. London and New York: The Guilford Press.
40. Bloch, S. (1996). *Supportive psychotherapy*. In S. Bloch (Ed.), An introduction to the psychotherapies (3rd Edition, pp. 294–319). Oxford: Oxford University Press.
41. Gilbert, S. and Ugelstad, E. (1994). Patients own contributions to long-term supportive psychotherapy in schizophrenic disorders. *British Journal of Psychiatry*, 164(23), 84–88.
42. Bancroft, J. (1989). *Human sexuality and its problems* (2nd Edition). Edinburgh: Churchill Livingstone.
43. Murphy, T. and Llewelyn, P. J. (2004). Psychological therapies. In E. Johnstone, D. C. Owens, S. Lawrie, M. Sharpe and C. P. Freeman (Eds.), *Companion to psychiatric studies* (7th Edition, pp. 295–318). Edinburgh: Churchill Livingstone.
44. Lemma, A. (2003). *Introduction to the practice of psychoanalytic psychotherapy*. West Sussex: John Wiley and Sons.
45. Holmes, J. and Crown, S. (1996). Individual long-term therapy. In S. Baloch (Ed.), *An introduction to psychotherapies* (3rd Edition, pp 21– 51). Oxford: Oxford Medical Publications.
46. Lemma, A. (2003). *Introduction to the practice of psychoanalytic psychotherapy*. West Sussex: John Wiley and Sons.
47. Hughes, P. and Kerr, I. (2000). Transference and countertransference in communication between doctor and patient. *Advances in Psychiatric Treatment*, 6, 57–64.
48. Hollender, M. H. and Ford, C. V. (1990).*Dynamic psychotherapy*. Washington: American Psychiatric Press.
49. Holmes, J. and Crown, S. (1996). Individual long-term therapy. In S. Bloch (Ed.), *An introduction to the psychotherapies* (pp. 21–51). New York: Oxford Medical Publications.
50. Malan, D. (1979). *Individual psychotherapy and the science of psychodynamics*. London: Butterworths.
51. Mace, C. and Binyon, S. (2005). Teaching psychodynamic formulation to psychiatric trainees. Part 1: Basics of formulation. *Advances in Psychiatric Treatment*, 11, 416–423.
52. Valiant, G. E. (1977). *Adaptation to life*. Boston: Little and Brown.
53. Lubrosky, L. (1984). *Principles of psychoanalytic psychotherapy*. New York: Basic Books.
54. Klerman, G. L., Budman, S., Berwick, D., et al. (1987). Efficacy of a brief psychosocial intervention for symptoms of stress and distress among patients in primary care. *Med Care*, 25, 1078–1088.
55. Leichsenring, F. and Leibing, E. (2007). Psychodynamic psychotherapy: A systematic review of techniques, indications and empirical evidence. *Psychology and Psychotherapy: Theory, Research and Practice*, 80, 217–228.
56. Leichsenring, F. and Leibing, E. (2007). Psychodynamic psychotherapy: A systematic review of techniques, indications and empirical evidence. *Psychology and Psychotherapy: Theory, Research and Practice*, 80, 217–228.
57. Lambert, M. J. and Ogles, B. M. (2003). The efficacy and effectiveness of psychotherapy. In M. J. Lambert (Ed.), Bergin and Garfield's *Handbook of psychotherapy and behaviour change*. Sussex: John Wiley.
58. Paul, G. L. (1967). Strategy of outcome research in psychotherapy.*Journal of Consultant Psychology*, 3, 109–118.
59. Roth, A. and Fonagy, P. (2005). What works for whom? *A critical review of psychotherapy research* (2nd Edition). New York: The Guildford Press.

20 Drugs and Other Physical Treatments

For psychiatric disorders or symptoms, psychotropic medications are extensively used. Psychotropic treatment is based on treating symptoms, which have a heterogeneous aetiology. It is important to appreciate the wide variability in drug concentrations that occurs in individual patients, given the same dose of a medication. There are a host of factors that will confound the individual patient's actual exposure to a particular medication and thus contribute to variable therapeutic and adverse effects. These drugs are grouped under the headings of their respective clinical applications: antidepressants, antipsychotics, mood stabilisers, anxiolytics and hypnotics, etc. However, this classification is not entirely satisfactory as many of these drugs have more than one indication.

Although some common side effects, important interactions and contraindications of classes of psychotropic medication or individual drugs are given here, for comprehensive information about a particular medication, the readers are suggested to consult an up-to-date book on psychopharmacology, or the latest version of British National Formulary (BNF). It is assumed that students and trainee doctors would already have read the basic pharmacology, therefore, a very brief and essential account is given in this chapter.

Pharmacokinetics and Psychodynamics

Pharmacokinetics describes the way the body handles the drug and distributed to its site of action. It involves absorption, distribution, metabolism and elimination. Pharmacokinetics has bearing on dose-response relationships, drug interactions, the risk of discontinuation and the frequency of administration. For a good and safe clinical practice, it is imperative to have this knowledge. Psychodynamics is the study of the mechanism of drug action, that is, the effect of the drug on the body.

Absorption

Absorption is influenced by the route of administration and drug properties. The bioavailability of a drug is the fraction of the administered dose reaching the systemic circulation. Most psychotropic drugs are lipophilic and are therefore easily absorbed from the gut.

Distribution

Once absorbed, a drug is distributed to the various tissues of the body. The rate of this process depends upon how each tissue is perfused with blood, the binding of the drug to plasma proteins, and the permeability of tissue membranes. Most psychotropic drugs have large volumes of distribution.

Metabolism and Excretion

Most psychotropic drugs are metabolised in the liver, but some in plasma, lung and kidney. Excretion by the kidneys is most important but may occur through the lungs or in bile, sweat, milk and saliva.

Elimination

During the distribution phase, change in drug concentration primarily reflects the movement of the drug within the body, rather than elimination from it. However, once distribution equilibrium is reached, the body acts kinetically as a single compartment, and a change in plasma concentration of the drug is observed (1).

First-order kinetics occurs with most psychotropic medications. In this, the rate of absorption or elimination is directly proportional to the amount of drug remaining.

In zero-order kinetics, a fixed amount of drug is absorbed or eliminated for each unit of time independent of drug concentrations, because of some other rate-limiting factor. Examples are alcohol and phenytoin.

Plasma Half-Life and Steady State

Plasma half-life is an important pharmacokinetic measure. It indicates how long it takes for the concentration of drug in the plasma to decline to half of its previous level. This has implications for the frequency of dosing. It is only useful for describing first-order kinetics, as the half-life remains the same whatever the concentration. Through half-life of a drug, it can be predicted how long it will take for a steady state to be reached after the start of regular dosing.

Tolerance, Dependence and Addiction

Tolerance occurs when the same drug effect can be obtained only by increasing the dose. It occurs with opiates, alcohol and benzodiazepines.

One explanation for this phenomenon is that the drug is metabolised more rapidly when the body has been exposed to it for a longer period. Tolerance may also represent an adaptation to the action of the drug, so a high concentration is needed to bring about the same effect.

Dependence occurs when there are physical or psychological symptoms because of discontinuation of the drug and there is a compulsion to have the drug reinstated.

Drug addiction is characterised by craving and drug-seeking behaviour. There are both physical as well psychological symptoms on withdrawal.

Potency

The potency of a drug is determined by the proportion of the drug reaching the receptor, its affinity for the receptor and its efficacy. Drugs that produce the same maximal effect have equal efficacy, but a drug which produces the maximum effect at a lower dose is considered to have a higher potency. Haloperidol, for example, is more potent than chlorpromazine because 5 mg of haloperidol and 100 mg of chlorpromazine achieve the same therapeutic effect.

Therapeutic Index

It is a relative measure of the toxicity or safety of a drug and is defined as the ratio of the median toxic dose to the median effective dose. Some drugs such as lithium have a narrow therapeutic range.

Use of Medication in Children

Although children and adolescents suffer from nearly all kinds of psychiatric illnesses, there are limited drug trials in children, and very few drugs are licensed for use. Drugs should be prescribed very selectively and cautiously in this group.

Use of Medication in Medically ill and Elderly Patients

When there are concomitant medical illnesses in psychiatric patients, especially in the elderly, caution needs to be exercised and the number and dosages of psychotropic drugs should be as low as possible. In elderly patients, there is relative metabolic impairment. Drugs, therefore, last longer, accumulate more and have more side effects. Consequently, there are higher chances of toxic reactions and accidental overdosing. Finally, as this group of patients might have cognitive impairment, their dosing regimes should be very simple and clear.

Use of Medication in Pregnancy and Breastfeeding

Psychotropic drugs may harm the developing fetus, so it is imperative to ascertain the pregnancy status of the patients before prescribing drugs. For women who are pregnant, the risks to the fetus must be balanced against the consequences of relapse of mental illness. A drug is more of a risk to the fetus in higher doses and in the first trimester. New drugs and drugs like carbamazepine and lithium, whose risks are known, should be avoided. Most drugs cross the placental barrier and also appear in breast milk.

Receptors and the Agonist Spectrum

Receptors are peptide structures to which neurotransmitters and some drugs attach, and which initiate their effects.

Agonist

A drug that attaches to the receptor and activates is called an agonist.

Partial Agonist

A compound which possesses an affinity for a receptor, but unlike a full agonist, will elicit only a small degree of the pharmacological response peculiar to the nature of the receptor involved, even if a high proportion of receptors are occupied by the compound. Partial agonists (such as buspirone, aripiprazole, buprenorphine, or norclozapine) also bind and activate a given receptor, but have only partial efficacy at the receptor relative to a full agonist.

Inverse Agonist

These are drugs that produce the opposite effect to that of an agonist.

Antagonist

A drug that attaches to the receptor and produces no activation is called an antagonist. In the presence of an agonist, an antagonist will block the actions of that agonist but do nothing itself. An antagonist will also block the actions of a partial agonist. Antagonists have no activity of their own even in the absence of an agonist.

Antidepressant Drugs

Antidepressants can be classified in a number of ways: Historical classification, structural classification, clinical classification (sedative and non-sedative), classification on the basis of pharmacokinetics properties (elimination half-lives), and finally pharmacological classification.

Pharmacological Classification of Antidepressants

- Tricyclics (TCAs)
- Monoamine Oxidase Inhibitors (MAOIs)
- Reversible inhibitors of monoamine oxidase Type A
- Second generation antidepressants
- Selective Serotonin Reuptake Inhibitors (SSRIs)
- Serotonin and Noradrenaline Reuptake Inhibitors (SNRIs)
- Noradrenergic and Specific Serotonergic Antidepressants (NASSAs)
- Noradrenaline Reuptake Inhibitors (NARIs)
- Antipsychotics used as adjunctive antidepressants

Tricyclic Antidepressants (TCAs)

This class of antidepressants is named for its characteristic three-ring structure which is closely related to that of the antipsychotic drugs in the phenothiazine class. The drugs in this class act by binding to the presynaptic transporter proteins and inhibiting reuptake of neurotransmitters into the presynaptic terminal. Inhibition of the reuptake prolongs the duration of transmitter action at the synapse, ultimately producing changes in both pre- and post-synaptic receptors. Although many of the drugs in this class are equally effective in inhibiting the reuptake of NE and 5-HT, some are more effective on one transmitter than the other. Although this difference does not change their antidepressant action, it does determine the drugs' side effects.

Histamine receptor blockade is responsible for sedation and fatigue. Anticholinergic side effects include dry mouth, constipation, urinary retention, dizziness, confusion, impaired memory, and blurred vision. Endocrine effects include breast enlargement, galactorrhoea, and gynaecomastia. Sexual dysfunction may occur. Side effects also include changes in blood sugar, increased appetite, weight gain, hepatic and haematological reactions, and hyponatraemia (particularly in the elderly). Some patients may have anorexia and weight loss.

The alpha 1 blockade in combination with the NE reuptake-blocking effects lead to several potentially dangerous cardiovascular side effects, including orthostatic hypotension, tachycardia, and arrhythmias. This particular set of side effects makes it especially difficult to treat depression in elderly patients with known cardiac disorders. In addition, toxicity following overdose causes cardiovascular depression, delirium, convulsions, respiratory depression, and coma. Heart arrhythmias may produce cardiac arrest. Tertiary amines (amitriptyline and imipramine), have more side effects because of having active metabolites.

Amitriptyline

The dose of amitriptyline in adults is 75 mg daily in single or divided doses, increased gradually to 200 mg daily if needed. The initial dose for adolescents and the elderly is 25 mg. For neuropathic pain, 10 mg is the starting dose, and 75 mg is the maximum dose. Amitriptyline is also used for migraine prophylaxis (usual dose ranges being 10 mg to 75 mg, and 150 mg maximum as a night dose).

Imipramine

Initial dose of imipramine is 75 mg in divided doses, increased gradually to 200 mg daily. In hospital patients, the maximum dose can be 300 mg. In elderly, the dose range is 10 mg to 50 mg. Imipramine is not recommended for depression in children.

Nortriptyline

The initial daily dose of this drug (25 mg) should be gradually increased to 75 mg in divided doses, the maximum daily dose being 150 mg. For adolescents and elderly patients the dose range is 25 mg–75 mg daily in divided doses.

Trimipramine

Initial starting dose is 50–75 mg daily in divided doses or as a single dose at bedtime. The maximum dose is 300 mg. In elderly 25 mg to 75 mg in divided doses is the starting dose, the maximum is 150 mg daily. Trimipramine is not recommended for children.

Trazodone

Initial dose for adults is 100 mg, and in the elderly 50 mg in divided doses or as a single bedtime dose. 300 mg daily is the maximum dose, but for in-patients, it can be given up to 600 mg daily. In smaller doses (from 50mg to 100mg) trazodone is also used for insomnia.

Dothiepin Hydrochloride

This medication has a high rate of fatality in overdose. The initial daily dose is 25 mg, the maximum being 150 mg. For in-patients, it can be 225 mg. In elderly, 75 mg is the usual maximum recommended dose.

Clomipramine

Clomipramine is a more selective inhibitor of the reuptake of serotonin, amitriptyline and imipramine. It is specific for blockade of the reuptake of 5-HT, as opposed to noradrenaline or dopamine. For depressive illness, 10 mg is the starting dose, which can be increased to 150 mg in divided doses. 200 mg daily is the maximum dose. The dose range for the elderly is 10 mg to 75 mg.

For phobias and obsessive-compulsive disorder the dose range is 25 mg to 250 mg. In the elderly the initial dose is 10 mg.

Doxepin

The dose range is 75 mg to 300 mg.

Monoamine Oxidase Inhibitors (MAOIs)

This group of drugs have an important place for atypical depression, treatment-resistant depression, and depression associated with panic and phobias. The more common side effects of MAOIs include changes in blood pressure, sleep disturbances including insomnia, and overeating, which may lead to excessive weight gain. There is an increased risk of neonatal malformations when MAOIs are used during pregnancy.

MAOIs are much less used in clinical practice because of their potential drug and dietary interactions, the most serious being tyramine- induced hypertensive crises. This occurs when certain foods and drinks are consumed. MAOIs inhibit monoamine oxidase, thereby causing an accumulation of amine neurotransmitters. The interaction with some amine drugs such as indirect acting sympathomimetics (present in many cough preparations) is also inhibited and their pressor action may be potentiated. Similarly, the pressor effect of tyramine present in certain foods and drinks may also be potentiated.

Some of the common dietary restrictions for patients taking MAOIs are as follows: Unpasteurised milk and yoghurt; aged cheese; Stilton; aged game; liver; canned meats; yeast extracts; salami; dry sausage; salted, dried, smoked, or pickled fish such as herring, cod, and caviar; peanuts, homemade yeast bread with substantial quantities of yeast; bread or crackers containing cheese; Italian broad beans; sauerkraut; bananas, red plums; avocados and raspberries; alcoholic beverages including red and white table wines, ale, beer, champagne and sherry.

Phenelzine

Phenelzine is rapidly absorbed after oral administration and has a short half-life. It is contraindicated in patients with cerebrovascular disease, phaeochromocytoma, and in the manic phase of bipolar affective disorder. Common side effects include postural hypotension. Dose is 15 mg 3 times daily, increased if necessary to 4 times daily after two weeks. In-patients can be given 30 mg 3 times daily. The dose should be gradually reduced, the usual maintenance dose being 15 mg on alternate days.

Tranylcypromine

Tranylcypromine carries the risk of dependence because of its amphetamine like action. The initial dose is 10 mg twice daily not later than 3 pm. After one week the second dose can be increased to 20 mg. Contraindications are the same as that of phenelzine.

Isocarboxazid

The initial dose is 30 mg in single or divided doses. After four weeks, it can be increased to 60 mg daily for 4–6 weeks. The dose should be then reduced to 10–20 mg daily. In some patients, 40 mg may be required. Contraindications are the same as that of phenelzine.

Reversible Inhibitors of Monoamine Oxidase Type A (RIMAs)

Moclobemide

It selectively and reversibly inhibits monoamine oxidase type A. Moclobemide causes less potentiation of the pressor effect of tyramine than the traditional or irreversible MAOIs. It is indicated for social anxiety as well. The initial dose is 300 mg in divided doses taken after food, and the maximum dose is 600 mg. Not recommended in children. Contraindications are acute confusional state and haemochromocytoma.

Second Generation Antidepressants

Lofepramine

Lofepramine lacks the anticholinergic, antihistamine and cardiotoxic properties of the traditional TCAs. Lofepramine is therefore less sedating and is comparatively safer in overdose. Usual dose range is 140 mg to 210 mg. For the elderly, a lower dose is advised, but for patients under 18 years, it is not recommended.

Amoxapine

This is usually started at 100 mg to 150 mg per day and increased to 200 to 300 mg daily by the end of the first week. If no improvement is seen at this dose after two weeks, it may be increased up to 400 mg per day in outpatients and up to 600 mg per day in hospitalised patients. Doses up to 300 mg may be given in single or divided doses. Doses of more than 300 mg per day should be divided in two or three doses daily.

Mianserin

It is structurally a tetracycle antidepressant. Mianserin is a presynaptic alpha-2 receptor antagonist, with no significant effect on the reuptake of monoamines. There is minimal cardiotoxicity and is therefore safe in overdose. The usual dose range is 30 mg to 90 mg daily.

Selective Serotonin Reuptake Inhibitors (SSRIs)

Highly selective serotonin reuptake inhibitors have little or no effect on noradrenergic or dopamine neurotransmission. They, moreover, have no affinity for cholinergic, muscarinic, histaminergic, or alpha-adrenergic receptors. They exert their therapeutic effects through selective blockade of the reuptake of serotonin into the presynaptic neurons. Because of the different receptor profile than the tricyclics, SSRIs produce a different pattern of side effects. While the antidepressant action may be related to increased 5-HT function at serotonergic receptors, increased 5-HT activity at other receptors causes side effects: anxiety, restlessness, movement disorders, muscle rigidity, nausea, headache, insomnia, gastro-intestinal disturbances, and sexual dysfunction.

Although the SSRIs are generally safer than the older drugs, they have serious interactions when combined with other serotonergic agonists or with drugs that interfere with the normal metabolism of the SSRIs. These effects, referred to as the serotonin syndrome, are characterised by severe agitation, disorientation and confusion, ataxia, muscle spasms, and exaggerated autonomic nervous system functions including fever, shivering, chills, diarrhoea, elevated blood pressure, and increased heart rate. One other distinctive characteristic of the SSRIs compared with the older antidepressants is their ability to cause physical dependence. As many as 60% of patients suffer withdrawal effects following drug termination. The withdrawal symptoms, which can last for several weeks, include dizziness and ataxia, nausea, vomiting and diarrhoea, fatigue, chills, sensory disturbances, insomnia, vivid dreams and increased anxiety, agitation, and irritability.

SSRIs should not be discontinued abruptly as there have been many reports that sudden cessation leads to various discontinuation symptoms. It is, moreover, recommended that SSRIs should be intiated in lower doses so that patients can tolerate them gradually and this will also improve adherence.

Fluvoxamine

This antidepressant has a high incidence of nausea and vomiting. There is no active metabolite but it is less suitable for liver impairment. Its half-life is 17–22 hours. For depression, the initial dose is 50–100 mg daily in the evening, increased gradually if necessary to max. 300 mg daily (over 150 mg in divided doses); usual maintenance dose 100 mg daily. For obsessive-compulsive disorder, initially, 50 mg in the evening increased gradually if necessary after some weeks to a maximum of 300 mg daily (over 150 mg in divided doses); usual maintenance dose 100–300 mg daily. In children over 8 years initially 25 mg daily increased if necessary in steps of 25 mg every 4–7 days to a maximum of 200 mg daily (over 50 mg in 2 divided doses).

Fluoxetine

This has a half-life of 2–4 days and its active metabolite is norfluoxetine. Fluoxetine is less suitable for liver impairment. It increases plasma concentration of haloperidol, phenytoin, clozapine, warfarin and TCAs. For depression, 20 mg daily is the starting dose increased after 3–4 weeks to a the maximum of 60 mg daily. For elderly patients usual maximum dose is 40 mg daily. In children (8–18 years) 10 mg daily is the initial dose, increased after 1–2 weeks if necessary to 20 mg.

For bulimia nervosa, 60 mg daily as a single or divided dose. For elderly the usual maximum dose is 40 mg daily. In obsessive-compulsive disorder, 20 mg daily is the initial dose; increased gradually if necessary to max. 60 mg daily. 40 mg is the usual maximum dose for elderly patients. Consider the long half-life of fluoxetine when adjusting dosage (or in overdosage).

Sertraline

Its active metabolite is desmethysertraline. It has a lower potential for drug interaction. In depressive illness, initially, 50 mg daily is recommended, increased if necessary by increments of 50 mg at intervals of at least 1 week to a maximum of 200 mg daily. The usual maintenance dose is 50 mg daily.

In obsessive-compulsive disorder, for both adults and children over 12 years, the initial dose is 50 mg daily, increased if necessary in steps of 50 mg at intervals of at least one week, the maximum dose being 200 mg daily. For children 6–12 years, start initially at 25 mg daily, increase to 50 mg daily after one week, further increase if necessary in steps of 50 mg at intervals of at least one week. The maximum recommended dose is 200 mg daily. For panic disorder, post-traumatic stress disorder, or social anxiety disorder, 25 mg daily is the initial dose, increased after one week to 50 mg daily. If there is a partial response, increase the dose in steps of 50 mg at intervals of at least one week to a maximum of 200 mg daily.

Paroxetine

Paroxetine has a half-life of 24 hours, and it is an antidepressant of choice in liver impairment. In depression, social anxiety disorder, post-traumatic stress disorder, generalised anxiety disorder, 20 mg is the recommended dose. In adults maximum dose is 50 mg daily, and in elderly patients 40 mg. Paroxetine is not recommended for patients under 18 years.

In obsessive-compulsive disorder, 20 mg daily is the initial dose. It is to be increased gradually in steps of 10 mg to a maximum of 60 mg daily. For elderly patients, 40 mg is the maximum dose. For panic disorder, 10 mg is the initial dose, and can be increased gradually in steps of 10 mg to a maximum of 60 mg daily. In elderly, 40 mg daily is the maximum dose.

Citalopram

Citalopram also has no active metabolite and it has a low potential for drug interactions. For depressive illness, initiate as 20 mg once daily, and increase if necessary in steps of 20 mg daily at intervals of 3–4 weeks, to a maximum dose of 40 mg daily. For the elderly, the maximum dose is 20 mg daily.

For panic disorder, 10 mg daily is the initial dose to be increased gradually if necessary in steps of 10 mg daily, to the maximum 40 mg daily. For the elderly 20 mg is the maximum dose.

Escitalopram

This is S-enantiomer of citalopram. It is more selective than citalopram and by removing R-citalopram (at the synapse) escitalopram functions more effectively. Escitalopram increases serotonin levels more than citalopram For depressive illness, generalised anxiety disorder, and obsessive-compulsive disorder, 10 mg once daily is the initial dose. It can be increased if necessary to a maximum of 20 mg daily. In the elderly patients, 10 mg daily is the maximum dose.

For panic disorder, 5 mg once daily is the initial dose, increased to 10 mg daily after 7 days, with 20 mg daily being the maximum dose. 10 mg daily is the maximum dose in the elderly.

For social anxiety disorder, 10 mg once daily is the initial and can be increased after 2–4 weeks to 20 mg daily.

Norepinephrine and Dopamine Reuptake Inhibitors (NDRIs)

Bupropion

Bupropion is an atypical antidepressant, with dopaminergic and nor-adrenergic actions. It is used for smoking cessation and is useful for patients who do not respond to SSRIs or as an adjunctive who have symptoms suggestive of a norepinephrine or dopamine deficiency (psychomotor retardation, anhedonia, hypersomnia, cognitive slowing and food craving etc.). Side effects include agitation, insomnia, nausea, and seizures. The risk of seizures is about 1 in 1000 cases. It is contraindicated in patients with a history of seizures, eating disorders, bipolar disorder, pregnancy, and breastfeeding.

Serotonin and Noradrenaline Reuptake Inhibitors (SNRIs)

Venlafaxine

A low dose (75 mg) predominantly acts on serotonin inhibition. At moderate to higher dose its acts equally as both a serotonin and noradrenaline reuptake inhibitor. Blood pressure measurement is recommended. Specialist supervision is only required for the severely depressed or hospitalised patients on doses >300 mg. Smaller packs are recommended for those at the risk of overdose. Venlafaxine remains contraindicated in patients with an identified high risk of serious cardiac ventricular arrhythmia and uncontrolled hypertension. Common side effects are constipation, nausea, anorexia, weight changes, vomiting; hypertension, palpitation, vasodilatation, changes in serum cholesterol, chills, yawning; dizziness, dry mouth, insomnia, nervousness, drowsiness, asthenia, headache, abnormal dreams, anxiety, confusion, hypertonia, sensory disturbances, tremor, difficulty with micturition, sexual dysfunction, menstrual disturbances and mydriasis.

For depressive disorder, the initial dose is 75 mg daily in 2 divided doses increased if necessary at intervals of at least 2 weeks; a maximum of 375 mg daily. It is not recommended for patients under 18 years. For generalised anxiety disorder, 75 mg once daily is the commencing dose, increased if necessary at intervals of at least 2 weeks, to 225 mg maximum dose. For social anxiety disorder, recommended initial dose is 75 mg once daily, which may be increased at intervals of at least 2 weeks; 225 mg being the maximum dose.

Duloxetine

This is a relatively balanced inhibitor of both neurotransmitters as compared with venlafaxine. There is no significant affinity for dopaminergic, adrenergic, muscarinic or histaminergic receptors. Side effects include nausea, vomiting, dyspepsia, constipation, diarrhoea, abdominal pain, weight changes, decreased appetite, flatulence, dry mouth; palpitation, hot flush; insomnia, abnormal dreams, paraesthesia, drowsiness, anxiety, headache, dizziness, fatigue, weakness, tremor, nervousness, anorexia, sexual dysfunction, visual disturbances, sweating, and pruritus.

For depression, 60 mg once daily is the initial dose, the maximum being 120 mg daily. For generalised anxiety disorder, the initial dose is 30 mg daily, to be increased if necessary to maximum 120 mg daily.

Serotonin Antagonist/Reuptake Inhibitors (SARIs)

Nefazodone

Nefazodone transiently inhibits the reuptake of serotonin. It is distinguished from SSRIs by its effect on the Serotonin 2A receptors (blocks them). Sexual dysfunction and anxiety are caused by stimulation of 5-HT 2A receptors, so nefazodone is less likely to cause these side effects. Rare cases of hepatic toxicity have been reported with nefazodone. It has been withdrawn in the UK.

Noradrenaline Reuptake Inhibitors (NARIs)

Reboxetine

It may cause side effects that mimic anticholinergic symptoms because increasing norepinephrine at alpha receptors outside the brain reduces acetylcholine at muscarine receptors.Side effects include nausea, dry mouth, constipation, anorexia; tachycardia, palpitation, vasodilation, postural hypotension; headache, insomnia, dizziness; chills; impotence; urinary retention; impaired visual accommodation; sweating; lowering of plasma-potassium concentration on prolonged administration in the elderly. Some other adverse effects are: vomiting, hypertension, paraesthesia, agitation, anxiety, irritability, hallucinations, aggression, Raynaud's syndrome, hyponatraemia, and testicular pain 4 mg twice daily is the starting dose, and can be increased if necessary after 3–4 weeks to a maximum of 12 mg daily in divided doses. It is not recommended in children and elderly patients.

Atomoxetine

Although atomoxetine has an antidepressant affect, it is predominantly used in Attention Deficit Hyperactive Disorder (ADHD).

Noradrenergic and Specfic Serotonergic Antidepressants (NASSAs)

Mirtazapine

Mirtazapine has actions on both norepinephrine and serotonin systems but is not a reuptake inhibitor. Therapeutic effect mainly exerted through antagonism of alpha receptors, which leads to increased serotonin and norepinephrine release.

Side effects profile is influenced by its antagonism of 5-HT2A, 5-HT2C and 5-HT3 receptors. Unlike SSRIs which stimulate these receptors, mirtazapine blocks them, and thus avoids the majority of the side effects of SSRIs such as sexual dysfunction, anxiety, insomnia, and gastrointestinal effects. The potent antagonist effect on histamine type 1 (H1) receptors results in somnolence-induction.

Side effects include increased appetite, weight gain, dry mouth; postural hypotension, peripheral oedema; drowsiness, fatigue, tremor, dizziness, abnormal dreams, confusion, anxiety, insomnia; arthralgia, myalgia; less commonly syncope, hypotension, mania, hallucinations, movement disorders; rarely myoclonus; very rarely blood disorders, convulsions, hyponatraemia, suicidal behaviour, and angle-closure glaucoma. A large meta-analysis concluded that mirtazapine has the highest efficacy among the 12 antidepressants in the various studies. The starting dose is 15 mg at bedtime and can be increased to 45 mg. Not recommended for patients under 18 years.

Noradrenaline Reuptake Inhibitors (NARIs)

Agomelatine

It is an antagonist at melatonin MT1 and MT2 receptors. Side effects include nausea, vomiting, diarrhoea, constipation, abdominal pain, headache, dizziness, drowsiness, agitation, sleep disturbances, fatigue, anxiety; back pain and sweating. Starting dose is 25 mg at bedtime, increased if necessary after 2 weeks to 50 mg.

Pindolol

It has a role in treatment-resistant depression as an adjunctive treatment.

Thyroxine

It is used to augment antidepressant drug therapy.

Antipsychotics used as Adjunctive Antidepressants

Aripiprazole is licensed in the United States, whereas Quetiapine XL is licensed in the UK, as adjunctive antidepressant medication.

The starting dose for Quetiapine XL is 50 mg in the evening which can then be increased to a maximum dose of 300 mg daily.

Fluanxol has been used in lower doses as an antidepressant.

Antipsychotics

Antipsychotics constitute a class of drugs to treat schizophrenia, delusional disorders, mania and psychotic symptoms of major depression. They relieve psychotic symptoms like thought disorder, hallucinations, and delusions they are also used to prevent relapse of psychotic illnesses. The antipsychotics should be used for at least 4–6 weeks (in optimal dosages) before they are disregarded as ineffective. Doses of antipsychotics vary around the world. Similarly, there is a significant difference in the rate of use of injectable or long-acting medication (being higher in Europe than in the USA).

The antipsychotic potency of antipsychotics is directly proportional to their ability to block dopamine receptors. Antipsychotics also act on acetylcholine, norepinephrine, histamine and serotonin receptors, resulting in various side effects.

The term 'major tranquillisers' is no longer used but 'neuroleptic' is still used in some countries. The typical antipsychotics are also referred to as conventional, traditional, standard, classical or first-generation antipsychotics. These antipsychotics are effective for alleviating positive symptoms of schizophrenia and in preventing their recurrence. They have no significant effect on the negative symptoms, mood symptoms and cognitive symptoms of schizophrenia. Typical antipsychotics are also effective in controlling and preventing episodes of mania.

Atypical antipsychotics (second generation antipsychotics) are a group of drugs which have at least equal efficacy (compared to conventional antipsychotics) for alleviating positive symptoms, increased efficacy for negative symptoms, decreased tendency to cause extrapyramidal symptoms (EPS) and tardive dyskinesia. They have a lower or negligible propensity to raise prolactin levels.

Atypical antipsychotics are increasingly being used for their mood stabilising efficacy in bipolar affective disorder.

The various antipsychotics differ in their predominant actions and side effects. Because the various antipsychotics seem to be of comparable efficacy (2), the side effects are usually considered in determining the choice of antipsychotic drug. Side effects are modified by patient characteristics such as age, gender, ethnicity and comorbid physical illness. There is a wide variation in patients' responses.

A large meta-analyses of 52 randomised trials comparing atypicals (clozapine, risperidone, quetiapine, sertindole and amisulpride) with conventional antipsychotics (haloperidol or chlorpromazine) demonstrated no difference in efficacy and overall tolerability between typical and atypical antipsychotics if adequate dosage adjustments are made (3). However, one risk-benefit analysis of the typical versus the atypical antipsychotics favours the use of the newer agents as first-line drugs in treating schizophrenia (4). Their use may increase patients acceptability and compliance which may have possible benefits regarding relapse rates (5).

Second-generation antipsychotic drugs differ in many properties and are not a homogeneous class. This meta-analysis provides data for individualised treatment based on efficacy, side effects, and cost (6). Combination of two antipsychotic is not generally recommended and in case this is required the cumulative side effects and total doses of the two drugs should be carefully considered.

Typical Antipsychotics

Typical antipsychotics specifically block D2 receptors in the mesolimbic dopamine pathway and also block D2 receptors in the mesocortical dopamine (DA) pathway. This can cause or worsen negative and cognitive symptoms. When D2 receptors are blocked in the nigrostriatal DA pathway, EPS (Parkinsonism, acute dystonia and akathisia) are produced. Other acute side effects of typical antipsychotics include postural hypotension, anticholinergic side effects (like dryness of mouth and urinary hesitancy), impotence and cardiotoxicity.

Acute dystonic reactions like abnormal face and body movements, tongue protrusion or torticollis may be seen with drugs like phenothiazines and butyrophenones. Features suggestive of Parkinsonism, like tremors, rigidity, mask-like expressions and pill-rolling movements of the fingers are also seen.

If the blockade of D2 receptors is on a long-term basis, it can produce tardive dyskinesia. Other long-term side effects include hyperprolectinaemia (leading to galactorrhoea, amenorrhoea, and low libido), weight gain, and tardive dystonia.

Neuroleptic malignant syndrome, rash, hepatitis and agranulocytosis are idiosyncratic reactions. Antipsychotics should be used with caution in patients with cardiovascular disease, severe respiratory disease, and severe renal impairment. All antipsychotics can precipitate coma if used in hepatic impairment.

Typical antipsychotics are classified according to their chemical group. Phenothiazines are sub-grouped into aliphatics (chlorpromazine and promazine), piperidines (thioridazine and pipotiazine) and piperazines (trifluoperazine and fluphenazine).

Butyrophenones include haloperidol and benperidol, whereas flupenthixol and zuclopenthixol are examples of thioxanthenes group. Diphenylpiperidines group include pimozide, and sulpiride is a benzamide. Some authors classify sulpiride as an atypical antipsychotic.

Chlorpromazine

Apart from treating schizophrenia, chorpromazine is used for a wide variety of other conditions including mania, insomnia, anxiety, control of a violent patient, nausea and vomiting, and as an appetite stimulant in anorexia nervosa. Previously 1000 mg daily was the maximum dose in schizophrenia and other psychotic disorders. Now 400–600 mg daily is recommended as a maximum dose.

Common early side effects are sedation, hypotension (it is dose-related and causes dizziness), dry mouth, indigestion and blurred vision—all usually improving over 2 weeks. Uncommon early side effects include dystonia, torticollis, arching of the back, tongue protrusion, and oculogyric crises. Later on mild rash, weight gain, galactorrhoea, amenorrhoea, reduced libido, ejaculatory problems, erectile impotence, photosensitivity pigmentation of exposed skin, frostbite, epileptic fits (dose-dependent), and jaundice may occur. Tardive dyskinesia can occur as a late side effect. Agranulocytosis occurs rarely. Chlorpromazine interferes with the metabolism of morphine, pethidine, tricyclics (TCAs), and therefore, increases their blood levels. It is contraindicated in hypothyroidism, cirrhosis, after a recent attack of hepatitis and in a patient who is semi- comatose.

Promazine

Promazine is much less potent as an antipsychotic than chlorpromazine and is not effective in schizophrenia (7). It is occasionally used by the elderly as a hypnotic or sedative. Its potential for non-dependence is an advantage. It may cause urinary and faecal incontinence, disorientation and lowered temperature. For the elderly, the usual dose is 25–100 mg daily once or in divided doses (4 times/day).

Thioridazine

The side effect profile of thioridazine is similar to chlorpromazine. It has been withdrawn in the UK because of the potential serious affect on the heart. There are, however, two serious exceptions. First, a high dose of this drug can cause retinal pigmentation and secondly it has got the propensity to prolong QTc interval. After its implication in a number of unexplained deaths, it was withdrawn in the UK. If used, ECG should be recorded before starting and for any dose increase, and electrolytes should also be checked. It is contraindicated in patients with cardiac disease, in those having an abnormal ECG and when patients are using other drugs which may cause ECG changes.

Levomepromazine

Initial dose 25–50 mg/daily in divided dosages, the maximum dose is 1g daily. It is very sedative.

Pericyazine

Pericyazine is less likely to cause EPS, is very sedative and is rarely prescribed. Starting dose in schizophrenia is 75 mg /day in divided doses, increased at weekly intervals by 25 mg, the maximum dose being 300 mg/day.

Pipotiazine

Pipotiazine is also less likely to produce EPS and is only available in depot form.

Perphenazine

Perphenazine is quite effective, and is not very sedating but EPS especially dystonia is more frequent at high doses.

Initial dose 4 mg three times a day, maximum dose 24 mg/day.

Prochlorperazine

This is licensed for both schizophrenia and mania. It is less sedating and EPS, particularly dystonias more likely. The dose starts at 12.5 mg BD for one week, later increased gradually to a maximum of 100 mg/day.

Fluphenazine

The oral preparation has been discontinued in UK and it is only available in depot formulation.

Haloperidol

Haloperidol has little antihistamine action and therefore has less sedation. Similarly, haloperidol is less likely to cause autonomic disturbances because of little anticholinergic activity. It has, however, a high propensity for extrapyramidal symptoms as it is a potent blocker of D2 receptors. It is being used commonly for states of severe agitation and excitement.

Haloperidol is also increasingly being used by the elderly because of their risk of stroke with atypical antipsychotics (risperidone and olanzapine). Maximum dose is now 15 mg/day and in treatment-resistant schizophrenia, it is 30 mg/ day.

Droperidol

Droperidol is no longer available in the UK because of its association with QTc prolongation.

Benperidol

Benperidol is now rarely prescribed for psychoses. It is a potent D2 blocker and has been used for antisocial sexual behaviour although the evidence for its efficacy is not sufficient.

Trifluoperazine

Trifluoperazine is a high potency phenothiazine (20 times more so than chlorpromazine). It causes little sedation or hypotension but is associated with a high risk of EPS including tardive dyskinesia. Starting dose is 5 mg BD, but there is no agreement on the maximum dose.

Flupenthixol

This is mostly used in depot form. In small doses flupenthixol is sometimes used as an antidepressant, but it is not used routinely for treatment of depression.

Zuclopenthixol

As compared to flupenthixol, zuclopenthixol has a sedative effect. The initial dose is 20–30 mg daily in divided doses, the maximum being 150 mg/day. It is more commonly used in depot formulation.

Pimozide

Pimozide is a relatively specific D2 antagonist and the side effects, therefore, consist of EPS and increased prolactin related problems. It has the potential for QTc prolongation and baseline ECG is essential before its commencement. Then an annual ECG is mandatory.

Pimozide should not be used with other antipsychotic drugs (including depot preparations), and tricyclic antidepressants. It is also contraindicated in patients who are taking other drugs which prolong QTc interval (e.g., certain antimalarials, antiarrhythmic drugs and certain histamines) or those which cause electrolyte disturbances (especially diuretics). Pimozide is claimed to be particularly useful in delusional disorders especially monosymptomatic hypochondriacal psychosis. The evidence for this is debatable. 16 mg daily is the maximum dose.

Sulpiride

Sulpiride is a specific D2 plus some D3 and D4 receptor blockers. 800 mg/day in divided doses is the maximum dose for negative symptoms and 2.4 g /day for positive symptoms.

Amisulpride

It is often classified as atypical. In low doses, amisulpride blocks presynaptic D2 and D3 oms. It has a low propensity for EPS, causes less weight gain compared with risperidone or olanzapine and at higher doses increases prolactin levels. Other side effects include insomnia, anxiety and dry mouth.

Atypical Antipsychotics

In the last decade there has been an increasing tendency among clinicians to use atypical antipsychotics more than the traditional antipsychotics. The main rationale is to avoid extrapyramidal side effects of typical antipsychotics. It is, however, important to remember that the atypical antipsychotics also have side effects, although different from typical antipsychotics. Moreover, it has not been proven definitely that atypicals are more efficacious than the typical antipsychotics.

Risperidone

Risperidone is a potent dopamine D2 receptor antagonist, a potent serotonin 5HT2A receptor antagonist, and potent alpha-1-adrenergic receptor antagonist. It has low affinity for serotonin 5HT2C receptors, low afffinity for histamine Hi receptors and negligible affinity for muscarinic M1 receptors. Maximum recommended dose is 6 mg daily. Doses above this are likely to cause EPS.

Common side effects of risperidone include hypotension, headache, weight gain, sedation and prolactin increase.

Olanzapine

Olanzapine is a potent dopamine D2 receptors and serotonin 5HT2A antagonist. It has a high affinity for serotonin 5HT2C-receptors, muscarine M1 receptors, and histamine H1 receptors. Olanzapine has a moderate affinity for alpha-1–adrenergic receptors.

The optimal dose range is 5–20 mg/day. There are some anecdotal reports that 30–40 mg/day may be more beneficial in some patients who fail to show adequate response with optimal dose (8). There is a low incidence of TD, EPS and no significant increase in prolactin levels. Weight gain is the most problematic side-effect which is not necessarily dose-dependent. Diabetes and raised triglycerides have been reported which is not only seen with those with weight gain. Other side effects include dry mouth, somnolence and constipation.

Quetiapine

Quetiapine has a weak affinity for dopamine D2 receptors, low affinity for serotonin 5HT2A and 5HT2C receptors, and very low affinity for muscarinic M1 receptors. Its affinity for alpha-adrenergic and histaminic H1 receptors is very high.

Maximum daily dose of Quetiapine XL for schizophrenia and bipolar affective disorder is 800 mg (as a single dose in late evening/night). Quetiapine causes low EPS and prolactin increase is also low. It causes less weight gain than olanzapine and risperidone. There are some reports of QTc prolongation but ECG is not a requirement. Common side effects include somnolence, dry mouth, headache, postural hypotension, dyspepsia, dizziness and constipation.

Aripiprazole

Aripiprazole is a D2 receptor and 5HT1A partial agonis, and a 5HT2A receptor antagonist. Whether or not aripiprazole acts as an antagonist or as an agonist depends on the extracellular concentration of dopamine. In areas where there is dopaminergic hyperactivity (the mesolimbic pathway) it may act as a dopamine antagonist, while in areas in which there is dopaminergic hypoactivity (the mesocortical pathway), aripiprazole may act as a dopamine agonist.

Its long-term efficacy is equal to olanzapine (9). Another study showed consistent and robust efficacy comparable to both conventional and atypical antipsychotics (10). The starting dose in schizophrenia is 10 mg/day whereas for mania it is 15 mg/day. The maximum daily dose for both disorders is 30 mg. It is not associated with hyperprolactinaemia, QTc prolongation, impaired glucose tolerance or weight gain. Common side effects include headache, agitation, akathisia, anxiety, insomnia, dyspepsia, and nausea. In general, it is better tolerated than most other atypical antipsychotics (11).

Sertindole

Sertindole has a high affinity for 5HT2, D2 and alpha-1 receptors. Because of its association with prolonged QTc interval, it is available in the UK only on named-patient basis but is not commonly used. ECG and electrolyte monitoring is required as well due to which its use is quite restricted. Side effects include postural hypotension, decreased ejaculatory volume, nasal congestion, weight gain and dry mouth.

Ziprasidone

Ziprasidone has a high affinity for 5HT2 and D2 receptors and moderate affinity for alpha 1, alpha 2 and H1 receptors. It also exhibits 5HT1A antagonism. It is not available in the UK. Its doses range from 40 mg to 160 mg/day. Common side effects include insomnia, headache, and nausea. There is no weight gain and no anticholinergic side effects.

Zotepine

Zotepine is an antagonist at 5HT2A, 5HT2C, D2 and H1 receptors. It is rarely prescribed in the UK. It is associated with a significant reduction in seizure threshold (risk is increased at doses above 300 mg/day) and may prolong QTc interval. ECG is required before its initiation and after every dose increment. Dose range from 150 mg–300 mg.

Side effects include dry mouth, insomnia, drowsiness, both hypo-and hyperthermia, blood dyscrasias, constipation, raised prolactin levels and weight gain.

Paliperidone

Paliperidone is an active metabolite of risperidone. It shares the characteristic D2, 5HT2A antagonism of atypical antipsychotic drugs, and a receptor-bind profile similar to risperidone.

Almost negligible liver metabolism and sustained release. The dose range is 3–12 mg/daily. Side effects include headache, weight gain and EPS at 9 mg and above.

Asenapine

This has an affinity for D2, 5HT2A, 5HT2C, alpha 1 and alpha 2 adrenergic receptors and relatively low affinity for H1 and anticholinergic receptors. The usual dose is 5 mg twice daily. Asenapine has less potential to increase prolactin levels than risperidone and may also be associated with a lower risk of weight gain.

Clozapine

Clozapine has a relatively low affinity for D2 receptor, but a high affinity for serotonin 5HT2A and 5HT2C receptors, a high affinity for alpha-adrenergic receptors, a high affinity for Muscarine M1 and M4 receptors, and high affinity for histamine H1 receptors. It does not cause tardive dyskinesia and is sometimes used to treat this condition. It does not elevate prolactin levels.

Clozapine is licensed for treatment-resistant schizophrenia and patients selected for treatment should have had an unsatisfactory improvement despite the use of adequate doses of at least two antipsychotics. Most improvement occurs in the first 12 weeks which continues for up to one year. It is recommended that clozapine should be used for more than 4–6 months if there is no response.

Since the pivotal study (12) in which the antipsychotic efficacy of clozapine was established, other meta-analysis have sustained its superior clinical efficacy. Clozapine also reduces suicidality. However, the liability of clozapine to cause agranulocytosis, and mandatory blood count monitoring, together with its propensity to induce seizures, sedation, hypotension, hypersalivation and weight gain limits its use as a frontline antipsychotic. Apart from these side effects, diabetes may develop in 30% of patients in five years. The claim of its efficacy for negative symptoms is not substantiated. The risk of agranulocytosis is 3% but is reduced to about 0. 6% if weekly blood counts are performed to detect the onset of neutropenia.

Before initiating clozapine it is mandatory to register the patient with the Clozaril Monitoring Service (or equivalent body). Full blood count is performed weekly for the first 18 weeks (when the risk of neutropenia/agranulocytosis is greatest), fortnightly until 52 weeks of treatment and then monthly thereafter. The stating dose is 12.5 mg daily, increasing by 25–50 mg daily to 300 mg within two weeks or longer. This strategy minimises the incidence of side effects. The dose is then adjusted to 450 mg in majority of cases, the maximum daily dose being 900 mg. If clozapine is stopped for any reason for 48 hours, it has to be recommenced at small doses.

Combinations of Antipsychotics

When there is failure to respond to clozapine or clozapine needs to be given in lower doses, combination of clozapine with other antipsychotic is used sometimes. The various combinations include: Clozapine and aripiprazole, clozapine and amisulpride, clozapine and lamotrigine, clozapine and olanzapine, clozapine and quetiapine, clozapine and risperidone, clozapine and sulpiride, and clozapine and ziprasidone.

Apart from these, other combination and augmentation strategies that have been tried are: amisulpride and aripiorazole, amisulpride and risperidone, amisupride and ziprasidone, olanzapine and quetiapine, olanzapine and sulpiride and finally risperidone and olanzapine.

Depot and Long-Acting Injections

Although these injections can improve overt compliance, pain at the site of injection is the most common problem. Nodules and occasionally abscesses may occur. Persistence of a steady state drug level results in patients experiencing side effects and may continue to do so for some time even after a dose reduction has been undertaken. There is no evidence to suggest that shortening the licensed dosing intervals will enhance efficacy. A small test dose is essential to avoid severe side effect. Typical depot injections may give rise to a higher incidence of EPS than oral preparations. EPS occur less frequently with atypical depot injections. There are no clear indications for using different depots, but zuclopenthixol may be more suitable for the treatment of aggressive patients whereas flupenthixol is generally used for an alerting affect.

Flupenthixol Decanoate

Following a test dose of 20 mg, the dose can then be gradually titrated. The maximum BNF dose is 400 mg every week. The dosing interval is 2–4 weeks. It is contradicted in patients with circulatory collapse or depressed consciousness due to any cause e.g., intoxication with alcohol or opiates.

Zuclopenthixol Decanoate

The test dose is 100 mg and the maximum is 600 mg every week. The dosing interval is 2–4 weeks. It is useful in controlling aggression and agitation.

Fluphenazine Decanoate

The test dose is 12.5 mg, the maximum dose 50 mg every week. Dosing interval is 2–5 weeks.

Fluspirilene

This is a water-based weekly injection. It has no advantage over other depots.

Haloperidol Decanoate

Test dose is usually 25 mg, the maximum weekly dose being 75 mg. Because of its long half-life, it can be given every 4–6 weeks.

Pipothiazine Palmitate

The test dose is 25 mg. This injection can be given every four weeks, the maximum weekly dose being 50 mg.

Olanzapine Embonate

It is licensed for deep IM gluteal use in patients who have previously received oral doses of olanzapine. This does not need oral supplementation. There have been reports of idiosyncratic excessive sedation and due to this, it is mandatory to observe the patients in a healthcare facility for at least two hours. Dose conversion is as follows:

For oral dose of 10 mg daily, starting dose is 210 mg every 2 weeks or 405 mg every 4 weeks. Maintenance dose after 2 months is 150 mg every 2 weeks or 300 mg every 4weekly. For dose of 15 mg/daily, starting dose of the injection is 300 mg every 2 weeks and after 2 months of initiation, the maintenance dose is 210 mg every 2 weeks or 405 mg every 4 weeks. For 20 mg/ daily, the starting dose is 300 mg every 2 weeks and after 2 months, the maintenance dose is 300 mg every 2 weeks.

Risperdal Consta

The test dose is 12.5 mg, and the maximum is 50 mg every two weeks. This has recently been licensed for deltoid site as well. Patients should be first preferably treated with oral risperidone for at few days before commencement of this injection, to have an idea about side effects like severe EPS and hypotension, etc. Oral cover is needed for some weeks and then tapered off. Since steady-state occurs about 6–8 weeks after each dose change, it is recommended that dose increases only every 8 weeks.

Paliperidone Palmitate

This has recently been licensed in the UK. It is given on 4 weekly basis and treatment should be initiated with a dose of 234 mg on treatment day one and then 156 mg one week later, with both injections administered in the deltoid muscle. The recommended monthly maintenance dose is 117 mg; some patients may benefit from lower or higher maintenance doses within the recommended range of 39 to 234 mg based on individual tolerability and/or efficacy. Monthly maintenance doses can be administered in either the deltoid or gluteal muscle. Adverse events most commonly reported in paliperidone-treated patients (incidence ≥ 5% and occurring twice as often vs placebo) were injection site reactions, somnolence/sedation, dizziness, akathisia, and extrapyramidal disorder.

Zuclopenthixol Acetate

This is available as clopixol acuphase and the dose range is 50–150 mg (as a single dose). The maximum cumulative dose is 400 mg over two weeks with no more than four injections. There is no convincing evidence that it works better than haloperidol IM injection.

Aripiprazole

The IM preparation is for calming down agitated patients. Initially 5.25 mg–15 mg (usual dose is 9.75 mg) as a single dose. This is followed by 5.25–15 mg after 2 hours if necessary, maximum daily injections being three. The maximum daily combined oral and IM dose is 30 mg.

The long-acting depot (Abilfy Maintena) is given on a monthly basis (400 mg usually but for some patients 300 mg may be sufficient).

There is ample evidence of its superior side effect profile, its role in minimising hospitalisation, and enhancing the quality of life.

In USA it is also licensed for Bipolar disorder.

Side effects of Antipsychotic Medication

Extrapyramidal Side Effects (EPS)

Although EPS usually result because of typical antipsychotics, they can also occur as side effects of atypical antipsychotics, and more rarely, from high doses of certain antidepressants especially SSRIs, and from lithium. Among atypicals, relatively high rates occur with amisulpride and with risperidone at doses above 6 mg/day.

Acute Dystonia

This occurs soon after treatment begins. Risk factors include: Male gender, age under 40 years, high doses of high potency typical antipsychotics (e.g., haloperidol, trifluoperazine), history of dystonia, hypothyroidism and hypoparathyrodism. Among depot preparations, fluphenazine decanoate has been associated with dystonia. Acute dystonia is uncommon in elderly.

Acute dystonia is characterised by involuntary muscle spasms that produce briefly sustained or fixed abnormal postures. These can include bizarre positions of limbs and trunk, oculo- gyric crises, tongue protrusion, trismus, torticollis and laryngeal-pharyngeal constriction. The head and neck muscles are the most commonly affected. Due to the bizarre and dramatic presentation, the patient may look histrionic. It is sometimes very painful and frightening. Acute dystonia can be reversed in 15 minutes or so by procyclidine 5–10 mg given intravenously or intramuscularly, or by 1–2 mg of benztropine or benzhexol.

Drug-Induced Parkinsonism

The diagnosis of drug-induced parkinsonism may be missed as the clinical picture may sometimes be taken for apathy or even depression. It is more common in the elderly and in females. It usually develops after several days to weeks of continuous treatment with antipsychotics. The classic triad of tremor, rigidity and bradykinesia is present. Tremor is of two types, a postural tremor of high frequency and low amplitude, usually seen in the hands with arms outstreched and the resting tremor, which is of low frequency and high amplitude. Rigidity is of two types, lead pipe type and cog- wheel rigidity.

Bradykinesia is the most common manifestation of drug-induced parkinsonism. Bradykinesia (also known as akinesia) is slowing of motor movements and in addition to voluntary actions, speech and facial muscles may also be affected.

Akathisia

Approximately 20–25% of patients prescribed typical antipsychotics are affected, and it is one of the major reasons of non-compliance (13). This is a subjectively unpleasant state of generalised motor restlessness, with a need to move. This leads to an inability to keep still. Although it may occur after some months of initiating antipsychotic treatment, the usual onset is within two weeks. Akathisia may be mistaken for worsening of psychotic symptoms and the dose of the antipsychotic may be inadvertantly increased. Akathisia has been linked to violence and suicide (14).

Reducing the dose of typical antipsychotics may alleviate symptoms of akathisia. If this fails, switch to an atypical antipsychotic e.g., Quetiapine. If akathisia persists, benztropine (6 mg/day), propranolol (10–20 mg TDS) or the antihistamine cyproheptadine (4–8 mb BD) may be helpful. Failing this strategy, diazepam (5 mg TDS) or clonidine (0.2 mg–0.8 mg/day) is recommended.

Tardive Dyskinesia (TD)

Tardive dyskinesia is a movement disorder occuring in some patients who are chronically (for some years) exposed to antipsychotic medications. It is a serious complication that, unlike the other EPS, does not always recover when the drugs are stopped. The movements usually affect the face, but the limbs and the muscles of respiration may also be involved. Symptoms include grimacing, chewing and sucking movements, tongue rolling, choreoathetoid movements of the fingers and toes and slow, writhing movements of the trunk. In a minority of patients, TD can affect walking, breathing, eating and talking. TD movements are not present during sleep. TD needs to be distinguished from tardive dystonia which is the long-term persistence of a dystonic movement disorder.

Studies indicate that approximately 5% of patients taking typical antipsychotics develop TD each year (15). Patients over the age of 65 have a marked increase in rates of TD. It is more common among women, diabetics, and those with diffuse brain pathology. Newer antipsychotics (atypical) have a lower risk of causing TD and clozapine has even been recommended for treating TD. TD may worsen during the weeks following the discontinuation of antispychotics and there is improvement later on (16). Agents used for treating TD include Vitamin E, botulinum toxin, nifedipine, reserpine, tetrabenazine, alpha-methyldopa, apomorphine, bromocriptine and levodopa. Clonidine has produced promising results (17) and propranolol has also been recommended (18). As mentioned above, clozapine has demonstrated good efficacy in the treatment of TD (19).

Tardive Dystonia

It is late-onset persistent dystonia which occurs in some patients. Unlike acute tardive dyskinesia, tardive dystonia may respond to anticholinergic medication. It may also respond well to clozapine.

Tardive Akathisia

This is late-onset persistent akathisia. In this the accompanying subjective sense of restlessness. Treatment is the same as that for acute akathisia.

Autonomic Effects

Anticholinergic Effects

Apart from aliphatic phenothiazines, atypical antipsychotics drugs like clozapine and olanzapine (which have significant M1 receptors affinity) cause anticholinergic effects like dry mouth, urinary hesitancy, and constipation.

Adrenergic Effects

Peripheral vasodilation due to antagonism of post-synaptic alpha-1 and alpha-2 adrenoreceptors, leads to orthostatic hypotension.

Chlorpromazine, clozapine, risperidone and quetiapine are associated with this common side effect. Incidence is low with ziprasidone and aripiprazole. Blockade of above mentioned receptors can also cause miosis, nasal congestion, and sexual dysfunction. Clozapine can cause urinary incontinence which can be treated with desmopressin in tablet form or ephedrine nasal drops. Clozapine can also cause tachycardia in the initial stages of treatment.

Cardiovascular Side Effects

Sudden Death

Thioridazine, sertindole, and clozapine have been implicated in sudden death. The first two antipsychotics are associated with prolongation of QTc interval, while clozapine may cause death through myocarditis or cardiomyopathy.

Cerebrovascular Accident or Stroke

Risperidone and olanzapine have been contraindicated for use in elderly people for the treatment of behavioural problems in dementia.

Other Cardiovascular Effects

Prolongation of QTc interval can predispose some patients to torsades de pointes which is a dangerous ventricular tachycardia. If untreated, it may lead to ventricular fibrillation and cardiac arrest. QTc intervals above 440 ms in men and 470 ms in women are considered critical and require action (dose reduction or change of drug etc.).

Apart from clozapine, chlorpromazine, haloperdol, fluphenazine, risperidone and quetiapine can cause myocarditis. Symptoms include unexplained fatigue, fever, chest pain, palpitations or breathlessness. Myocarditis usually starts in the first 6–8 weeks of treatment, while cardiomyopathy may occur later (20).

Metabolic Side Effects

Diabetes and Hyperlipidaemia

Metabolic syndrome constitutes abdominal obesity (waist to hip ratio), plus two out of the following factors: Elevated triglycerides, reduced HDL cholesterol, raised blood pressure and elevated fasting glucose.

Diabetes can be either induced or exacerbated with atypical antipsychotics (21). This side effect is associated with clozapine and olanzapine (22) and to a lesser extent with risperidone and quetiapine (23).

Weight Gain

Clozapine is the biggest culprit regarding weight gain, followed by olanzapine, thioridazine, sertindole, chlorpromazine, quetiapine, and risperidone (24). Medications with relatively low tendency to induce weight gain include: amisulpride, aripiprazole, ziprasidone, haloperidol, fluphenazine and trifluoperazine.

The risk of weight gain is greater in females and individuals with the lowest baseline BMI are at the greatest risk of antipsychotic-induced weight gain (25).

Hyperprolactinaemia

Risperidone, amisulpride and zotepine are the more potent D2 antagonist and have the highest risk of inducing hyperprolactinaemia. High doses of olanzapine can also increase prolactin levels. Ziprasidone, clozapine and quetiapine are not usually associated with this problem. Aripiprazole not only does not elevate prolactin levels but is reputed to reduce pre-existing hyperprolactinaemia.

Hepatic, Dermatological and Ocular Side Effects

Chlorpromazine, clozapine and olanzapine may be associated with mild elevation of liver enzymes during the first month of exposure which appear to be benign and usually return to normal despite continued treatment. Apart from this side-effect, cholestatic jaundice and hepatocellular toxicity may occur Phenothiazines can cause allergic and photosensitive rashes and occasionally exfoliative dermatitis, generalised urticaria and angioneurotic oedema may occur. Allergic rashes are very rare with atypical antipsychotics. Antipsychotic medications which have anticholinergic profile can commonly cause impairment of accomodation. These drugs are contraindicated in close-angle glaucoma. Long-term exposure to phenothiazines may also cause lenticular and corneal deposits.

Haematological Side Effects

Neutropenia, thrombocytopenia agranulocy- tosis and thrombocytopenic purpura have been described with antipsychotics. Agranulocytosis is the most severe adverse reaction to clozapine. It is not dose dependent.

Sedation

Clozapine, olanzapine and quetiapine are the most sedative atypicals. Sedation can contribute to weight gain.

EEG and Seizures

Antipsychotics can cause EEG changes and lower the seizure threshold. The risk of seizures is increased in those with a history of epilepsy, or previous drug-induced fits, head trauma, or other cerebral pathology. The risk is greatest with clozapine, reaching an estimated frequency of 10% in patients receiving the drug for 3. 8 years (26). It is also significantly high with chlorpromazine, intermediate with thioridazine and trifluoperazine, and lowest with pimozide, haloperidol, sulpiride and fluphenazine.

Temperature Dysregulation

Clozapine can cause hyperthermia whereas hypothermia can be caused by chlorpromazine.

Neuroleptic Malignant Syndrome (NMS)

This is a rare but very serious side effect of antipsychotic drugs. It is associated with 15% mortality and is a medical emergency. If NMS develops, the antipsychotic drug should immediately be discontinued and the patient hospitalised. Most cases occur during the first two weeks of exposure to antipsychotic medication but they can occur anytime (27). There is alteration in the level of consciousness, fever, rigidity, and autonomic instability (tachycardia, diaphoresis, hypersalivation, incontinence, labile blood pressure).

Risk factors include: Male gender, dehydration, an intramuscular route of antipsychotic, rapid dose escalation, poorly controlled EPS, alcoholism, iron deficiency anaemia, presence of organic brain disease or mental retardation, concomitant lithium administration, and use of physical restraint.

Neuroleptic-induced heat stroke may also be present with fever and elevated CPK, but can usually be distinguished from NMS by the presence of agitation, muscle flaccidity and dry skin (28). Another condition to consider in the differential diagnosis is lethal catatonia. This is a febrile form of catatonia which occurs in medication-free patients and which often has similar clinical signs to NMS.

Mood Stabilisers

Lithium

Lithium remains a key drug in the treatment of bipolar disorder (29). Due to its established efficacy, it has continued to hold its place firmly as for many decades as a prophylactic treatment of bipolar affective disorder. It is also used in the augmentation of antidepressant treatment and, less frequently, in the augmentation of antipsychotic treatment of schizophrenia. It is reported to have specific antisuicidal effects.

There is a lot of evidence regarding lithium's efficacy in preventing recurrence of mood disorders (30). One study showed that lithium had prophylactic efficacy against mania, prolonging the time to intervention in a pooled analysis of two placebo-controlled 18-month trials of lamotrigine and lithium in bipolar I disorder. Although both lithium and lamotrigine delayed the time to treatment for any mood episode, lamotrigine showed a more robust effect in preventing depression than mania (31).

There is no evidence that lithium monotherapy is an effective treatment for schizophrenia. The evidence available on augmentation of antipsychotics with lithium was inconclusive. However, a trial of lithium has been recommended for treatment and prophylaxis if a patient has a recurrent episode of schizophreniform disorder. The antisuicidal effect of lithium treatment was studied in people with bipolar disorder, major affective disorder and schizoaffective disorder. The suicide rate in the groups receiving lithium treatment was significantly lower than that in groups without lithium (32). It is thought that this benefit is because of a reduction in impulsivity by lithium.

A recent meta-analysis of 12 randomised studies reporting suicide rates in people with mood disorders provides new support for the protective effect of lithium in this context (33).

However, lithium use is associated with a range of tubular and glomerular disorders resulting in chronic kidney disease and more rarely renal failure (34). It remains unclear who remains at the risk of either milder degrees of renal impairment or specific renal lesions and the influence of other factors like age, hypertension, and diabetes are also debatable. Screening for risk of renal disease is essential before prescribing lithium.

Lithium has a narrow therapeutic index (ratio of therapeutic dose to toxic dose), and acute toxicity is more likely in those with an already diminished glomerular filtration rate (35). It needs to be borne in mind that in some patients lithium may still be the only suitable mood stabiliser despite an abnormal estimated glomerular filtration rate. Because of the narrow therapeutic index and a number of adverse effects, there may be poor adherence to treatment (36).

Lithium toxicity (lithium intoxication) varies in presentation. Acute toxicity can occur in lithium naïve individuals or after a long, uneventful course of treatment. It can occur at therapeutic serum levels, and it can arise following a change in dose or the introduction of new medication. Chronic toxicity can be insidious but its effects are potentially serious. Mild toxicity is characterised by nausea, diarrhoea, blurred vision, polyuria, dizziness, a fine resting tremor, muscle weakness or drowsiness. Cerebellar signs are a core feature of lithium neurotoxicity. With increasing severity, parkinsonism and chorea may occur, indicating basal ganglia involvement. Confusion, blackouts, fasciculation, hyper-reflexia, incontinence and hypernatraemia may develop. In severe cases, acute renal failure, hypotension or hypertension occur. Electrocardiogram changes include sinus and junctional bradycardia and heartblock. Impaired consciousness, seizures and coma may progress to death.

Neurotoxic effects may be insidious in onset. A persistent cerebellar ataxia has been reported in the absence of overt toxicity.

Drug Interactions with Lithium

There are numerous drugs which interact with lithium. Thiazides should be avoided as they will raise serum lithium concentrations and extreme caution is needed with loop diuretics.

Angiotensin-Converting Enzyme inhibitors (ACE inhibitors) and Non-Steroidal Anti- Inflammatory Drugs (NSAIDs) reduce the excretion of lithium, whereas sodium bicarbonate increases lithium's excretion.

There are possible increased serotonergic effects with venlafaxine and lithium toxicity has been reported with SSRIs and tricyclics. When given with methyldopa, clonazepam, carbamazepine, phenytoin, olanzapine, clozapine, flupenthixol, haloperidol, phenothiazines or zuclopenthixol, neurotoxicity may occur. There is also an increased risk of extrapyramidal side effects with antipsychotics.

Side Effects of Lithium

Early side effects are nausea, vomiting, abdominal discomfort, diarrhoea, fine tremor, polyuria and thirst. If vomiting and diarrhoea are severe and persistent, then toxicity should be suspected. Late side effects are weight gain, nephrogenic diabetes insipidus, thyroid enlargement (goitre) occurs in 5% of patients and hypothyroidism in 5–10%. Treatment with thyroxine is indicated and lithium does not have to be discontinued. When lithium is stopped, thyroid function usually returns to normal within two months. Lithium can cause benign reversible T-wave flattening or inversion. It can also produce or exacerbate acne and psoriasis. Other late effects are teratogenic effects, and toxicity.

In therapeutic doses lithium does not impair psychomotor coordination and driving private motor vehicles is not a bar. Driving certain public vehicles is however excluded with a diagnosis of bipolar affective disorder and after an admission for mania, the patient may not drive for 6–12 months.

The therapeutic range is from 0.4 to 1.2 mmol/L. Some authors insist that the minimum effective plasma level should be 0.6 mmol/L. The blood sample is taken 12 hours after the dose. The dose ranges from 600–1200 mg/day. While there is no established evidence for withdrawal or rebound psychoses, there is likelihood of relapse of mania if lithium is abruptly stopped. It is therefore essential that if lithium is to be discontinued it should be gradually reduced over a period of four weeks, and preferably up to three months, before stopping.

Carbamazepine

Carbamazepine is superior to lithium in rapid cycling (more than four episodes per year) and is also indicated in patients who have failed to show response to lithium (37). Although carbamazepine is effective in bipolar disorder, its overall efficacy is probably a little less than lithium. The starting dose is 400 mg daily, and the maximum is 1600 mg/day.

Common side effects include dry mouth, nausea, vomiting, oedema, ataxia, dizziness, drowsiness, fatigue, headache, hyponatraemia, eosinophilia, leucopenia, thrombocytopenia, dermatitis, and urticaria.

Carbamazepine increases the metabolism of tricyclic antidepressants, benzodiazepines, haloperidol, oral contraceptive agents, thyroxine, warfarin and other anticonvulsants. Neurotoxicity has been reported with a combination of lithium and carbamazepine even with normal lithium levels.

Valproate

Valproate has been shown to be efficacious for mania (38). It is generally well tolerated but side effects include vomiting, and tremor. Weight gain, rash, transient hair loss and potentially acute liver damage. It is advisable to monitor liver function tests every 3–6 months. For sodium valproate (which is not licensed for bipolar disorder) the starting dose is 600 mg daily or 500 mg modified release, increasing to 2000 mg according to the clinical response. Semi-sodium valproate is licensed and its starting dose is 750 mg daily in divided dose, the maximum being 2G daily. It should not normally be prescribed for women of childbearing age.

Lamotrigine

Although lamotrigine is not licensed in the UK for treating mood disorders, however it is used, as some studies have shown its efficacy. It is effective in the acute treatment of bipolar depression (39) and also in the long-term prevention of this disorder (40). As a monotherapy, lamotrigine does not have a significant anti-manic effect in manageing acute mania or in the prophylaxis of bipolar affective disorder. Apart from skin eruptions, nausea, headache, diplopia, blurred vision, dizziness, ataxia, and tremors are common side effects.

The recommended starting dose is 25 mg for the first two weeks, and then 50 mg daily for the next two weeks. The maximum dose is 300 mg per day.

Gabapentin

It is not licensed for the treatment of mood disorders and as with lamotrigine, gabapentin is sometimes used in bipolar disorder in patients who have not responded to standard treatments. The most common side effects are somnolence, dizziness, fatigue, and nystagmus. The usual dose range is between 600 mg and 2400 mg daily.

Antipsychotics Used in Bipolar Disorder

Typical antipsychotics like haloperidol and chlopromazine have been used for decades to treat mania. The atypicals which have shown efficacy for mania include olanzapine, risperidone, quetiapine, ziprasidone and aripiprazole.

The efficacy of aripiprazole in the treatment of acute mania and prevention of manic relapse has been well-established. In a placebo-controlled combination treatment study with either valproate or lithium, aripiprazole was superior to valproate or lithium alone (41). Because of the good tolerability side effect profile, aripiprazole has been given recommendation grade 1 in the guidelines of the world federation of societies of biological psychiatry (42).

Olanzapine has shown superiority over placebo in four double-blind placebo-controlled monotherapy studies (43). It has also exhibited superiority over valproate and lithium but more patients have reported adverse events which may limit the use of olanzapine. Weight gain, increased glucose levels, and increased lipids levels, are serious side effects of olanzapine. Studies have shown the efficacy of quetiapine (44) and risperidone (45) but like olanzapine, these two atypical antipsychotics have also been implicated in causing metabolic side effects. Risperidone, in addition, also causes prolactinoma.

Hypnotics

Diazepam and Other Benzodiazepines

Benzodiazepines are effective anxiolytics and hypnotics. They are safe from overdose when taken alone. Deaths from benzodiazepine overdose are very rare and patients have survived overdose of up to 2 g. Benzodiazepines can be taken with most other drugs as they have very little interactions. Benzodiazepines work by potentiating the inhibitory neurotransmitter γ-aminobutyric acid (GABA) in the CNS.

They differ in potency, the high potency benzodiazepines being alprazolam, clonazepam and lorazepam. Diazepam has low potency. Lorazepam, oxazepam, and temazepam have half-lives averageing 12 hours or less. Alprazolam has a half-life of 9 to 16 hours. When taken orally, the bioavailability of diazepam is almost complete and peak plasma concentrations are reached in 30–90 minutes. The presence of food reduces the rate but not the extent of absorption. Absorption following intramuscular administration is erratic and often slower than after oral dosing. In adults, the elimination half-life is around 20 hours, but over 65 years of age it is 40 hours. As it takes approximately five half-lives to wash a drug out of the plasma, for diazepam it is between 4 to 10 days on average.

The common side effects of benzodiazepines are cognitive and psychomotor impairment, metallic taste, sleep disturbance, agitation, restlessness, blurred vision, sore eyes, headache, tremor, and photophobia. The amnesia caused by benzodiazepines is of anterograde type, with no impairment of retention or retrieval of previously stored information. Moreover, they can have paradoxical reactions (e.g., aggressive behaviour), tolerance, and dependence. Benzodiazepines are best avoided during pregnancy as there have been reports of cleft lip and cleft palate.

Benzodiazepines used as hypnotics include nitrazepam and flurazepam which have a prolonged action. Loprazolam, lormetazepam and temazepam are short-acting and have little hangover effect. The dose of nitrazepam is 5–10 mg at bedtime. Lormatazepam's maximum dose is 1.5 mg and that of loprazolam is 2 mg. The dose range of flurazepam is 15–30 mg at bedtime. Temazepam is usually given as 10–20 mg but in exceptional circumstances can be given up to 40 mg. The maximum dose of chlordiazepoxide is 120 mg. Withdrawal symptoms of benzodiazepines include confusion, toxic psychosis, and convulsions.

Other Hypnotics

Zopiclone

Although zopiclone is structurally different from benzodiazepines and barbiturates, it interacts with the GABA-A receptors. It has sedative, hypnotic, anticonvulsant and muscle-relaxant properties. It has a short half-life and is used for night sedation. It should not be used for more than four weeks. Hangover effects, effects on alcohol and the interaction with alcohol, are less marked than for most benzodiazepines. It should, however, not be prescribed for those patients who are abusing alcohol or other substances. Side effects include a bitter taste, nausea, vomiting, irritability, and depression. Rarely zopiclone can cause confusion, amnesia, nightmares, and hallucinations. The usual dose is 7.5 mg and the maximum is 15 mg at night.

Zolpidem

Zolpidem is very fast-acting and begins to act within half to one hour. There are no significant side effects but lightheadedness may occur. Four weeks use does not result in withdrawal or dependence. Side effects include, diarrhoea, nausea, vomiting, dizziness, headache, drowsiness, agitation, amnesia, depression, confusion, perceptual disturbances or diplopia, tremor, ataxia, skin reactions, changes in libido, and muscular weakness. The usual daily dose range is 5–10 mg.

Zaleplon

Zaleplon is short-acting and its elimination half-life is around one hour. There are, therefore, no hangover effects in the morning and four weeks use is quite safe. Side effects include amnesia, paraesthesia, and dysmenorrhea. Less common side effects are: Anorexia, incoordination, confusion, impaired concentration, depression, depersonalisation, dizziness, and hallucinations. The usual daily dose is 10 mg.

Chloral hydrate

The use of chloral hydrate has significantly declined although it is associated with very few side effects and is short-acting. It is contraindicated in severe cardiac disease, gastritis and acute porphyria. Side effects include gastric irritation, abdominal distention, flatulence, headache, excitement, delirium, ketonuria and rash. The hypnotic dose is 1–2 g.

Clomethiazole

Like chloral hydrate, the use of clomethiazole is now very limited. This is contraindicated in acute pulmonary insufficiency, and in patients who are dependent on alcohol and continue to drink. Side effects include nasal congestion, irritation, and headache. Rare side effects are gastrointestinal disturbances, paradoxical excitement, confusion, rash, and urticaria. For severe insomnia, 1–2 capsules (192 mg each).

Antihistamines (Promethazine Hydrochloride)

Promethazine is available over the counter for insomnia. Because of its prolonged action, it can cause drowsiness the following day. The side effects include headache, psychomotor impairment, urinary retention, dry mouth, blurred vision and gastrointestinal disturbances. Rare side effects include hypotension, palpitation, arrhythmias, extrapyramidal effects, dizziness, confusion, depression, tremor, bronchospasm, rashes and liver dysfunction. The dose range is 25–50 mg/day.

Barbiturates (Amylobarbitone Sodium and Paraldehyde)

The use of barbiturates as hypnotics and anxiolytics is now significantly decreased. Barbiturates are very strong respiratory depressants and unsuitable in chronic bronchitis. They are not used in elderly because of the possibility of causing disorientation. Their main adverse effects are on psychomotor function. Cognitive performance and motor skills are both impaired, and this can occur as a hangover effect following a single night-time dose. With chronic use, tolerance develops to their effects.

They are contraindicated with alcohol use as alcohol potentiates their effect. They should be used with care as they have a serious risk of dependence, and there is a risk of death from accidental poisoning, and of suicide. In renal or liver disease, amylobarbitone has to be used with caution but paraldehyde is safe in poor renal function (as it is excreted in the breath). Amylobarbitone is started with 400 mg or 600 mg orally and then 200 mg every four hourly. More rapid control of severe emotional and behavioural disturbance is gained by a single intramuscular or slow intravenous dose of 250 mg or more (up to 0.5 g intramuscularly and 1g intravenously). The use of paraldehyde in controlling excitement is now obsolete as it is quite unpleasant in smell, and injection of more than 5 ml at one site can cause local necrosis and sterile abscess formation. The dose is 5–10 ml.

Anxiolytics

Benzodiazepines

Benzodiazepines are very effective in alleviating anxiety symptoms but because of the dependence potential they should be prescribed in the smallest possible doses and for the shortest possible time. Diazepam, alprazolam, chlordiazepoxide hydrochloride, lorazepam, and oxazepam are all effective in anxiety states. Diazepam, alprazolam, chlordiazepoxide and clobazam have a longer action, while lorazepam and oxazepam are short-acting. Maximum dose of diazepam is 30 mg/day, of chlordiazepoxide 120 mg/day, lorazepam 4 mg/day, and oxazepam 30 mg/day. Alprazolam is given as 250–500 micrograms 3 times daily.

Beta-Blockers (Propranolol Hydrochloride)

Propranolol is only useful in reducing the somatic symptoms of anxiety (palpitation and tremors, etc.) and does not alleviate the psychological symptoms of anxiety. Propranolol is contraindicated in asthma, marked bradycardia, hypotension, metabolic acidosis and severe peripheral arterial disease. Side effects include gastrointestinal disturbances, hypotension, bronchospasm, dyspnoea, headache, fatigue, dizziness, paraesthesia, vertigo, and sleep disturbances. Initiating dose is 40 mg, increased to 40 mg three times a day.

Buspirone

Buspirone is helpful in generalised anxiety disorder but not in panic disorder. Unlike benzodiazepines, buspirone takes 1–2 weeks to have its effect. It does not have an affinity for benzodiazepine receptors but stimulates 5HT1A receptors and is also an antagonist at D2 receptors. Early side effects associated with buspirone are lightheadedness, nausea, nervousness and headache. It does not cause sedation and tolerance and dependence does not usually occur. It is not indicated for treating benzodiazepine withdrawal. Buspirone should not be used in combination with MAOIs as this can result in hypertensive crises. There are no signficant interactions with trcyclic antidepressants and antipsychotics. However, as buspirone has pro-convulsant effects, it is contraindicated in patients with epilepsy. The recommended dose is 5–10 mg three times a day.

Meprobamate

This is contraindicated in acute pulmonary insufficiency, respiratory depression and acute porphyria. Side effects are similar to those with diazepam but their incidence is greater with meprobamate. Drowsiness is the most common side effect. Other common side effects include hypotension, weakness, gastrointestinal disturbances, and paraesthesia. Dose is 400 mg 3–4 times a day.

Barbiturates (see above)

Anticholinergic Drugs

Antimuscarinic drugs are used to treat the extrapyramidal symptoms caused by antipsychotic medication. Their routine use with antipsychotic medication (without the presence of EPS) is not recommended. It needs to be borne in mind that they are not useful to treat tardive dyskinesia. Apart from procyclidine, orphenadrine, and benzhexol hydrochloride (trihexyphenidyl hydrochloride) are also used to manage EPS. There is no significant difference between these drugs except different patients vary in their tolerability profile.

Side effects include constipation, dry mouth, nausea, vomiting, tachycardia, dizziness, confusion, euphoria, hallucinations, impaired memory, anxiety, urinary retention, blurred vision, and rash.

The maximum dose of procyclidine is 30 mg in divided doses. Orphenadrine is started at 150 mg in divided doses, the maximum daily dose being 400 mg daily. Benzhexol hydrochloride is commenced as 1 mg daily, the usual maintenance dose is 5–15 mg in divided doses. The maximum is 20 mg daily.

Electroconvulsive Therapy (ECT)

ECT continues to remain a debatable treatment option especially because of the significant concern about its association with memory loss. Moreover, it has also been used in certain disorders without any evidence of its efficacy. ECT involves the application of electrical current to the head. In contrast to the past, when sine wave current was used, modern ECT machines deliver alternating current, the magnitude of which is constant in brief pulses (1–2 milliseconds). This results in less electrical current delivered and fewer cognitive deficits after the treatment. Electrode placement may be either bilateral or unilateral. Different recommendations have been made regarding the relative merits and disadvantages of unilateral versus bilateral ECT. Unilateral ECT produces less confusion and memory disturbance. It is, however, less effective in severe illnesses and may require more applications. The dose of ECT requires clinical judgement because efficacy and adverse cognitive effects both increase along with the intensity of the stimulus. The seizure duration should be more than 20 seconds to ensure optimal efficacy. The seizure threshold is the minimum charge required to induce a seizure and can vary 40–fold between individuals. The current recommendations are that the charge should exceed the seizure threshold by 150–250% for unilateral non-dominant ECT and by 50–100% for bilateral EC (46). Factors raising the seizure threshold are male sex, advanced age, administration of bilateral ECT, anticonvulsants, benzodiazepines and general anaesthesia.

ECT is usually administered twice weekly in the UK and three times a week in the USA. There is no evidence to suggest that giving ECT three times weekly has more benefits as compared to twice weekly. The number of ECT treatments required also remains a matter of debate and clinical judgement has to be exercised for this. Generally, 6–12 treatments are given.

The NICE guidelines advocate the restriction of the use of ECT 'only to achieve rapid short- term improvement of severe symptoms after an adequate trial of other treatment options has proven ineffective and/or when the condition is considered potentially life-threatening'. According to NICE guidelines, even those patients who have been detained under the mental health act, cannot be given ECT without their consent. Moreover, as the long-term benefits and risks of ECT have not been clearly established, NICE guidelines do not recommend ECT as a maintenance therapy for depressive illness or the use of ECT in schizophrenia.

In spite of the controversy, electroconvulsive therapy is an important treatment option for major depression and is indicated for life- threatening symptoms of depressive illness. It is particularly indicated in cases of severe psychomotor retardation in which there are immediate concerns about the patient's physical well-being, for example if their fluid intake is poor. It may be used urgently when there is an acute risk of harm to the individual or to other people, due to the patient acting on psychotic delusions or hallucinations. However there is no direct evidence that ECT prevents suicide. Remission rates are higher and remission occurs earlier in patients with psychotic as opposed to non-psychotic depression (47). Studies suggest that major depression with psychotic features and patients in the depressive phase of bipolar affective disorder respond very well to ECT (48). Although the effectiveness of ECT in depression is well-established (49) there is less evidence that short-term benefits are maintained in the long-term.

ECT may be effective in the management of puerperal psychosis, especially when affective symptoms predominate. ECT is also safe and effective in pregnancy, the risk being associated only with anaesthesia. In recent years there has been some renewed interest in the use of ECT in mania, but the supporting evidence is small. In cases of severe manic illness, where there is severe exhaustion, excitement or manic stupor, it has the advantage of producing a rapid response. Patients with mixed affective states, who usually show poor response to drug therapy, may respond better to EC (50). Electroconvulsive therapy has traditionally been recommended for acute catatonic symptoms associated with both schizophrenia and affective disorders. Classic cases of catatonia have become much less frequent with the introduction of neuroleptic drugs, but cases of catatonia still occur.

The efficacy of ECT in schizophrenia has been the subject of many critical reviews and the administration of ECT to those with schizophrenia lacks a strong research base (51). In fact, some authors have even warned against the use of ECT in schizophrenia (52). ECT, however, has a role in catatonic schizophrenia and when there is prominent affective symptomatology. Lithium is occasionally used for lethal catatonia and neuroleptic malignant syndrome. Lethal catatonia is a syndrome described by some investigators as clinically similar to the neuroleptic malignant syndrome. However, other authors insist that there are differences in mode of onset, signs and symptoms and outcome. Lethal catatonia often begins with extreme psychotic excitement, which, if persistent, can lead to fever, exhaustion, and death. Neuroleptic malignant syndrome begins with severe extrapyramidally induced muscle rigidity (53).

ECT is a safe treatment, having a mortality rate no greater than that associated with the administration of a general anesthetic for minor surgery. There are no absolute contradictions to it (54) and all patients should be individually assessed and the benefits of ECT weighed against its potential hazards. However, recent cerebral infarction, increased intracranial pressure, unstable angina, uncomplicated congestive cardiac failure, severe cardiovascular or pulmonary disease and fragile vascular aneurysms place patients at risk with ECT. Common side effects associated with ECT include headache, nausea, dizziness, short-term retrograde amnesia, muscular aches, transient confusion and cognitive side effects. Recent evidence has suggested that some patients may suffer from long-term memory deficits.

Psychosurgery

Psychosurgical techniques involve lobotomies, cingulotomies, tractotomies and cingulotomies. The major indication for psychosurgery is the presence of a debilitating, chronic mental disorder that has not responded to any other treatment. Patients suffering from chronic intractable major depressive disorder and OCD, have responded to psychosurgery. Psychosurgery is also done in some neurological disorders such as epilepsy and chronic pain disorder. Although psychosurgery is now rarely done in many countries (including the UK), interest in psychosurgical approaches has recently been rekindled in the USA (55).

Other Somatic Treatments

Repetitive Transcranial Magnetic Stimulation (RTMS), deep brain stimulation and vagus nerve stimulation are new techniques that are being tried in various psychiatric disorders. The RTMS technique involves repeated short bursts of magnetic energy to stimulate nerve cells in the brain. There are encourageing reports that this technique is effective for mania and depression. It cannot, however, be used in patients with psychotic features and those who are suicidal or very dangerous (56). Moreover, very few places have the facility of this technique as well as for deep brain stimulation and vagus nerve stimulation.

In deep brain stimulation, an electrode is implanted at a specifically designated area of the brain depending upon the disorder being treated. Electric impulses are then sent to that area via a wire. Blockade of the electrical signals generated in that area reportedly results in improvement of symptoms. Vagus nerve stimulation has been tried for depressive disorder (57).

REFERENCES

1. Hindmarch, I. and Currie, D. J. (1995). In D. J. King (Ed.), *Seminars in clinical psychopharmacology*. London: The Royal College of Psychiatrists.
2. Lieberman, J. A., Stroup, T. S., mcevoy, J. P., et al. (2005). Effectiveness of antipsychotic drugs in patients with chronic schizophrenia. *New England Journal of Medicine*, 353, 1209–1223.
3. Geddes, J., Freemantle, N., Harrison, P., et al. (2000). Atypical antipsychotics in the treatment of schizophrenia: systematic overview and meta-regression analysis. *British Medical Journal*, 321(7273), 1371–1376.
4. Lieberman, J. A. (1996). Atypical antipsychotic drugs as a first-line treatment of schizophrenia: A rationale and hypothesis. *Journal of Clinical Psychiatry*, 57(11), 68–71.
5. Sharif, Z. A. (1998). Common treatment goals of antipsychotics: acute treatment. *Journal of Clinical Psychiatry*, 59(19), 5–8.
6. Leucht, S., Corves, C., Arbter, D., Engel, R. R., et al. (2009). Second-generation versus first-generation antipsychotic drugs for schizophrenia: A meta-analysis *The Lancet*, 373(9657), 31–41.
7. Taylor, D., Paton, C. and Kerwin, R. (2007). *The Maudsley Prescribing Guidelines* (9th Edition). UK: Informa Healthcare.
8. Reich, J. (1999). Use of high dose olanzapine in refractory psychosis. *American Journal of Psychiatry*, 156, 661.
9. Chrzanowski, W. K., Marcus, R. N., Torbeyns, A., et al. (2006). Effectiveness of long-term aripiprazole therapy in patients with acutely relapsing or chronic, stable schizophrenia: a 52– week, open-label comparison with olanzapine. *Psychopharmacology*, 189, 259–66.
10. Ozdemir, V. (2000). Aripiprazole. *Current Opinion in CPNS Investigative Drugs*, 2, 105–111.
11. Mir, A., Shivakumar, K., mcallister, V., et al. (2006). Change is sexual dysfunction on switching to aripiprazole. *Schizophrenia Research*, 81, 137–138.
12. Kane, J., Honigfield, G., Singer, J., et al. (1988). Clozapine for the treatment-resistant schizophrenic. *Archives of General Psychiatry*, 45, 789–796.
13. Owens, D. G. C. (1988). Clinical Psychopharmacology. In C. Johnstone, C. P. L. Freeman and A. K. Zealley (Eds.) *Companion to psychiatric studies* (6th Edition). Edinburg: Churchill Livingstone.
14. Van Putten, T., et al. (1987). Behavioural toxicity of antipsychotic drugs. *Journal of Clinical Psychiatry*, 48, 13–19.
15. Kane, J. M. and Lieberman, J. (1992). Tardive dyskinesia. In J. M. Kane and J. A. Lieberman (Eds.), *Adverse effects of psychotropic drugs*. New York: Guildford Press.
16. Glazer, W. M., Bowers, M. B., Charney, D. S., et al. (1989). The effect of neuroleptic discontinuation on psychopathology, involuntary movements, and biochemical measures in patients with persistent tardive dyskinesia. *Biological Psychiatry*, 26, 224–233.
17. Freedman, R., Kirch, D., Bell, J., et al. (1982). Clonidine treatment of schizophrenia. Double blind comparison to placebo and neuroleptic drugs. *Acta Psychiatrica Scandinavia*, 65, 35–45.
18. Perenyi, A. and Farkas, A. (1983). Propranolol in the treatment of tardive dyskinesia. *Biological Psychiatry*, 18, 391–394.
19. Lieberman, J. A., Saltz, B. L., Johns, C. A., et al. (1991). The effects of clozapine on tardive dyskinesia. *British Journal of Psychiatry*, 158, 503– 510.
20. Killian, J. G., Kerr, K., Lawrence, C., et al. (1999). Myocarditis and cardiomyopathy associated with clozapine. *The Lancet*, 354, 1841–1845.
21. Liebzeit, K. A., Markowitz, J. S., Caley, C. F. (2001). New onset diabetes and atypical antipsychotics. *European Neuropsychopharmacology*, 11, 25–32.

22. Haddad, P. M. (2004). Antipsychotics and diabetes: review of non-prospective data. British *Journal of Psychiatry*, 184, 80–86.
23. Melkersson, K. and Dahl, M. L. (2004). Adverse metabolic effects associated with aypical antipsychotics: literature review and clinical implications. *Drugs*, 64, 701–723.
24. Allison, D. B., Mentore, J. L., Heo, M., et al. (1999). Antipsychotic-induced weight gain a comprehensive research synthesis. *American Journal of Psychiatry*, 156, 1686–1696.
25. Findling, R. L., Steiner, H., Weller, E. B. (2005). Use of antipsychotic in children and adolescents. *Journal of Clinical Psychiatry*, 66(7), 29–40.
26. Devinsky, O., Honigfeld, G. and Patin, J. (1991).Clozapine-related seizures. *Neurology*, 41, 369–371.
27. Addonizio, G., Suman, V. L. and Roth, S. D. (1987). Neuropleptic malignant syndrome: review and analysis of 115 cases. *Biological Psychiatry*, 22, 1004–1020.
28. Lazarus, A. (1989). Differentiating neuroleptic- related heatstroke from neuroleptic malignant syndrome. *Psychosomatics*, 30, 108–110.
29. National Institute for Health and Clinical Excellence. (2006). *The management of bipolar disorder in adults, children and adolescents, in primary and secondary care*. Leicester: The British Psychological Society.
30. Burgess, S., Geddes, J., Hawton, K., et al. (2001). Lithium for maintenance treatment of mood disorders. *Cochrane Database of Systematic Reviews*, 3, CD003013.
31. Goodwin, G. M., Bowden, C. L., Calabrese, J. R., et al. (2004). A pooled analysis of 2 placebo- controlled 18-month trials of lamotrigine and lithium maintenance in bipolar I disorder. *Journal of Clinical Psychiatry*, 65, 432–441.
32. Tondo, L., Hennen, J., Baldessarini, R. J., et al. (2001). Lower suicide risk with long-term lithium treatment in major affective illness: A meta-analysis. *Acta Psychiatrica Scandinavica*, 104, 163–172.
33. Cipriani, A., Wilder, H., Hawton, K., et al. (2005). Lithium in the prevention of suicidal behaviour and all-cause mortality in patients with mood disorders: A systematic review ofrandomised trials. *American Journal of Psychiatry*, 162, 1805–1819.
34. Schreiner, A, Waldherr, R., Rohmeiss, P. and Hewer, W. (2000). Focal segmental glomerulosclerosis and lithium treatment. *American Journal of Psychiatry*, 157, 834.
35. Oakley, P. W., Whyte, I. M. and Carter, G. L. (2001). Lithium toxicity: An iatrogenic problem 8 in susceptible individuals. *Australian and New Zealand Journal of Psychiatry*, 35, 833–840.
36. Mccreadie, R. G., mccormick, M. and Morrison, D. P. (1985). The impact of lithium in South- West Scotland. The discontinuation of lithium. *British Journal of Psychiatry*, 146, 77–80.
37. Greil, W. and Kleindienst, N. (1999). Differential response to lithium and carbamazepine in the prophylaxis of bipolar disorder. *Journal of Clinical Pharmacology*, 18, 455–460.
38. Bowden, C. L., Brugger, A. M., Swann, A. C., et al. (1994). Efficacy of divalproex v. Lithium and placebo in the treatment of mania. The Depakote Mania Study Group. *JAMA*, 271, 918–924.
39. Calabrese, J. R., Bowden, C. L., Sachs, G. S., et al. (1999). A double-blind placebo controlled study of lamotrigine monotherapy in outpatients with bipolar depression I depression. *Journal of Clinical Psychiatry*, 60, 79–88.
40. Bowden, C. L., Calabrese, J. R., Bowden, C., et al. (2003). A placebo-controlled 18-Month trial of lamotrigine and lithium maintenance treatment in recently manic or hypomanic patients with bipolar I disorder. *Archives of General Psychiatry*, 60(4), 392–400.
41. Vieta, E., Tjoen, C., mcquade, R. D., Carson, W. H. Jr., Marcus, R. N. Sanchez, R., et al. (2008). Efficacy of adjunctive aripiprazole to either valproate or lithium in bipolar patients partially non-responsive to valproate or lithium monotherapy: A placebo-controlled study. *American Journal of Psychiatry*, 165, 1316–1325.
42. Grunze, H., Vieta, E., Goodwin, G. M., Bowden, C., Licht, R. W., Moller, H., Kasper, S., et al. (2009). Guidelines for the biological treatment of bipolar disorders. Update 2009 on the treatment of acute mania. *The World Journal of Biological Psychiatry*, 10(2), 85–116.
43. Tohen, M., Sanger, T. M., mcelroy, L., Tollefson, G. D., Chengappa, K. N., Daniel, D. G., et al. (1999). Olanzapine versus placebo in the treatment of acute mania. Olanzapine HGEH Study Group. *American Journal of Psychiatry*, 156, 702–709.
44. Mcintyre, R. S., Brecher, M., Paulsson, B., Huizar, K. and Mullen, J. (2005). Quetiapine or haloperidol as monotherapy for bipolar mania—a 12 week, double blind, randomised, parallel group, placebo-controlled trial. *European Neuropsychopharmacology*, 15, 573–585.
45. Khanna, S., Vieta, E., Lyons, B., Grossman, F., Eerdekens, M. and Kramer, M. (2005). Risperidone in the treatment of acute mania: Double-blind, placebo-controlled study. *British Journal of Psychiatry*, 187, 229–234.
46. Weiner, R. D. (1994). Treatment optimisation with ECT. *Psychopharmacology Bulletin*, 30, 313–320.
47. Petrides, G., Fink, M., Hussain, M., et al. (2001). Electroconvulsive therapy remission rates in psychotic versus non-psychotic depressed patients: a report from CORE. *Journal of ECT*, 17, 244–253.
48. Mintel, R. E. and Mandel, M. R. (1979). The treatment of psychotic major depressive disorder with drugs and electroconvulsive therapy. *Journal of Nervous and Mental Disease*, 167, 726–733.
49. UK ECT Review Group. (2003). Electroconvulsive therapy-systematic review and meta-analysis of efficacy and safety in depressive disorders. *The Lancet*, 36, 799–808.
50. Ciappareli, A., Dell'Osso, L., Tundo, A., et al. (2001). Electroconvulsive therapy in medication non-responsive patients with mixed mania and bipolar depression. *Journal of Clinical Psychiatry*, 62, 552–555.
51. Tharyan, P. (2000). Electroconvulsive therapy for schizophrenia. *Cochrane Database System Review*, 2, 1469–1493.
52. Hamilton, M. (1986). Electroconvulsive therapy.Indications and contraindications. *Annals of the New York Academy of Sciences,* 462, 5–11.
53. Castillo E, Rubin RT, Holsboer-Trachsler E (1989) clinical differentiation between lethal catatonia and neuroleptic malignant syndrome. *Am J Psychiatry*. 146(3), 324–8.
54. Kelly, K. G. and Zisselman, M. (2000). Update on electroconvulsive therapy (ECT) in older adults. *Journal of the American Geriatric Society*, 48, 560–566
55. Sadock, B. J. and Sadock, V. A. (2008). *Kaplan and Sadock's Concise textbook of clinical Psychiatry* (3rd Edition). Philadelphia: Lippincott Williams and Wilkins.
56. Abrams, R. (2002). *Electroconvulsive therapy* (4th Edition). New York: Oxford University Press.
57. Christmas, D., Morrison, C., Eljamel, M. S., et al. (2004). Neurosurgery for mental disorder. *Advances in Psychiatric Treatment*, 10, 189–199.

Index

U

V

W

Z

www.ingramcontent.com/pod-product-compliance
Lightning Source LLC
Chambersburg PA
CBHW080536250926
51846CB00016B/1367
* 9 7 8 9 6 9 2 1 0 7 8 8 4 *